Marriage and Fertility

Studies in Interdisciplinary History

Edited by
Robert I. Rotberg and Theodore K. Rabb

Contributors
Stanley Chojnacki
Miriam Cohen
Emily R. Coleman
Cissie Fairchilds
Jean-Louis Flandrin
Susan Grigg
Barbara A. Hanawalt
Michael S. Hindus
William L. Langer
Peter Laslett
William Robert Lee
Robert V. Schnucker
Joan W. Scott
Edward Shorter
Daniel Scott Smith
George D. Sussman
Louise A. Tilly

Princeton University Press
Princeton, New Jersey

The articles included in this reader are reprinted by permission of the authors and the
editors of the *Journal of Interdisciplinary History*.
They originally appeared in the *Journal* as indicated below:
Coleman, "Medieval Marriage," *JIH* II (1971),
205-219: copyright © the JIH & MIT
Hanawalt, "Childrearing," VIII (1977), 1-22:
copyright © the JIH & MIT
Chojnacki, "Dowries," V (1975), 571-600:
copyright © the JIH & MIT
Schnucker, "Elizabethan Birth Control," V
(1975), 655-667: copyright © the JIH & MIT
Shorter, "Illegitimacy," II (1971), 237-272:
copyright © the JIH & MIT
Lee, "Bastardy," VII (1977), 403-425:
copyright © the JIH & MIT
Shorter/Lee, "Comment and Reply," VIII
(1978), 459-476: copyright © the JIH & MIT
Fairchilds, "Female Sexual Attitudes," VIII
(1978), 627-667: copyright © the JIH & MIT
Flandrin/Fairchilds, "Comment and Reply,"
IX (1978), 309-321: copyright © the JIH &
MIT
Tilly, Scott, and Cohen, "Women's Work,"
VI (1976), 447-476: copyright © the JIH &
MIT
Sussman, "Wet Nurses," VII (1977), 637-653:
copyright © the JIH & MIT
Langer, "Birth Control," V (1975), 669-686:
copyright © the JIH & MIT
Laslett, "Menarche," II (1971), 221-236:
copyright © the JIH & MIT
Grigg, "Remarriage," VIII (1977), 183-220:
copyright © the JIH & MIT
Smith, Scott, and Hindus, "Premarital Preg-
nancy," V (1975), 537-570: copyright © the
JIH & MIT

FIRST PRINCETON PAPERBACK, 1980

Contents

Introduction

With this volume the editors of the *Journal of Interdisciplinary History*, in association with Princeton University Press, launch a series of readers in interdisciplinary history. All will be designed to make investigations of specific themes more easily accessible for students at all levels. Two such collections have been published before, one on the history of the family, the other on the American Revolution, but we hope that henceforth these publications will be more regular and thus more comprehensive.

Since the first collection derived from the *Journal*'s articles was devoted to the history of the family, it is appropriate that this new series should begin on a related theme, Marriage and Fertility. This has been one of the *Journal*'s most persistent interests, linking historians, demographers, and economists on topics that have ranged from early medieval France to modern America and Japan. The articles which follow are primarily on European history, but their subject matter indicates the remarkable variety, both of the marriage and fertility patterns of past societies, and of the methods scholars have used to investigate them.

The first four papers deal with the period before 1600, when the statistical series that are so often the basis for studies of marriage and fertility are not available. Accordingly, ingenious use has to be made of the sparse documents that have survived. As Emily Coleman demonstrates, even a single major source can be sufficient to yield information about marriage patterns in as dimly understood a period as the ninth century. She arrives at revealing statistics and important conclusions about the nature of familial and social change from a survey of the holdings of a single French monastery. What she finds—as is often true in this type of study—is a unique situation, unlike any in European history.

Other unlikely sources—English coroners' reports from the thirteenth to the fifteenth centuries, and the records of dowries in Renaissance Venice—are exploited by Barbara Hanawalt and Stanley Chojnacki for similarly unexpected ends. Hanawalt is able to trace the stages of childhood development, the variety of household structures, and the importance of women's contributions in a period when concrete information has been rare and elusive. Chojnacki, also dealing with the fourteenth and fifteenth centuries, albeit in the more richly documented setting of Venice, assembles extensive statistical evidence to reach equally startling conclusions about the position of women and changes in kin relationships during the early Renaissance. A final essay on the pre-modern era, by Robert Schnucker, uses traditional documentary sources, but for non-traditional ends: to show the degree to which birth control was already an issue in sixteenth-century England, long before the time when, according to the standard historiography, family limitation became a central feature of the transition of Western society to modernity.

That transition, especially the change in sexual attitudes and in female roles that it entailed, is the subject of a cluster of articles. The stimulus to this flurry of research was a provocative and forcefully argued essay by Edward Shorter on the reasons for the rise in illegitimacy in nineteenth-century Europe. Asserting that a new "sense of self," as opposed to acceptance of community standards, emerged among the lower classes, especially among women, Shorter claims that the result was a liberation of behavior that was abetted by improved education and was given opportunities for expression in the rapidly growing cities of the time. He sees the increasing transiency of relations between men and women as a consequence of this new outlook, and not of purely economic or social forces.

Three of the articles in this collection are essentially replies to Shorter. William Robert Lee takes the position that, although bastardy became more prevalent in southern Germany around 1800, the change was not accompanied by a "sexual revolution." Instead, it was accommodated within the traditional social and moral assumptions of the region. Both Lee and Shorter clarify their positions in a subsequent exchange. Cissie Fairchilds moves the spotlight to the area around Aix-en-Provence in France, where the shift of the late eighteenth and early nineteenth centuries is explained in terms of the economic situation rather than moral attitudes. The traditional outlook, she argues, persisted well beyond 1800. Even though exploitation by their social superiors did decline, the women who were abandoned by their babies' fathers were scarcely enjoying a new freedom of self-expression. They had expected marriage, as they had for centuries, but had been forsaken because of the growing economic hardship of the period. Challenged in her interpretations by Jean-Louis Flandrin, Fairchilds responds in a brief exchange, although both writers take a position opposed to Shorter.

The final response to the Shorter thesis in this collection is the article by Louise Tilly, Joan Scott, and Miriam Cohen. They take issue with the notion that the work that became available to women during the Industrial Revolution, and the move to the city that was required by the new jobs, were liberating forces. They emphasize the burdens and traditional nature of women's work in the nineteenth century; the loss of communal protection in the urban setting; the disruption of expectations of marriage by economic change; and the persistence of traditional sexual attitudes. There the matter currently rests—the basic facts of a fundamental transformation in behavior generally accepted, but with their meaning still in dispute.

A special aspect of the move of working mothers to the city is examined in the article on Paris by George Sussman. He shows the effects of their recourse to wet nurses, particularly on infant mortality, and indicates how the system changed and eventually died out in the nineteenth century. Poverty was one of the determinants of the pattern of wet nursing, and it was also a major influence on the growing interest in birth control. William Langer's article takes us back to England, where the resistance to family limitation described in Schnucker's article on the Elizabethan period was finally overcome in the nineteenth century by publicists who became convinced that overpopulation was the main cause of the misery of the lower classes. Although practical measures remained elusive, Langer demonstrates that the change in attitude brought about by writers and reformers is at the heart of the transformation that created modern marriage and fertility patterns. An essential element in those patterns was, of course, the age of menarche, before which marriage could not take place, and after which sexual tensions could rise if marriage were postponed too long. This is the subject of Peter Laslett's article, which provides both an overview of recent research and some telling evidence from Yugoslavian sources.

The final two articles are based on American evidence. Susan Grigg, studying Newburyport materials, offers a comprehensive account of the influences at work in remarriage. She argues that age and sex, and thus attitude rather than need, were the chief determinants of the decisions by widows and widowers to remarry. Daniel Scott Smith and Michael Hindus, placing the arguments raised by Shorter in a larger perspective, survey the incidence of premarital pregnancy from the seventeenth to the twentieth centuries. They detect a succession of cycles and fluctuations, and suggest that there was not just one major nineteenth-century shift in outlook, but a series of periods when pregnancy outside wedlock seemed to become more acceptable and common. Their explanations rely on the state of relations within the family and on social change, not on Shorter's "sense of self."

Taken together, these articles outline the ways in which human behavior before, during, and after marriage has varied and altered in Western society during more than a millennium. A constant theme is the interaction between attitudes and social and economic forces; as the relationship among these influences becomes more fully comprehensible in the eighteenth and nineteenth centuries, thanks to the availability of abundant evidence, we can begin to appreciate the complexity of the transition to "modern" forms of married life. That it is essential for historians to understand this transformation if they are to assess the origins of the modern world, and that they will have to use the methods of a number of disciplines to advance their understanding, are the two prime reasons for launching this series of readers in interdisciplinary history with a volume on marriage and fertility.

—R.I.R., T.K.R.

Marriage and Fertility

Emily R. Coleman

Medieval Marriage Characteristics: A Neglected Factor in the History of Medieval Serfdom

Only recently have historians come to appreciate the role which demographic factors have played in the social history of the Middle Ages. In the traditional view, medieval society remained rigidly stratified and static; change, when it came, was attributable largely to external factors playing upon the medieval world—the opening of frontiers, the expansion of trade, and the growth of towns. All of this is true, but it does not represent a complete picture of the forces working to transform medieval society. This paper examines another factor, hitherto neglected by scholars, which apparently played a major role in the social history of the Middle Ages, and, particularly, in the history of medieval serfdom: the marriage patterns characteristic of the servile population.

I have utilized one of the magnificent documents of medieval social history—the Polyptych of the Abbot Irminon, redacted probably between c. 801 and c. 820. It describes the lands and the some 2,000 families belonging to the monastry of Saint Germain-des-Prés near Paris. This polyptych of Saint Germain-des-Prés is an extraordinary example of the medieval *censier* or manorial extent of the estates and benefices which comprised and/or were dependent upon an abbey or church. There is a *breve*, or chapter, describing each part of the seigneury, relating in some detail the type and size of the elements of the demesne, the amount of arable tenanted land, the number of people on the land, the dues they owed, and information on mills and churches.

The polyptych has been the worthy object of intense and careful study for over a century. The manuscript, which is preserved in the Bibliothèque Nationale (*Fonds latin*, manuscript no. 12832), has been edited twice. The first edition (1844) was by Guérard, whose detailed introduction has become a starting point for all studies of the document.[1] Fifty years later Longnon revised some of Guérard's paleographic interpretations and reduced the introduction to more manageable

Emily R. Coleman is currently preparing a social-demographic study of the Carolingian peasantry in the Île-de-France.

The author wishes to express her gratitude to David Herlihy of the University of Wisconsin for his guidance and encouragement. She also wishes to thank Maureen F. Mazzaoui of Indiana University.

1 Benjamin Guérard, *Polyptyque de l'Abbé Irminon ... avec des Prolégomènes* (Paris, 1844), 2v.

proportions.[2] Since then, the document has revealed and confirmed numerous findings for its patient researchers.[3] It is interesting to note, however, that these diligent scholars have concentrated almost wholly upon the tenurial aspect of the document.[4] The material that it contains on early ninth-century demography has not been systematically analyzed.[5]

The document is unusually rich in demographic information. It is not a total census for the Île-de-France, but it is far more than a tenurial document (in the sense of being concerned more with property than with people). The redactors were closely interested in the people who lived on the monastery's land and/or who owed personal dues to Saint Germain-des-Prés.[6] Even a cursory glance at some of the *brevia* reveals the strict attention given in the census to the dependents on those ecclesiastical lands. Each fisc (villa) is broken down by manse (the dependent family farm), and those on the manse are denoted individually, by status and by name—including, in most cases, the children.[7] Moreover, the census listed those peasants who lived on these

2 Auguste Longnon, *Polyptyque de l'abbaye de Saint Germain-des-Prés rédigé au temps de l'abbé Irminon* (Paris, 1886–1895), 2v.

3 The best bibliography for the monastery is still L. H. Cottineau, *Répertoire topo-bibliographique des abbayes et prieures* (Macon, 1939–40), 2v. The most recent general works of which I am aware are *Mémorial du XIVe Centenaire de l'Abbaye de Saint Germain-des-Prés* (Paris, 1959); L.-R. Ménager, "Considérations sociologiques sur la démographique des grands domaines ecclésiastiques carolingiens," in *Etudes d'histoire du droit canonique dédiées à Gabriel Le Bras* (Sirey, 1965), II. Unfortunately, these sources do not contain a bibliography of recently published works. For additional bibliography, see the *Cambridge Economic History* (Cambridge, 1966), I, or the concluding bibliography in Georges Duby, *Rural Economy and Country Life in the Medieval West* (Columbia, S.C., 1968). For sources on the use of land measures such as *aripenna* (arpents) and *bunuaria*, see Guérard, *Polyptyque*; P. Guilhiermoz, "De l'équivalence des anciennes mesures à propos d'une publication récente," *Bibliothèque de l'Ecole des Chartes* (Paris, 1913), LXXIV, 267–328; Lucien Musset, "Observations historiques sur une mesure agraire: le bonnier," *Mélanges d'histoire du Moyen Age dédiés à Louis Halphen* (Paris, 1951), 535–541.

4 For an exceedingly fine example of the type of work that has been done, as well as an additional bibliographical source, see Charles-Edmund Perrin, "Observations sur le manse dans la région parisienne au début de IXe siècle," *Annales d'Histoire Sociale*, VII (1945), 39–52.

5 The most ambitious attempt at a demographic analysis was by Ferdinand Lot, "Conjectures démographique sur la France au IXe siècle," *Le Moyen Age*, XXXII (1921), 1–27, 107–137. This study has been acutely and variously criticized by Henri Sée, "Peut-on évaluer la population de l'ancienne France," *Revue d'Économie Politique*, XXXVIII (1924), 647–655; Charles-Edmund Perrin, "Note sur la population de Villeneuve-Saint-Georges au IXe siècle," *Le Moyen Age*, LXIX (1963), 75–86; Ménager, "Considerations sociologiques," 1316–1335.

6 For example, see Perrin, "Note sur la population," 80–81.

7 Longnon, *Polyptyque*, Brevia I, II, III, IV, *passim*.

lands, even if they belonged personally to other seigneuries.[8] The monastery's interest in more than just a head count is also made clear by the attention paid to familial relationships, noting even when children had a mother different from the woman with whom they were living.[9] If we utilize the available data, we find a wealth of information dealing with sex ratios, family size, and, especially, medieval marriage characteristics.

The working and personal relationships associated with the seigneurial regime of Saint Germain-des-Prés display a hierarchical society with subtle, but important, distinctions in rank. These range from the descendants of simple slaves to the descendants of purely free men, and cover most of the ground in between. In an entirely predictable manner, the 9,219 peasants composed four main categories: *liberi* (making up a diminutive 1.30 per cent of the total census), *coloni* (82.74 per cent), *lidi* (3.17 per cent), and *servi* (comprising a surprisingly small 5.02 per cent), with 7.77 per cent of the population of undeterminable status.[10] Although these groups were in theory supposed to have their own rather distinct set of responsibilities and taxes due to their various positions in the social and economic hierarchy, a close examination of the polyptych reveals that the different types of tenures basically determined the redevances (dues) that their inhabitants, of whatever status or varieties of status, had to pay.

By the ninth century, the manse was no longer the area delegated to one family. There was no determinable relationship between the size of the plots and the services due from the peasants, and still less relationship between the size and the number of villein households that they supported.[11] In Abbot Irminon's polyptych, the number of manses supporting more than one family ranged from about 8 per cent to about 67 per cent; 701 out of 1,726 manses had multiple households

8 For instance, *Polyptyque*, IX: 145, 157, 289, 290; XXI: 1, 3, 81, 82, 86; XXII: 53, 72, 84; and other examples might easily be found.
9 For example, *ibid.*, XXI: 25, 27, 33; XXIV: 25.
10 The *liberi*, technically, were legally free individuals. They were, for the most part, the descendants of Roman peasants who were tied to the land they worked by the late imperial legislation of Constantine and Diocletian. The *lides* are believed to have originally been *laeti*—the barbarians introduced into Gaul as auxiliaries during Diocletian's reign. They came as both farmers and soldiers but, during the decline of the Roman world by the barbarian invasions, they became servile laborers. The *servi* were simply the descendants of slaves. For more on these groups and the redevances owed by them, see Guérard, *Polyptyque . . . Prolégomènes*; Longnon, *Polyptyque*, Introduction; Henri Sée, *Les classes rurales et le régime domanial en France au Moyen Age* (Paris, 1901).
11 Duby, *Rural Economy*, 51; Perrin, "Observations sur le manse," 47.

—equaling 40.61 per cent of the total population.[12] The fact that over 40 per cent of the manses were supporting at least twice the number of people than was originally intended would be explained, at least in part, by a growth in population which exceeded the ability of the seigneury to clear new lands and create new manses quickly enough.[13] This picture of a dense population and vigorous expansion is substantiated and reinforced by what seems to have been a definite upward demographic trend during the Carolingian period.[14]

Yet, while there was an increase in population, the manors belonging to Saint Germain-des-Prés did not show a trend toward large families. The average number of children ranged from slightly more than one child per couple to slightly over three children per couple.[15] Rarely did the households include other than those in the immediate family.[16]

However, although familial characteristics were surprisingly modern, Saint Germain's seigneuries showed a startlingly high sex ratio, quite unlike that which one would ordinarily expect. The sex ratio is generally defined as:

> the number of men to each 100 women in a population. The normal [modern] ratio at birth is about 105. However, this declines with the greater mortality of males until most [modern] populations show an equal number of men and women in the total.[17]

12 See Appendix I for a more visual demonstration of the following statistics: Breve I had 12.20 per cent of its manses supporting multiple households. Breve II: 44.34 per cent; III: 34.29 per cent; IV: 19.35 per cent; V: 58.88 per cent; VI: 25.00 per cent; VII: 29.87 per cent; VIII: 8.34 per cent; IX: 63.74 per cent; X: no demographic information; XI: 66.67 per cent; XII: no demographic information; XIII: 67.61 per cent; XIV: 56.66 per cent; XV: 53.36 per cent; XVI: 27.27 per cent; XVII: 11.11 per cent; XVIII: 66.67 per cent; XIX: 67.39 per cent; XX: 30.95 per cent; XXI: 14.12 per cent; XXII: 19.23 per cent; XXIII: 8.34 per cent; XXIV: 30.17 per cent; XXV: 30.95 per cent; *Fragmento Duo*: 33.34 per cent.

13 This demographic evidence is also supported by the prevalence of demi-manses. See, for example, Perrin, "Observations sur le manse."

14 This phenomenon has been noted by B. H. Slicher van Bath, *The Agrarian History of Western Europe, A.D. 500–1850* (London, 1966), 77ff, esp. fig. 9; Perrin, "Observations sur le manse"; David Herlihy, "The Agrarian Revolution in Southern France and Italy, 801–1150," *Speculum*, XXXIII (1958), 23–41, for southern Europe.

15 *Polyptyque*, I: 2.53 children per couple; II: 2.32; III: 2.82; IV: 1.92; V: 2.73; VI: 2.30; VII: 2.81; VIII: 2.04; IX: 2.60; XI: 2.60; XIII: 2.59; XIV: 2.41; XV: 2.20; XVI: 2.18; XVII: 1.12; XVIII: 1.08; XIX: 2.54; XX: 2.40; XXI: 2.72; XXII: 3.03; XXIII: 2.13; XXIV: 1.70; XXV: undeterminable; *Fragmento Duo*: 2.78.

16 Duby, *Rural Economy*, 53. *Polyptyque*, VIII, I, XVIII, XI, IV, *passim*.

17 J. C. Russell, *Late Ancient and Medieval Population* (Philadelphia, 1958), XLVIII, Pt. 3, 13–14.

The polyptych shows different characteristics. The ratios among the adult populations on the manors of Saint Germain-des-Prés ran from 110.3 to 252.9 men for each 100 women; if the entire population (where determinable) is taken into account, the ratio still ranged from 115.7 to 156.2—both of which may be seen in Table 1 below.[18]

The causes for such a marked predominance of men, especially in certain areas, are difficult to determine; we must assume that more factors are involved than a communal genetic freak. It is probably safe to discount the under-reporting of women, however. Polyptychs were relatively sophisticated and carefully constructed tax rolls. They gave information relevant to manorial income with a uniformity that would suggest methodical planning. It is unlikely that a monastic management possessing the ability to conceive and execute a project on so large a scale, and employing what appears to have been a definite basic formula of inquisition, would have simply neglected real taxable units in the form of some women. The redactors took care to mention those women who did not belong to Saint Germain-des-Prés when they were married to the monastery's peasants; and women not tied to any particular manse were mentioned regularly among those who paid the head tax at the end of the *brevia*.[19] The importance of women in a peasant society was undeniable; they made up an important labor source, aside from their more obvious role in childbearing. Moreover, women were of especial importance in Saint Germain-des-Prés because it was they who passed on the status valuation to their children.[20]

There are several plausible reasons for the unbalanced sex ratio. Certainly, one must not ignore the possibility of female infanticide. That, and the death of many women during parturition, would account for a certain disequilibrium in the sex ratio. Undoubtedly, ninth-century midwives and medical practices produced many widowers. This might also account for the marked inequality we find generally, or for the inequality apparent in children's sex ratios. It is possible,

18 This male preponderance, as anomalous to modern times as it is, was not peculiar to the estates of Saint Germain-des-Prés. The Salic Law, both in its first redaction under Clovis and in the more extensive version under Charlemagne, stipulates a *wergeld* three times higher for a woman of childbearing age than for an adult male—which suggests a scarcity of women. See Andrée Lehmann, *Le rôle de la femme dans l'histoire de France au moyen âge* (Paris, 1952), 42.

19 See above, note 9; Perrin, "Note sur la population," 80–81; *Polyptyque*, III: 61; V: 94–116; VII: 81; IX: 30; *passim*.

20 See below, 214.

however, that the estates which showed a definite preponderance of men as opposed to women may have been in the process of clearing the forest for cultivatable fields. In those areas, women would have been of less use. They would have followed the men and boys to the untamed regions slowly, as conditions of life gradually softened and their skills and abilities could be more profitably utilized. In other words, the sex ratio might be an indication of an internal frontier clearance in the Île-de-France that provided more fields and food to supply the rising population of the ninth century.[21] Yet, it is also possible that the numerical masculine superiority was the result of an immigration of men who had hoped to find work and protection on these monastic lands.[22] Taken together, infanticide, maternal mortality, frontier clearance, and masculine mobility suggest a possible complex of factors explaining the high sex ratios displayed by the polyptych.

What is important is the indisputable fact of the high sex ratio, for whatever reason. The important point to note about this preponderance of men is that, as a result, the marriage market should have been auspicious for women. Since the number of men to each woman was so high and the economic advantages of a wife in a peasant society were so obvious, one would have expected the women to make excellent marriages in terms of both economics and status. Yet these two assumptions seem to be erroneous.

Many of the scholars who have studied the polyptych have noted, in passing, the odd marriage characteristics of the inhabitants.[23] There was, in addition, an unusually high proportion of socially unequal marriages—among the different peasant statuses—for which no apparent reason has hitherto been suggested. In 251 out of a total of 1,827 marriages, or 13.74 per cent, in which the statuses of both spouses were determinable, that of the man and woman were different. On the individual estates, the percentages ran from 1.28 per cent to 80 per cent, as seen in Table 1.

In 61 out of 251 cases, the man married beneath himself. In 190 cases or 75.69 per cent of the unequal matches, it was the woman, who may be assumed to have been in an ideal position, who married below her status. And it is interesting to note that in these cases, the average

21 This is a highly theoretical suggestion. The subject of sex ratios deserves more detailed treatment.
22 Ménager, "Considerations sociologiques," 1334–1335, and n. 66.
23 Among them, Longnon, *Polyptyque*, Introduction; Duby, *Rural Economy*; Guérard, *Polyptyque . . . Prolégomènes.*

Table 1 ·Sex Ratios and Marriages

Breve	TOTAL SEX RATIO	ADULT SEX RATIO	ADULT *Coloni* SEX RATIO	UNEQUAL MARRIAGES		
1.	177.1	252.9	207.6	21.40% or	3 out of	14
2.	133.3	136.6	129.6	10.17%	12	118
3.	148.6	150.0	152.19	18.87%	10	53
4.	153.1	126.6	106.66	10.70%	3	28
5.[a]	146.9?	146.9	135.5	1.28%	1	78
6.[a]	115.8?	115.8	101.81	6.38%	3	47
7.[a]	149.24?	149.24	124.07	15.00%	9	60
8.	130.6	140.0	119.23	25.93%	7	27
9.	128.0	125.38	112.14	8.94%	32	358
11.[b]	143.3	112.5	no male coloni	80.00%	12	15
13.[b]	141.6	119.8	91.86	37.19%	61	164
14.	124.3	125.8	115.12	3.64%	4	110
15.	131.6	114.6	106.48	9.18%	9	98
16.	125.3	125.84	116.25	8.86%	7	79
17.	134.3	125.0	127.77	5.41%	2	37
18.	118.1	142.8	257.14	38.48%	5	13
19.[a]	110.3?	110.3	110.99	4.31%	4	93
20.	144.0	123.3	119.23	20.69%	6	29
21.	128.8	121.5	104.76	24.00%	18	75
22.	128.6	112.1	107.06	18.63%	19	102
23.	122.7	118.1	141.17	15.00%	3	20
24.	115.7	120.2	122.92	12.65%	22	174
25.[a]	145.6?	145.6	123.07	11.92%	5	42
Fragmento Duo	156.2	133.3	123.07	9.09%	1	11

a The sex ratio among children is undeterminable.
b Brevia 10 and 12 contain no demographic materials.

number of children per couple ran to 2.04 as opposed to 1.76 where the man was the socially superior partner.

Why would so many of the available women—almost one sixth of the married population—marry men socially inferior? It could not have been due merely to a lack of eligible men of the same status. As was noted, the vast majority of people on the seigneuries were *coloni*, and it was the *colonae* who took the major role in this social transformation when the sex ratio averaged 117.06 among adults.[24] Even so, there was no dearth of marriageable *servi*. For example, in the Breve

24 See Table 1.

de Gaugiaco, there were four unmarried *servi* and only one unmarried *ancilla* (female *servus*). In the Breve de Nuviliaco, there were two to one. In fact, the overall sex ratio among *servi* adults was an incredible 297.56. Furthermore, it is unlikely that the unattached men of the corresponding status would be in the wrong age group. This was the least important of qualifications in an age untouched by concepts of "romantic love." Also, in some cases, the sex ratio was even more favorable among the children—which would indicate a rough similarity of age—than among adults.

We can rule out, too, any connection between personal and tenurial status as a factor in marriage. Unequal marriages appeared on free manses[25] and servile manses.[26] The extent of the holding made no difference, either. They occurred on manses whose territory ranged from twenty-eight *bunuaria* of arable land and four arpents of vineyards to eight *bunuaria* of arable land, one and one-half arpents of vineyards, and one and one-half arpents of meadow to two *bunuaria* of arable alone, with gradations in between, above, and below.[27]

It has been suggested, by Bloche among others, that by the time when the polyptych was redacted, social stratifications had become devoid of practical significance.[28] He suggested that the classes found within the manorial surveys were administrative anachronisms. In the day-to-day life of the individual they were meaningless, and were kept alive only by the fact that scribes and other servants of administration usually utilized terminology and categories of social analysis that were at least a generation behind the times. To an extent, this was certainly true. The dues relevant to personal service had generally fallen into disuse. Yet this unfortunately does not explain the marital mismatching that occurred on the manors of Saint Germain-des-Prés. If the solution were simply that no one really took the status hierarchy seriously, there would inevitably have been a statistically parallel number of cases of men making misalliances; and the average number of children in both groups would have been more evenly balanced. Yet this was not so—over three-fourths of these mixed marriages show that the women married below their status. Thus, while the social hierarchy had less and less meaning in economic life, it apparently retained some importance within a hierarchically-conscious society; every group had

25 For example, *Polyptyque*, VII: 7, 14, 15, 42; I: 6; XVIII: 6, 7, 8; *passim*.
26 See, for instance, *ibid.*, I: 13, 14; IV: 28; *passim*.
27 See, for example, *ibid.*, XI: 4; VII: 14; XVIII: 6; I: 13; etc.
28 Marc Bloch, *French Rural History* (Berkeley, 1966), 70.

its own "pecking order"—in fact, this was of particular psychological importance when the distinctions came to mean very little in practical life.

It is nevertheless possible to suggest a hypothesis as to the cause of the peculiar situation. On the manors of Saint Germain, the status of the mother decided the condition of the children, as prescribed in the laws of the Emperors Gratian, Valentinian II, and Theodoric.[29] Now this may not have always held true, but it apparently was a general rule, enhanced by the occasional exception. If the difference in status between husband and wife were very large, the position of the children sometimes became a compromise; this unusual situation was specifically mentioned by the redactors of the document. In the rules of inheriting status, however, Longnon agrees with Guérard that the condition of the mother seems to have been the determining factor. Their interpretation, as one would expect, is verified by an examination of the polyptych itself, in such passages as: "Frotcarius, Frudoldus, Frotbertus. These three are *lidi* because they were born of a *lida* mother; Martinus, a *servus*, and his wife, an *ancilla*, named Frotlindis, are people of Saint Germain. These are their children: Raganbolda, their daughter, is an *ancilla*, Faregaus, Widericus, and Winevoldus are *lidi* because their mother was a *colona*" (an example of the occasional compromise); or "These are the children of Dudoinus by another woman, and they are *servi*: Berhaus, Aclevertus, Dodo, Faregaus, Acleverga, Audina," or "Witbolda, an *ancilla*, and her sons, who are *servi*. . . ."[30]

There are many more examples.[31] In the Breve de Murcincto, on the eighth manse, the redactors took unusual care in recording the status of the children: "Alveus, a *colonus*, and his wife, a *colona*, named Ermoildis, are people of Saint Germain; they have four children—also *coloni*. . . ."[32] The reason would seem to be that the scribe had

29 P. Krueger (ed.), *Corpus Juris Civilis* (Berlin, 1959); *Codex Justinianus*, XI, 68, 4. "Ex ingenuo et colonis ancillisque nostris natasve origini, ex qua matres eorum sunt, facies deputari."

30 "Frotcarius, Frudoldus, Frotbertus. Isti tres sunt lidi, quoniam de lida matre sunt nati, Martinus servus et uxor ejus ancilla, nomine Frotlindis homines sancti Germani. Isti sunt eorum infantes: Raganbolda, filia eorum, est ancilla; Faregaus, Widericus, Winevoldus sunt lidi, quoniam de colona sunt nati. Isti sunt filii Dudoini de alia femina, et sunt servi: Berhaus, Aclevertus, Dodo, Faregaus, Acleverga, Audina. Witbolda ancilla et filii ejus servi. . . ."

31 *Polyptyque*, IX: 25; XIII: 65, 67, 68; also see, e.g., XIX: 18; XVII: 45; XXIV: 3, 169; XXV: 42.

32 "Alveus colonus et uxor ejus colona, nomine Ermoïldis, homines sancti Germani, havent secum infantes IIII, *similiter coloni* . . ." *Polyptyque*, XVII: 8. Italics mine.

initially mistaken the status of Ermoildis; originally he had recorded her as an *ancilla*, caught the error, and corrected it by replacing that word with "*colona.*" [33] As always, the names of the children followed their parents' names and statuses. But here the uncommon step was taken of adding "*similiter coloni*" so that there would be no error in calculating the children's status by misreading Ermoildis as an *ancilla*—because her condition devolved on her children. And, in other instances as mentioned above, the redactors carefully noted when children had mothers other than the women with whom they were living.[34]

Although social hierarchy made no effective difference in the life style of a couple, and mixed marriages were apparently not frowned upon, a consciousness of status did exist, and the woman herself passed on this status. This being so, one might suggest that the marriage characteristics exhibited by the polyptych represented a conscious pattern, if not a policy, on the part of at least some of the peasants. Is it not possible that men knowingly looked for a woman of higher social position for the psychological pride and prestige of an advantageous match and/or in order to improve the condition of his progeny? Certainly, the latter possibility was a result, whatever the original reason. This thesis can be graphically shown by both Appendix II and Table 2, where status comparisons for the children as opposed to adults show a trend toward higher status in the younger generation. Of the 8,377 people whose status is determinable, 87.81 per cent of the adults were *coloni* and 7.56 per cent were *servi*. In the next generation, however, their children were 90.34 per cent *coloni* and only 4.31 per cent *servi*.

This conclusion may be shown from another angle as well. The original status that a manse received corresponded to that of its original tenant and remained the same in perpetuity. It is extremely difficult to be definite because of the large number of manses of unspecified status and the possibility that old *hospicia*, or cottars' holdings, may have been absorbed into the seigneury as free manses. Yet, it would seem fair to posit that the entire population of the manors of Saint Germain-des-Prés at the time of the polyptych's redaction contained a larger proportion of *coloni* as compared to *servi* than at the time of the land's original division into free and servile manses.

In the overall picture of these medieval marriage characteristics,

33 See Longnon, *Polyptyque*, 250, n. 2.
34 See above, 209, and note 9.

Table 2   Status Change Comparison[a]

Breve	TOTAL ADULTS	TOTAL CHILDREN	ADULT Coloni		Coloni CHILDREN		ADULT Servi		Servi CHILDREN	
1.	53	34	40 or	75.47%	29 or	90.63%	6 or	11.32%	0 or	0.00%
2.	304	330	287	94.41%	320	96.97%	14	4.61%	5	1.52%
3.	130	134	116	89.23%	123	91.79%	8	6.15%	3	2.24%
4.	67	54	62	92.54%	54	100.00%	5	7.46%	0	0.00%
5.	221	226	219	99.09%	226	100.00%	2	0.09%	0	0.00%
6.	117	117	111	94.87%	114	97.44%	3	2.56%	0	0.00%
7.	138	147	121	87.68%	117	79.59%	17	12.32%	30	20.41%
8.	64	68	57	89.06%	58	85.29%	3	4.69%	4	5.88%
9.	816	812	734	89.95%	755	92.98%	35	4.29%	23	2.83%
11.	34	36	6	17.65%	5	13.89%	15	44.12%	9	25.00%
13.	353	415	237	67.14%	302	72.77%	51	14.45%	45	10.81%
14.	271	189	256	94.46%	183	97.34%	13	4.80%	1	0.53%
15.	256	196	223	87.11%	186	94.88%	29	11.33%	8	4.08%
16.	192	91	173	90.10%	79	86.81%	18	6.77%	8	8.79%
17.	88	51	82	93.18%	44	86.27%	4	4.55%	0	0.00%
18.	31	9	25	80.65%	6	66.67%	2	6.45%	2	22.20%
19.	198	237	192	96.97%	229	96.62%	0	0.00%	0	0.00%
20.	78	64	57	73.08%	55	85.94%	19	24.36%	6	9.38%
21.	157	195	129	82.17%	169	86.67%	17	10.83%	8	4.10%
22.	207	259	176	85.02%	250	95.53%	24	11.59%	0	0.00%
23.	46	46	41	89.13%	37	80.43%	3	6.52%	5	10.87%
24.	360	307	321	89.17%	285	92.83%	35	9.72%	18	5.86%
25.	101	undeterminable	96	95.05%	undeterminable		3	2.97%	undeterminable	
Frag. Duo	34	43	29	85.29%	41	95.35%	5	14.71%	2	4.65%
OVERALL	4,316	4,060	3,789	87.81%	3,667	90.34%	326	7.56%	175	4.31%

a Breve XI shows a loss in both coloni and servi; on this fisc the loss was absorbed by the more fluid intermediate group of lidi. Conceivably the trend could continue in the next generation or the lidi could buy their emancipation. Brevia VII, VIII, XVIII, and XXIII do not show the characteristic we have been tracing in the two to three generations which characterize the polyptych. There is no need to assume that the upward demographic spiral would have taken place consistently and at the same rate in all places. Again the trend could conceivably continue in the next generation. The overall characteristics for the polyptych are visually demonstrated in Appendix II.

women would not necessarily have resented or objected to marrying beneath themselves because, in essence, it made no effective change to their lives, nor would their children lose caste. But there could be a more positive reason. One can assume, with the sex ratio being as generally high as it was, that in many cases a woman would have had a fair number of brothers. While the number of children in a family averaged between two and three, there would obviously be cases of five, six, seven, even eight or more children in a ménage.[35] At the same time, on the lands belonging to Saint Germain-des-Prés, women could work and control their manses themselves if there were no men in the households; for the most part, we see this in the case of widows.[36] Therefore, it would appear reasonable to suggest that where a woman had a large number of brothers, the possibility of her attaining control of the family plot was slim. As a consequence, she would offer little economic incentive toward marriage to a man of her own status.[37] Yet, at the same time, her very status—without the economic inducement of land—would offer positive motivation to a man in a lower social position. In other words, a man would marry up for psychological reasons or with the conscious intention of improving the status of his progeny; a woman would marry down due to the force of economic circumstance. The result was the transformation of the class structure. One confirmation of this interpretation is the larger number of children in these families, by contrast with those in which the male was of a higher status. The hypothesis is reinforced, too, by the fact that— aside from discernible widows—the unmarried women of these fiscs were quite often, though not always, from a low social situation.

This explanation also helps to account for the fact noted above— the larger proportion of *coloni* as opposed to *lidi* and *servi*. *Lidi* could have bought themselves into a higher situation[38] and thereby reduced their numbers. But *servi* had no way of improving their positions in their lifetimes unless they successfully ran away and became *hôtes* on some other seigneury, as many of them undoubtedly did. Many more, however, must have found it difficult to leave; and is it not possible to suggest that while they could not ameliorate their own

35 *Polyptyque*, II: 30, 36; III: 12, 13; V: 15, 47, 62; VII: 16, 8, 40, 58; IX: 92, 119; XI: 3, 8; XIII: 5, 67, 81; XIV: 9, 11, 30; these are just isolated examples of which many more could easily be found.
36 See, for example, *ibid.*, XV: 66; XVI: 86, 41; XX: 38–41; *passim.*
37 This point was suggested by William Courtenay.
38 Longnon, *Polyptyque*, Introduction, 41.

plight economically, they might do so psychologically or even aid their children's condition by a judiciously chosen marriage.[39] The lords would not object, for they lost virtually nothing in personal dues (what they lost in *manoperae* [*corvées*], they made up in *censive*), and the dues of the tenure remained the same.

While it is impossible to argue back from a ninth-century document to a fourth-century situation, one may wonder if the thesis of virtual slave nonreproduction and mass manumission[40] is as satisfactory an answer to the problem of the decline of slavery as has been supposed. If one ventures to wander into the dubious world of pure hypothesis, the polyptych of Saint Germain-des-Prés might conceivably represent an indication—a link in a chain—of a gradual but persistent improvement in status through calculated marriage arrangements, by selection on a basis of heritable status. It is a thesis that certainly suggests another basis for future investigation into the fact that slaves declined in percentage and absolute numerical importance throughout most of the Middle Ages. There are obviously other problems which the polyptych suggests for investigation, but they are too diverse and detailed to be discussed here. One thing, at least, is clear: within Saint Germain-des-Prés, by slow degrees, a statistically interesting proportion of the peasantry moved up a rung of the status ladder.

39 This pattern of unequal marriages was not a situation unique to the ninth century or Saint Germain-des-Prés. Cinzio Violante, in his *La Società Milanese Nell'età Precomunale* (Bari, 1953), noted that clerics would marry free women so that their children would inherit the mother's free status and the father's ecclesiastical benefices. These clerics were *coloni* (159), and, c. 1000, Otto III questioned this abuse in a diploma to the Vercelli church: "Statuimus quoqui, ut omnes filii vel filie colonorum ex familia sancti Eusebii in servitute ecclesie maneant neque libertas matris, se colone servo adhesit, hiis qui nati fuerint, prosit volumus." Sickel [ed.], (*Monumenta Germaniae Historica, Diplomata regum et imperatorum Germaniae* [Hanover, 1888], II, pt. 2, 811–812, no. 383.)
40 Marc Bloch, "Le servage dans la société européenne," *Mélanges historiques* (Paris, 1963), I, 259–528.

Appendix I

Manses Supporting Multiple Households[a]

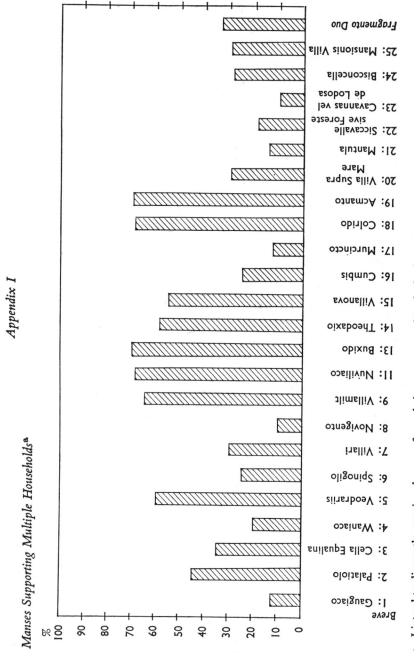

a   I intend to discuss the varying degrees of population pressure against the land at a later date.

Appendix II

Improvement in Status over the course of two to three Generations[a]

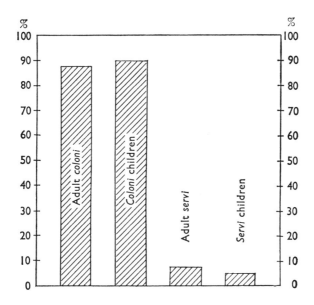

a   This chart represents the characteristics exhibited by 8,377 people whose status can be determined. Over the course of two to three generations, as determinable in the polyptych of Saint Germain-des-Prés, there has been a small but definite and significant improvement in the status of the monastery's peasants.

Journal of Interdisciplinary History, VIII:1 (Summer 1977), 1–22.

Barbara A. Hanawalt

Childrearing Among the Lower Classes of Late Medieval England

Anxiety about the breakdown of the modern family, the application of Freudian and Eriksonian models of child development to historical subjects, and the study of households by demographers combined to make Ariès' *Centuries of Childhood* the center of debate and the object of attack among social historians. Ariès suggested that the sentimental concept of the family existing for the sake of rearing children was a modern idea which developed in early modern Europe in response to the loss of other familial functions to the centralized state and the exigencies of industrialization. In the Middle Ages, he argued, the family had extensive kinship and community ties which shared and could outweigh the emotional bonds of the family to children.[1]

Although Ariès drew his data primarily from the upper class, his theory has raised issues which should be investigated for all ranks of society. First, he assumed that the medieval household was a large one in which both extended family and outsiders lived together, a view of the preindustrial family which Laslett has denied.[2] Second, he argued that children became valuable to society only when they reached the age of seven and could be sent out to another house to work, in other words, only when they became economically productive.[3] Third, he ignored the actual process of childrearing before the age of seven, leaving this issue unexplored. In this essay I have studied these three problems and have used coroners' rolls, a source often ignored by historians of the family,

Barbara A. Hanawalt is Assistant Professor of History at Indiana University and the author of *Crime in East Anglia in the Fourteenth Century: Norfolk Gaol Delivery Rolls* (Norwich, England, 1976).

The author would like to thank the Southeastern Summer Institute for Medieval and Renaissance Studies for the opportunity to join a seminar on the medieval household with David Herlihy in 1974. His direction and help during the seminar were very much appreciated.

1   Philippe Ariès (trans. Robert Baldick), *Centuries of Childhood; a Social History of Family Life* (New York, 1962), 368.
2   Peter Laslett, "The Comparative History of Household and Family," *The Journal of Social History*, IV (1970), 75–87.
3   Ariès, *Centuries of Childhood*, 128.

in order to move the investigation of childrearing away from the elite minority to the practices of the majority.

One of the central issues in the criticisms of Ariès and in the general discussion about childrearing in the Middle Ages and later has been that, although the literate upper classes left some records of childrearing, the lower classes, who comprised the bulk of society, did not.[4] The approaches of peasants and the lower urban class to raising children were usually not represented in artistic and literary remains. For the Middle Ages the problem is particularly difficult because many of these sources were the works of ecclesiastical writers who had little direct experience with normal family life. Even the usual sources of information on childrearing in the Middle Ages are inconclusive. For instance, medievalists have countered early modernists' contentions that the Middle Ages lacked a concept of childhood by indicating the instances in artistic representations, chronicles, saints' lives, and ecclesiastical pronouncements where children were treated as children. However, the mere representation of a child *qua* child rather than as a little man does not indicate a sentimental attachment to children. Injunctions of church synods and penitentials about infanticide may only indicate an extension of the commandment, "Thou shalt not kill," rather than a particular love for the children who might be killed.[5] In the hands of a skilled historian, such as McLaughlin, these literary sources become the basis for a serious discussion of trends in childrearing and attitudes toward childhood in the Middle Ages. She has shown that the attitudes of writers move from a threatening view of children in the ninth century to a greater interest and concern for children by the end of the thirteenth century. Understandably, however, works such as hers and Hunt's return repeatedly to the qualification that the literary remains of the upper classes of medieval and early modern Europe may or may

4 Lutz Berkner, "Recent Research on the History of the Family in Western Europe," *Journal of Marriage and the Family*, XXXV (1973), 395–405. Berkner provides an excellent survey of current literature on the history of the family. He emphasizes the lack of studies of peasant families.
5 Richard H. Helmholtz, "Infanticide in the Province of Canterbury during the Fifteenth Century," *History of Childhood Quarterly*, II (1975), 384. Helmholtz has shown that there was a legal punishment for infanticide which was no more or no less severe than, for example, sex offenses. The Church does not seem to have had any particular sentiment for childhood in pursuing the ecclesiastical court trials of those who killed their children.

not reflect what practices were used by the bulk of the population.[6]

The coroners' inquests are a unique source of information on the daily life of the peasants, villagers, and middle to lower classes in towns. The nobility and wealthier urban families seldom appeared because they were less likely to meet with ordinary accidents or homicides and because they would usually be exempt from most judicial procedures, including the coroners' inquests. The inquests record cases where conflicts among members of a community or family led to homicide and where work, play, or neglect led to accidental deaths. Evidence on the rolls which specifically relates to the family permits a study of the activities of children and other members of the household, an estimate of the types of family structures and number of people in the household, and, to a certain extent, the emotional relations of family members. For instance, if a child died in a cradle fire, the inquests indicated not only the cause of death but who first discovered the accident, how the fire got started, the people who were present or should have been, and the date on which it happened. The victims in a household struck by fire or attacked by robbers would all be listed along with their relationships to each other, their activities before death (if known), and the layout of the house. The most obvious bias in the source is that it is a sample of those people in society who were careless, accident prone, unfortunate, or violent. Nevertheless, an analysis of any accident or homicide statistics is a study of the practices and mores of the society. The people who appear in them are representative of their society; they are simply more unlucky or aggressive than their neighbors.

Each inquest reads like a vignette of medieval life, having freshness and immediacy because it was recorded so soon after death, in the language of the jurors and witnesses. When a person died violently or suddenly, i.e. by homicide, misadventure (accidental death), or suicide, the neighbors were required by law to summon one of the county coroners to come and view the body. The coroner empanelled a jury of the neighborhood in which the body was found and held an inquest to determine the cause of

6 Mary Martin McLaughlin, "Survivors and Surrogates: Children and Parents from the Ninth to the Thirteenth Centuries," in Lloyd de Mause (ed.), *The History of Childhood* (New York, 1974), 101–181; David Hunt, *Parents and Children in History* (New York, 1970).

death. Like the modern coroner, he inspected the wounds and inquired into the date and hour of death, the place and circumstances surrounding it, witnesses, the death instrument, suspects, the age of the victim if he were a minor, and perhaps even motivations in the cases of homicide. The information was recorded on pieces of parchment at the time of the inquest and later copied onto rolls which were presented to the king's justices upon demand.[7]

The coroners' rolls used in this paper give a sampling of different social and economic conditions in late medieval England. Urban life is represented by two series of published rolls: the London rolls, containing 205 cases, and the Oxford rolls, containing 110 cases from the fourteenth century. The data for rural society come from published Bedfordshire inquests, containing 189 cases, and from a run of over 100 years of Northamptonshire coroners' rolls in manuscript, yielding 1307 cases from the fourteenth and early fifteenth century.[8] Many of these cases deal with families. Children are specifically involved as victims in 17 percent of the Northamptonshire cases (214), 18 percent of the Bedfordshire cases (33), 6 percent in London, and .9 percent in Oxford. The ages of the children were recorded up to their twelfth birthday when they legally assumed adult responsibilities.

Since children are not reared without interaction with their environment, we will want to know the size of the household, its physical description, and the relationship of the occupants. Esti-

---

7 After the justices from the central court tried the homicide suspects who had been arrested and collected the money due from the *deodands* (i.e. the value of the death instrument in accidents), they deposited the rolls with the Exchequer, where they were preserved. The *deodand* was a revenue source for the king. Initially, the death instrument was to be sold and the money contributed to prayers for the soul of the victim. It later became a contribution to the royal treasury. The collection and preservation of the rolls was sporadic. Those counties which were visited most frequently by the justices of the king's bench have very good series, while those that had few visitations have poor ones. The amount of detail on the record depends very much on the interest an individual coroner took in recording information and how busy he was. For a complete description of the coroners see R. F. Hunnisett, *The Medieval Coroner* (Cambridge, 1961).

8 R. R. Sharpe, *Calendar of Coroners' Rolls of the City of London, A.D. 1300–1378* (London, 1913); H. E. Salter, *The Records of Medieval Oxford* (Oxford, 1912); Hunnisett, *Bedfordshire Coroners' Rolls* (Bedfordshire, 1960), XLI. I have also used a few examples from his *Calendar of Nottinghamshire Coroners' Inquests 1485–1558* (Nottingham, 1969), XXV; the Northamptonshire coroners' rolls are preserved in the Public Record Office in London under the classification of Just. 2. In addition to the coroners' rolls, I have used the jail delivery rolls of 1300–1348 for Northamptonshire, Yorkshire, and Norfolk, which are the records of trials for felonious offenses. The rolls examined contained about 10,500 criminal cases. They are preserved in the Public Record Office under the classification of Just. 3.

mates of the number of people living under one roof have varied somewhat depending on the nature of the source. Russell estimated 3.5 persons per household, but Hallam, working with more complete census data, placed the size at 4 people in the rather densely populated fenland area of Lincolnshire.[9] Both Russell and Hallam found that the nuclear family predominated, although in the fens of thirteenth-century Lincolnshire there were instances of single-person households and extended families. The coroners' rolls give some information, particularly in burglary cases, of the number of people living in a household. Yet the evidence is not entirely reliable because some members of the household, particularly young children, might have escaped attack from the burglary and therefore not be listed. Nevertheless, the Bedfordshire coroners' rolls, which are among the most detailed, show that the late thirteenth-century rural household was far from being a static unit. The sample is a small one, twenty-five cases, but of these just over half were nuclear families. The rest of the families were either extended families with the husband's mother living with her son's family, or two brothers or two sisters living together, or a single woman or man either living alone or with young children. The families had from one to four children. The number of children per household was probably greater after the Black Death because, prior to 1349, 24 percent of the accident victims were children. After the plague the percentage increased to 31 percent. The presence of more children per household is consistent with demographic studies which show that marriages and births tended to increase after a plague. In addition to immediate members of the family, some households also contained servants who lived with their master or guests who had been staying for extended periods of time.

Aside from a preference for living with family, convenience seemed to determine living arrangements in rural Bedfordshire.[10] The twenty-five cases indicate that there were upwards of 3.5 per-

9 Josiah Cox Russell, *British Medieval Population* (Albuquerque, 1948), 24–26; H. E. Hallam, "Some Thirteenth-Century Censuses," *Economic History Review*, X (1958), 352; Edwin D. DeWindt, *Land and People in Holywell-cum-Needingworth* (Toronto, 1972), 171, placed the size at 3.8; John Kraus, "The Medieval Household: Large or Small?" *Economic History Review*, IX (1956–57), 420, puts the household size at 4.5.

10 Hunnisett, *Bedfordshire Coroners' Rolls*, cases 20, 52, 71, 73, 102, 111, 179, 203, 224, 249. "Swetalys" had been staying at the house of Thomas Saly of Riseley throughout the autumn, before she was found dead.

sons per household, most of them related and part of the nuclear family. In London and Oxford the household picture was altogether different for the lower classes. The rolls speak more frankly about transitional relationships with concubines, and the nuclear families which do appear were limited to a husband, wife, and one child. The smaller number and size of nuclear families accounts for the very low percentage of children appearing in the urban coroners' rolls.[11]

The evidence of coroners' rolls on the composition of the households must remain more suggestive than conclusive, but lacking other reliable evidence, the tentative conclusions it suggests deserve comment. For instance, although the rural families seem to have lived in predominantly nuclear units at one hearth, other arrangements were common to the society. Because the coroners' rolls record deaths, they particularly draw attention to the transitory aspects of the family: if the grandmother died, it would become a simple nuclear family; if a wife died, the house would become that of a widower; and so on. Stepparents must have been common because of the tendency of widows and widowers to remarry in order to increase land holdings and insure labor on the land.[12] The evidence indicates that both Laslett's em-

An interesting sidelight which the Bedfordshire data suggest is that the theory of constant households does not hold for late thirteenth-century England. According to this theory, the number of households remains constant so that in periods of economic contraction a control will be maintained over the distribution of resources. If the number of hearths remains fixed, then around each hearth one might expect to find extended families with the married and single children living with their parents. Although the late thirteenth century was a time of scarcity and over-population in Bedfordshire, households there do not show any evidence of being impacted. On the contrary, the wattle and daub houses seem to have been easy to acquire. There are even cases of accidents occurring in vacant houses. The real shortage seems to have been food rather than housing, for a number of inquests mention poor people dying from exposure while returning to their homes from begging, or dying in their homes from accidents due to their weakened condition. One of the fallacies of the constant household theory is the assumption that because fields and food are in limited supply, housing is also limited and existing hearths will be called upon to accept more members. Housing was obviously available in thirteenth-century Bedfordshire, but not food.

11   The difference between the urban and rural household picture is similar to that which Herlihy is finding for rural and urban Florence. Cities have more single people and smaller nuclear families among the poorer classes, while the peasantry have larger families and fewer single people. David Herlihy, "Mapping Households in Medieval Italy," *Catholic Historical Review*, LVIII (1972), 1–22; Diane Hughes, "Urban Growth and Family Structure in Medieval Genoa," *Past & Present*, 66 (1975), 2–4.

12   J. Z. Titow, "Some Differences between Manors and the Effects on the Condition of the Peasant in the Thirteenth Century," *Agricultural History Review*, X (1962), 1–13, notes the demand for widows in marriage. The extensive remarriage may account for some of the medieval folk and fairy tales about wicked stepmothers and stepfathers.

phasis on the nuclear family and Ariès' assumption of an extended family were correct. Although the small nuclear family was the most common type of family, it was certainly not the only one with which a growing child would be acquainted. Furthermore, to list the number and relationships of the people living under one roof does not completely define "family." One also wants to know the extent to which relatives and communities assumed some of the social functions now normally associated with a family.[13] The size of the household in which the child grew up and the amount of community interaction in its rearing might depend on the wealth and status of its family. Wealthier families or those of greater status might have had more living family members due to better diet.

A physical description of the household in which the child was reared emerges from the evidence jurors gave to the coroner on the circumstances surrounding deaths. In the thirteenth century many peasant houses were made of wattle and daub so insubstantial that burglars pushed the walls down rather than enter through the doors. For the poorer members of the peasant community this type of housing must have continued well into the fourteenth century, but by the end of the century houses were more substantial. They had courtyards with walls or ditches surrounding them and wells and ovens within. There would probably be two rooms and often two floors. The floors, covered with straw, were highly flammable, as were the straw pallets used for beds. The main room contained a raised hearth in the center of the floor. The child spent the first years of life in a cradle near the fire. Also around the fire were pots, pans, and trivets. Tables, chairs, and beds were the only other furniture mentioned. During the day the open door provided light and children and animals wandered through freely. At night candles were used, which seem to have been left to burn all night, sometimes catching the houses on fire. In the city the child was raised in a shop or a tenement, the construction of which was better than wattle and daub, but they burned easily nonetheless.

A brief description of the roles of parents in the household is also essential, for they were the models of behavior for their offspring. In describing the different tasks of men and women in the

13 Familial compounds of peasant families linked by an overall family patriarch are not indicated in coroners' roll data. Italian peasant and patrician families had this structure. See Hughes, "Urban Growth and Family Structure," 4.

rural social order, historians have tended to follow John Ball's classification that Adam delved, Eve span, and all men and women since then have been locked into the first parental model.[14] The evidence from the coroners' rolls shows that the sexes were assigned distinct tasks, but these tasks cannot be divided between field and home with easy facility. Reaping and stacking of hay and straw were done by both men and women. Taking grain to the mill was also a task for either. By and large, the heavy work was done by men in both urban and rural society. In rural society men worked more outside than women and more of them died in work-related accidents.[15] An analysis of the instruments of their death shows that men's work was more dangerous. They did all of the digging in marl pits and quarries, and in both urban and rural society they did all of the masonry and carpentry. They also did the milling, carting (this was the most dangerous activity, accounting for a quarter of the accidents of rural men), barn work, herding of animals, and training of horses. In urban society the heavy work, with the exception of the shipping and building industries, was mostly carried on indoors in a variety of crafts or shops. The women in the rolls are pictured as working in kitchens or the courtyard or doing errands about the town or village. They also gathered herbs and wood, did the laundry, weaving, and, one of the most important tasks, the brewing (in London, this was done by men). Beyond those mentioned, there were many activities of both sexes which did not appear in the inquests because they were not dangerous. Nevertheless, certain patterns of fairly well-defined role structure emerge from the coroners' rolls. The children would be expected to imitate and eventually perform the tasks of their model parent. Because of the sex differentiation in division of labor in the household, we may expect that males were raised differently than female children.

The matrimonial pattern in the households seems to have been as traditional as the division of labor. The majority of references in the coroners' rolls are to husbands and wives. But as Sheehan has shown, the bond of marriage might be very loose and the possibility of bigamous unions common.[16] In addition to the

14 George C. Homans, *English Villages of the Thirteenth Century* (Cambridge, Mass., 1940), 353–381.
15 65 percent of the men compared to 48 percent of the women.
16 Michael M. Sheehan, "The Formation and Stability of Marriage in Fourteenth Century England, Evidence of an Ely Register," *Medieval Studies,* XXXIII (1971), 228–263.

children of legitimate marriages, manorial records indicate illegitimate children. The actual extent of illegitimacy is impossible
to measure. Women are mentioned in the coroners' inquests of
London and Oxford as concubines and more quaintly in the country as "entertaining" men. For instance Lucy Pofot, widow of
Thomas of Houghton, came from a local tavern accompanied by a
"ribald stranger" who asked for entertainment and Lucy com-
plied. The ungrateful guest murdered her in the night. The con-
cubine of a clerk in fifteenth-century Nottinghamshire sought a
solution to her unwanted pregnancy by swallowing poison to
cause an abortion, but it killed her instead.[17]

What happened to unwanted babies at birth? Given the nature
of the coroners' rolls, one would assume that they would be an
ideal source for studying the incidence of infanticide. However,
out of a sample of about 4,000 homicide cases taken from coroners' rolls and jail delivery rolls, there were only two cases of new-
born infants being murdered. In one case Alice Grut and Alice
Grym were indicted for drowning a three-day-old baby in a river
at the request of Isabell of Bradenham, her son, and her daughter.
They were all acquitted. In the other case, the jurors of Oxford
said that a baby girl, one-half-day old, was carried downstream,
and they knew nothing about the father or the mother. They assumed that she had not been baptized since the navel was not
tied.[18] The murder of toddlers and older children was also extremely rare in the circuit court records (2 percent of all
homicides). Some of these children were killed in accidental slay-
ings and some in the course of burglaries, but only three were
killed out of malice. Out of a sample of 2,969 homicide cases taken
from the jail delivery rolls, only nine involved the killing of young
children by an insane mother.[19] Even Helmholtz, looking through
ecclesiastical records for cases of infanticide, could find only a few
examples.[20]

The extraordinarily low incidence of recorded infanticide and
child murder does not necessarily mean that it was rare. A plausi-

17 Hunnisett, *Bedfordshire Coroners' Rolls*, cases 35 and 94.
18 Just. 3/48 m. 4d; Salter, *Oxford Coroners' Rolls*, 27.
19 This amounts to .03 percent of all the cases, hardly enough evidence to bear the weight
of the psychoanalytical superstructure which Barbara Kellum in "Infanticide in England in
the Later Middle Ages," *History of Childhood Quarterly*, I (1974), 371–75 tried to build on
evidence in my "The Female Felon in Fourteenth Century England," *Viator*, V (1974),
259–261.
20 Helmholtz, "Infanticide in Canterbury," 384.

ble argument can be made that infanticide was not consistently illegal in the Middle Ages. A statute law against mothers killing
their illegitimate children was not passed until 1623,[21] and Hurnard correctly observed that "women who killed in childbirth
were sometimes regarded as responsible and sometimes not."[22] In
any case, the crime was easily concealed, making criminal prosecution difficult. The Church was well aware of the methods of
concealment. In penitentials, and particularly in the English
synodal legislation of the thirteenth century, parents were told not
to sleep with children because they might smother them, not to
leave them alone, and not to leave them unattended near fires.
Helmholtz found that the Church heard cases involving accusa-
tions and confessions of these practices, but the extent of the practices remains a mystery.[23] One might argue that they were concealed through reporting them as accidental deaths. Among the
accidental deaths of infants in our sample, there were no reported
cases of overlaying, but 50 percent of the cases involving children
one year and under were caused by fire and 21 percent by drowning (see Tables 1 and 2). Was this neglect or premeditated murder?
A fairly consistent pattern associated with infanticide is that female
children were killed more frequently than male.[24] The coroners'
rolls, however, show that in Northamptonshire the percentage of
accidental deaths of boys of all ages was much higher than that of
girls—63 percent of all accidental deaths among children were
male and 37 percent were female (see Table 3).[25] In the age group of
one year and under, twenty-eight boys died compared to twenty
girls. The low discrepancy of death from accidents between male
and female children in this age group is consistent with modern
accident figures, which show male children having higher accident
rates than females in general, but the degree of excess of male
deaths over female deaths is lowest in infancy and increases with

21 William S. Holdsworth, A History of English Law (Boston, 1924), IV, 501.
22 Naomi D. Hurnard, The King's Pardon for Homicide before 1307 (Oxford, 1969), 169.
23 McLaughlin, "Survivors and Surrogates," 120–121; Helmholtz, "Infanticide in Canterbury," 380–382.
24 Emily R. Coleman, "L'infanticide dans le Haut Moyen Age," Annales Economic,
Société, Civilisations, XXIX (1974), 315–335. Richard C. Trexler, "Infanticide in Florence:
New Sources and First Results," History of Childhood Quarterly, I (1973), 98–116.
25 This is very close to modern figures, where 63.5 percent of all accidental death victims
fourteen and under are males: Accident Facts, 1968 Edition (Chicago, 1968), 14.

Table 1 Distribution of Causes of Accidents for Male Children by Age

| | AGE | | | | | | | | | | | | |
	1	2	3	4	5	6	7	8	9	10	11	12	UNSPECIFIED
Animals	1	3						2		1			
Water													
wells	3	13	11	4	1					2			
ditches	3	8	7	1	2							3	1
ponds	1	5	3		1					1			
streams		2	1		2	2	2	2	1			3	
Equipment													
cart			2			1							2
mill												1	1
knife	1					1							2
pot	6	5	4					1					2
arrow												1	1
hatchet													1
Fire	13	4	3	1	1						1		2
Heavy object	1	1			1		1					1	
Victim falls	1	1			1			1				1	1

Table 2 Distribution of Causes of Accidents for Female Children by Age

						AGE							
	1	2	3	4	5	6	7	8	9	10	11	12	UNSPECIFIED
Animals	1	2	2										
Water													
wells	2	5	1	1									2
ditches		6	3	1									4
ponds	1	1	1		1								2
streams		1			2	2		1					
Equipment													
cart		1											
mill			1										
knife	1												1
pot	3	6	5						1				3
arrow			1										
hatchet													
Fire	11	4											5
Heavy object			1	2	2								
Victim falls	3					1				1			

Table 3 Distribution of Children's Accidents by Age and Sex

	AGE												UNSPECIFIED
	1	2	3	4	5	6	7	8	9	10	11	12	
male	28	47	31	2	7	4	3	7	1	5	2	10	9
female	22	26	15	5	5	1	0	1	1	0	1	0	16
Total	50	73	46	7	12	5	3	8	2	5	3	10	25
Total n =	249												

age.[26] Concrete evidence for infanticide is still lacking. There are four possibilities: 1) infanticide was a widespread phenomenon but was accepted by society and, therefore, ignored in the records; 2) it was successfully concealed; 3) infant mortality being between 30 percent and 50 percent, willful murder was unnecessary; 4) all children were valued because of the need for laborers in peasant society of the fourteenth century.[27]

Those children who survived the dangers of birth, disease, and homicide had to be fed, sheltered, and attended to during the first years of their lives. When one looks at the accident pattern, the stages of the developing child fall into four clearly defined groups: birth to one year old, two to three years old, four to seven years old, and eight to twelve years old (see Tables 1 and 2). These four stages are remarkably close to those which Hunt has adapted from Erik Erikson's work on child development, and reference will be made to Hunt's *Parents and Children* throughout.

The first stage of the child's life was occupied with problems of feeding, warmth, and attention. We may assume, along with McLaughlin, that both peasant and urban lower-class mothers nursed their own children.[28] Probably the child was not given milk on demand because, as we shall see, the children seemed to be left alone for long periods. Peasant women occasionally nursed other children. In one inquest a husband lost his temper and killed his wife because he claimed that she spent too much time at his neighbor's house giving milk to Robert Asplon's son.[29]

When not being nursed, the baby was kept in a cradle by the fire. The most common accident for both male and female infants was to be burnt in the cradle (50 percent of female infants and 46 percent of male). There is no proof that children were swaddled, but they might have been.[30] As described in the coroners' rolls, a typical case showed a child lying in its cradle next to the hearth when a chicken or pig came in and knocked burning straw or an ember into the cradle. Since the infants were wrapped in linen,

---

26 Albert P. Iskrant and Paul V. Joliet, *Accident and Homicide* (Cambridge, Mass., 1968), 23. Indeed, the ratio is extremely close to the modern one they give on 138.
27 The percentages are from E. A. Wrigley, *Population and History* (New York, 1969), 116–131.
28 McLaughlin, "Survivors and Surrogates," 115–116. Nursing continued from one to three years.
29 Hunnisett, *Bedfordshire Coroners' Rolls*, case 255.
30 McLaughlin, "Survivors and Surrogates," 113–114.

linsey-woolsy, or wool, the smell of buring cloth, if not the cry of the child, would call attention to the accident if an adult were in the house. In one case a child's entire legs were burned. The extent of the burns seems to indicate that infants were often left alone in the house, and a few cases tells us this directly. In one inquest the jurors said that the father was in the fields and the mother had gone out to the well when the child was burned. In a London case of neglect Johanna, daughter of Bernard de Irlaunde, a child of one month, was killed in her cradle by a sow bite. Her mother had left her alone in their shop with the door open and a sow wandered in and bit her head. The jurors go on to say that "at length" her mother returned to the shop and found her.

By the third year of the child's life cradle deaths were no longer common and the children appeared to have entered into the second phase of development, reception to outside stimulus.[31] By the end of the first year swaddling cloths, if used at all, were not kept on children all the time, for they were mobile enough to get into trouble.[32] They wandered around courtyards and fell into wells, ponds, and ditches on their parent's property. They also got into accidents in the house, the most common of which was pulling pots off trivets and scalding themselves. Falls and playing with knives also brought death (see Tables 1 and 2).

The second stage of childhood in Hunt's Eriksonian model and the second readily definable accident grouping is from two to three, when children obviously have considerable motor skills and a lively interest in their environment.[33] Although cradle fires continued to be a hazard in the early stages of this period, the accident pattern indicates that the process of exploring, reaching out to the world around, and imitating adults became more intensified. Wells were the most dangerous object of the children's new lives as wanderers (25 percent of the deaths), but ditches (20 percent), ponds (8 percent), and streams and rivers (3 percent) also figured in their perambulations. For instance William, son of William

31 Just. 2/111 m. 17; 2/112, m. 38; 2/113 m. 27, 31; 2/255 m. 5; Sharpe, *Coroners' Rolls of London,* 56–7; Just. 2/113 m. 31 (a boy of three dies in a cradle fire).
32 Hunt found that young Louis XIII was sometimes free of swaddling cloths, and completely free by eight months: *Parents and Children,* 128.
33 *Ibid.,* 135–136. This is the period which Erikson describes: "The development of the muscle system gives the child a much greater power over the environment in the ability to reach out and hold on, to throw and to push away, to appropriate things and to keep them at a distance." It is also the stage at which the child learns about authority.

Faunceys (aged 3 ½), fell into a ditch at Robert Wreng's house while his mother was in Robert's house getting ale. In another case a father was going to the mill and did not know that his three-year-old son was following him. The child fell into the river and drowned. Children got into accidents which show an increased interest in the work of their parents. One little boy was killed watching his father cut wood.[34] Both boys and girls of this age group became interested in cooking, ale making, and laundry. In trying to stir the pots or look into them they fell into the pots or dumped the scalding liquid on themselves. Sex differentiation appeared early—27 percent of the girls and only 14 percent of the boys this age were involved in accidents playing with pots or cauldrons. In the accidents which occurred outside the home in bodies of water, only 44 percent of the girls met their death while 64 percent of the boys did. Modern studies of accidental death indicate that male children are more adventurous, take more fatal risks, and venture further from home.[35] Such developmental explanations for the greater death rate of boys and the statistics for drowning and other risk-taking adventures perhaps hold true for medieval children as well. The explanation may also have a psychological basis. According to the coroners' roll evidence, children of two and three were already identifying with the roles of their parents in the household and were imitating them—little girls copied their mothers by cooking and boys followed their fathers about their tasks.

Greater physical mobility without sufficient motor control caused many of the accidents of two- and three-year-olds. For instance, one child was playing with a duck and holding it in her arms. She wanted to put it into the river but fell in herself. Children would be attracted to feathers floating in the water and would drown trying to grasp them; or, in trying to throw an object into the water, would throw themselves in as well.

Toddlers, like infants, seemed to have been often left alone or in inadequate care. One child wandered off and drowned, having been left in the care of a blind woman while her parents were in the fields. In other cases, a child may have been left in the care of older

---

34 Hunnisett, *Bedfordshire Coroners' Rolls*, cases 18, 62, 77; Just. 2/106 m. 1d, m. 2; 2/107, 2/109 m. 8.

35 Iskrant and Joliet, *Accident and Homicide*, 23. In modern figures boys are predominant in drownings.

siblings. William Claunche's daughters, Muriel (almost six years old) and Beatrice (almost three), were left in his house in Great Barford while William and his wife were in the fields. A fire broke out and the younger girl was unable to escape. In another case two sisters, eight and four, were left home at night while their parents were in a tavern. A neighbor, committing a burglary in the house, killed the two girls. A little boy (two) was left at home apparently in the care of older children while his parents went to church. He went outside to look for the other boys and fell into a well. His sister found him.[36] Other accidents occurred when one or both parents were present but otherwise occupied.[37] Were these medieval parents negligent of their children's safety by leaving them unattended or inadequately supervised? If adults were present when children fell into water, they could be of little help because they themselves did not know how to swim—40 percent of all adult accidents were drownings, sometimes in shallow water. A comparison with modern figures would indicate, however, that medieval parents probably spent less time supervising children. In 1968 in the United States only 7.5 percent of all accident victims were children under four, although in our medieval sample 68 percent were children under four.[38] Furthermore, while the modern curve indicates infancy as the highest period for accidents, with a sharp decrease at two and three, the medieval pattern reverses this curve.[39]

In spite of their apparent negligence, the parents of these active two- and three-year-olds were obviously able to instill some sense of caution into their wandering children, for the number of

---

36 Hunnisett, *Bedfordshire Coroners' Rolls*, cases 14, 25, 109; Just. 2/109 m. 7.

37 One couple was trying to heat their oven in the courtyard when their son went to another part of the courtyard and drowned; *ibid.*, case 236. Another father was eating lunch when his child wandered outdoors and drowned; *ibid.*, case 33.

38 *Accident Facts,* 14. The validity of this comparison may be questioned because of the greater proportion of children in medieval society. Still, the difference in the number of children would have to be very great to account for a difference of almost 60 percent. Even if inaccurate, the comparison does provide some perspective in understanding the accidents of children in the middle ages.

39 Iskrant and Joliet, *Accident and Homicide,* 19, 22, 138. The death rate in infants is nearly three times that of children one to four. It is interesting that in folklore of this period two to three was considered to be the most dangerous age. It is in that period that children in northern mythology were most likely to be stolen by elves. Carl Haffter, "The Changeling: History and Psychodynamics of Attitudes to Handicapped Children in European Folklore," *Journal of the History of the Behavioral Sciences,* IV (1968), 55–61.

accidents dropped dramatically for both boys and girls after they reached the age of four: only 11 percent of children involved in misadventure died in the period of four to seven. What accounts for the drop in the number of accidents? According to Hunt's Eriksonian schema, this is supposed to be the age when children discover infantile sexuality, but the coroners' rolls give no evidence that children suddenly took their fingers out of the pots and put them on their genitals instead.[40] There is not a great deal of evidence on the disciplining of children or ways in which they were taught to be more responsible.

There are a few cases of children dying from extreme forms of discipline. An eleven-year-old boy was whipped to death by his enraged mother and a five-year-old London urchin who stole some wool died from a punch on the ear delivered by the woman keeping the shop.[41] But discipline alone did not bring about the reduction in the accident rate. From the age of four children began to spend more time with their parents. Ironically, in medieval society the children seemed to have had more adult supervision from the age of four to seven than they did from infancy through three years old. This greater supervision did not appear to come about because the children were suddenly more valuable to the parents, but because their greater mobility made it possible for them to be with adults more. Contrary to Ariès' assumption that the children suddenly became productive, their accident pattern indicates that they were doing little work. Their misadventures were still almost entirely related to playing children's games. The work which they did perform must have been rather minimal: some herding, babysitting, and perhaps some work in family gardens.[42]

The most striking change in the child's life in its progress to adulthood seems to have come at ages eight through twelve. The children during this period were independent from adults and were given tasks of their own to perform. They still lived at home for the most part, contrary to Ariès' belief that all children older

40 Hunt, *Parents and Children*, 159–179.
41 Just. 2/107 m. 5; Sharp, *Coroners' Rolls of London*, 83. It is interesting to note that the shopkeeper was not even indicted for the homicide. The coroners' jury returned a verdict of misadventure indicating that the discipline of killing a thief caught in the act, even if a child, was excusable.
42 Just. 2/109 m. 7.

than seven were sent to live in another person's home.[43] Boys from eight to thirteen were shepherds, mill hands, reapers, and servants.[44] Their tasks show that they were moving into adult life and were being trained for the work they would eventually perform as men. Their accident pattern both in work and play became much closer to that of men. They no longer chased feathers or played with ducks; they were learning to have mock fights with staffs, to shoot at targets with bows and arrows, and to play such games as getting an arrow to glance off the ground and rise up and hit a target.[45] In the urban setting as well, young boys were being groomed for adult life during the period of eight through twelve. In Oxford and London this meant school for some boys. The evidence is indirect, but it is there. In Oxford a school master fell from a willow tree into the river and drowned as he was cutting willow switches with which to beat his students. In London an eight-year-old boy on his way to school was crossing London Bridge and playing a game he had often enjoyed in which he caught hold of a projecting beam and swung on it. He fell into the Thames and drowned. Other boys appeared in the coroners' rolls as selling eels and other goods in the streets, as apprentices, and as beggars. The girls in both urban and rural society were approaching the adult female pattern of accidents. They took up the duties of gathering wood, minding children, and working in the fields at harvest.[46]

The coroners' rolls show that the children growing up in the medieval household went through distinct developmental stages closely compatible with those described by Erikson, but, in addition, the inquests tell us something about the emotional climate in the home. One would assume that the rolls would reflect only negative feelings within the family since they record homicides

43 Ariès, *Centuries of Childhood*, 365. Some lower-class children were sent away in fourteenth-century England. In London and other urban centers the pattern was different than that among the rural lower classes because of apprenticeship. Among the upper classes as well it was customary to send children to another family.

44 Hunnisett, *Bedfordshire Coroners' Rolls*, cases 31, 117, 119, 247, 252; Just. 2/106, 2/109 m. 1, 7.

45 Just. 2/109 m. 1; in the last case mentioned, the arrow hit a thirteen-year-old boy in the stomach: Just. 2/255 m. 6.

46 Salter, *Oxford Coroners' Rolls*, 60; Sharpe, *Coroners' Rolls of London*, 25, 61, 169; Hunnisett, *Bedfordshire Coroners' Rolls*, cases 58, 228; Just 2/109 m. 7.

and violent death. But the evidence raises the possibility that the medieval family was remarkably congenial: only 8 percent of all homicides involved intrafamilial murders. This is low compared to the 53 percent of all murders which are intrafamilial in modern Britain and 30 percent in the United States.[47] Does this low incidence of intrafamilial crime indicate remarkable domestic tranquility within the medieval home? The evidence which Raftis and his students have been accumulating from manorial court rolls indicates that the main village families were very much concerned with preserving peace within the family and thereby perpetuating their status and control in the community. The familial relationships which led most frequently to intrafamilial homicides were husbands and wives (55 percent), followed far behind by fathers and sons and brothers (about 11 percent each). The father-daughter and mother-son relationships each produced only about 8 percent of the homicides. In nonhomicidal disputes in manorial courts, the children tended to be pursuing actions against the parents, but in homicides, the parent was usually the slayer. On the whole, there is little evidence of homicidal violence within the family.[48]

But to argue a sentimental attitude toward children, there must be more than a forbearance in killing them. We would expect emotional outpourings from the parents upon finding a dead child. The rolls, unfortunately, stop short of the parents' lament. Certain indirect expressions of parental emotions are present, as in the case of the Nottinghamshire woman who tried to save her daughter from a beating. An Oxford mother gave her life in an attempted rescue of her twenty-week-old son.

> On Friday last [9 Aug. 1298] John Trivaler and Alice his wife were in a shop where they abode in the parish of St. Mary late at night, ready to go to bed, and the said Alice fixed a lighted candle on the wall by the straw which lay in the said shop, so that the flame of the

47 Barbara Hanawalt Westman, "The Peasant Family and Crime in Fourteenth-Century England," *The Journal of British Studies*, XIII (1974), 4.
48 J. Ambrose Raftis, *Tenure and Mobility* (Toronto, 1964), 32–63; *Warboys; Two Hundred Years in the Life of an English Medieval Village* (Toronto, 1974), 225–240; DeWindt, *Land and People*, 191. These works show that the family tended to be a cohesive unit, at least in the higher strata of peasant society. Indeed, only 2 percent of all assaults and bloodlettings involved a family in Wakefield manor courts. See Westman, "Peasant Family and Crime," 5–6, 17.

candle reached the straw before it was discovered and immediately the fire spread throughout the shop, so that the said John and Alice scarce escaped without, forgetting that they were leaving the child behind them. And immediately when the said Alice remembered that her son was in the fire within, she lept back into the shop to seek him, and immediately when she entered she was overcome by the greatness of the fire and choked.[49]

In another case, a father rushed to protect his young daughter from rape and was killed himself. Finally, there is the case of a boy ten years old who was shooting at a dung hill with his bow and arrow. Missing the dung hill, he shot a five-year-old girl instead. He fled from the scene because he was afraid of her father's anger.[50] These three cases indicate that the parents may have had a great love for their children, even enough to risk their own lives saving them, but they do not necessarily indicate sentimental love for children. Likewise, the fact that when a child was lost or killed the mother or father was almost always the first finder may not indicate anything more than that the community considered it the parent's responsibility to take on the burdens of being first finder.[51] None of the cases show parents playing with children when the accidents occurred. The coroners' rolls, therefore, tell us that the parents did not hate their children enough to kill them except in rare cases and that they often loved them enough to risk their own lives for them. They do not indicate one way or another a sentimental attachment to the state of childhood, which Ariès would find essential for the modern family.

The coroners' rolls provide solid information on the childrearing of the lower classes of society and additional information on the nature of the medieval household. The growing child of the lower classes lived in a household which was fairly small and may or may not have had servants and aged relatives living in it. While there is a tendency to look upon the lower class as monolithic, there were many gradations of wealth and status within rural and urban communities. It is possible that in cases where infants died of neglect, the household was a poor one which needed every

49 Salter, *Oxford Coroners' Rolls*, 7.
50 Hunnisett, *Bedfordshire Coroners' Rolls*, cases 58, 74.
51 The first finder had to find pledges and come to the court sessions. There is some evidence that the actual first finder went and told the parents about the death so that they could be the official first finders. *Ibid.*, cases 128, 197.

able-bodied hand in the field. Servants might have been out of the question or the parents may have been working for hire themselves and could only leave an infant with an older sibling or with the old and handicapped. The demand for labor may have been so great in these households that infanticide was not generally practiced. At two and three when the children were mobile they began to follow their parents about and to imitate them. The types of accidents of male and female children began to differentiate following the pattern of activities for adult men and women which the children saw in their home. Children from four through seven were less likely to have accidents but this seems to arise not from their usefulness to society but because they were more often in the company of responsible adults and their parents had, by this time, instilled some sense of caution and responsibility in them. After the age of seven the children did become a part of the productive economy of the household, but it was usually their own household rather than another.

The stages of child development indicated in the coroners' rolls are remarkably close to those blocked out by Erikson. Their motor development and, to a certain extent, their psychological development is reflected in the sorts of accidents that they encountered. But the emotional climate within the lower-class household continues to be elusive. Ariès' suggestions that children competed for their parents' affection with extended kin and neighbors may be correct. Homicide statistics certainly indicate that the emotional contacts which led to fatal attacks tended to be with fellow villagers and friends rather than family members.[52] Since homicide is seldom random and most often occurs between people who know each other well, it is possible that the strong ties were with the outside rather than with members of the immediate household.

52 Hanawalt, "Violent Death in Fourteenth and Fifteenth Century England," *Comparative Studies in Society and History*, XVIII (1976), 297–320.

Journal of Interdisciplinary History, v:4 (Spring 1975), 571–600.

Stanley Chojnacki

Dowries and Kinsmen
in Early Renaissance Venice
In the fifteenth canto of
the *Paradiso* (ll. 103–105) Dante wistfully observed that in contrast to
his own time, the epoch of his great-great-grandfather, Cacciaguida,
did not see fathers taking fright at the birth of daughters. In those good
old days, dowries had not yet "fled all limitation." Dante may have
been indulging in a familiar kind of romanticizing; certainly twelfth-
century Florentine fathers also had to face responsibility for their
daughters' dowries. But his laments about the rise in dowries had
plenty of echoes. In fact, the problems that the dowry institution itself,
and especially dowry inflation, posed in the early Renaissance (fourteenth–fifteenth centuries) are a familiar theme in the historical literature on the period.[1]

The fact of dowry inflation is fairly well documented. An example
from Venice can give a sense of the trend. In a sample of fifty mid-
trecento patrician dowries, the average was about 650 ducats and the
largest, about 1540 ducats.[2] By the fifteenth century, however, it was

Stanley Chojnacki is Associate Professor of History at Michigan State University and the
author of several articles on Renaissance Venice.

The author would like to thank the American Philosophical Society for a grant
which enabled him to collect much of the material for this article, and the Institute for
Advanced Study, Princeton, for providing a congenial setting in which to write it.

1   There is disagreement among historians of law about the degree to which Roman
dowry practice, as opposed to Germanic institutions such as the Lombard *faderfio*,
survived in the early Middle Ages. By the twelfth century, however, the Roman
institution seems to have regained ground lost in earlier centuries; and the comeback
involved more of a blending with Germanic law than a wholesale rejection of it. See
Francesco Brandileone, "Studi preliminari sullo svolgimento dei rapporti patrimoniali
fra coniugi in Italia," *Archivio giuridico,* LXVII (1901), 231ff; Francesco Ercole, "La dote
romana negli statuti di Parma," *Archivio storico per le province parmense,* n.s., VIII (1908),
21–23. For the early Renaissance, see Lauro Martines, *The Social World of the Florentine
Humanists, 1390–1460* (Princeton, 1963) 19, 37–38; Frederic C. Lane, *Andrea Barbarigo,
Merchant of Venice, 1418–1449* (Baltimore, 1944), 39.
2   The dowry figures are taken from Archivio di Stato, Venice (henceforth cited ASV),
Notarile, Cancelleria inferiore (all henceforth abbreviated CI and followed by the
bundle number and the notary's name) 114, Marino, S. Tomà, protocol (henceforth,
prot.) 1366–91, *passim.* This source records the repayment of dowries to widows or their
heirs upon the death of husband or wife. The entries usually mention the date on which
the dowry had been paid to the husband, normally at or around the time of the wedding.
The fifty cases studied represent marriages contracted between 1346 and 1366.

In this and in all other monetary references, the various Venetian moneys have
been converted into ducats, for purposes of uniformity and comparison. For these

a rare patrician dowry that fell below 1,000 ducats, and there was a strong tendency to go much higher.[3] This tendency was alarming enough to induce the Venetian Senate in 1420 to place a limit of 1,600 ducats on patrician dowries, a good indication that many dowries were larger. But such measures did no good. There are many instances of larger dowries in the years after 1420; and at the beginning of the sixteenth century the Senate passed another law reaffirming the principle of dowry restraint—but resignedly raising the ceiling to 3,000 ducats.[4]

It would be valuable to know whether the rise in dowries was greater, smaller, or about the same as price movements generally in the period. Were Dante and the Venetian senators alarmed because dowries were soaring out of all proportion to other expenses—and to incomes? Or were their laments over dowries just symptomatic of a general concern over a rising cost of living? Sketchy data, great variations year-to-year in the availability of articles of consumption, and a complex monetary system that fluctuated dizzily during the period make it impossible to plot with any precision general movements in prices or, on a broader level, in the overall cost of living—even without getting into the delicate and complex question of different levels of wealth in the consuming, and dowry-raising, population.[5]

---

conversions, see Nicolò Papadopoli-Aldobrandini, *Le monete di Venezia* (Venice, 1893–1907), I, 383–385; Frederic C. Lane, *Venetian Ships and Shipbuilders of the Renaissance* (Baltimore, 1934), 251–252. See also correspondences noted in the records of estates administered by the Procuratori di S. Marco. Thus, in 1347 the gold ducat was worth 2.63 lire *a grossi*, the Venetian money of account (ASV, Procuratori di S. Marco, Commissarie [hereafter abbreviated PSM], Miste, B. 70a, Nicolò Morosini, account book, fol. 2r).

3   We have been unable to find a fifteenth-century equivalent to the records in CI 114 cited above. However, already in the late fourteenth century the standard had risen. In 25 patrician marriages contracted between 1370 and 1386, the average dowry was 1,000 ducats (figures again taken from CI 114, Marino, prot. 1366–1391). It is clear that by the fifteenth century 1,000 ducats was something of a minimum for respectable patrician dowries. Cf., in addition to examples cited below, Lane, *Andrea Barbarigo*, 23–41, *passim*; Andrea da Mosto, "Il navigatore Alvise da Mosto e la sua famiglia," *Archivio veneto*, 5th ser., II (1927), 168–259, *passim*.

4   For the fifteenth-century law, see Marco Barbaro, "Libro di nozze patrizie," MS in Biblioteca Nazionale Marciana, Venice, MSS italiani, classe VII, 156 (8492), fol. a; the sixteenth-century law, dated 4 Nov. 1505, is in *Ibid.*, fols. a-b.

5   Jacques Heers, *L'Occident aux XIVe et XVe siècles: Aspects économiques et sociaux* (Paris, 1966), 294–299; Gino Luzzatto, "Il costo della vita a Venezia nel Trecento," in *idem*, *Studi di storia economica veneziana* (Padua, 1954), 285–287. A graphic picture of the changing relations between gold and silver in Venetian moneys can be found in Carlo M. Cipolla, *Studi di storia della moneta, I: I movimenti dei cambi in Italia dal secolo XIII al XV* (Pavia, 1948), 44–47.

In general, there seems to have been a rise both in prices, particularly in manufactured goods, and in the standard of living.[6] However, there has not been much research on this question in the Italian context. As a center of exchange Venice certainly escaped the worst of the "price scissors" that afflicted the agrarian sector. Yet, wheat prices appear to have risen during the period. In 1342–43, a *staio* (2.3 bushels) of wheat cost a Venetian householder 22 silver *grossi*, equal at the time to just under one ducat. By 1390 importers were selling wheat to the Venetian government's grain office at about 1.7 ducats per *staio*—a wholesale price that still prevailed, however, in 1432.[7] But wheat prices are a notoriously unrepresentative index of prices generally. Although other isolated bits of evidence testify to a rise in the cost of living, they do not add up to a clear enough picture against which we can gauge the relative impact of the dowry rise. Yet, the leading authority on medieval Italian dowries speculated that the increase in dowry levels could be attributed in large part to prospective bridegrooms' growing dowry pretensions in the face of the rise in the cost of living.[8]

But if we cannot be sure whether the increase in dowries was greater than general increases in the cost of living, there is good documentation of a development that helps to explain the concern of fathers in the fourteenth and fifteenth centuries. It is the great squeeze that governmental exactions, especially in the form of forced loans (*prestiti*), put on private wealth. This important question cannot be

6 The data are fragmentary, regionally selective, and sometimes contradictory. See Harry A. Miskimin, *The Economy of Early Renaissance Europe, 1300–1460* (Englewood Cliffs, N.J., 1969), 89–92; Robert S. Lopez, in *The Cambridge Economic History of Europe* (Cambridge, 1952), II, 343–347; Gino Luzzatto, (trans. Philip J. Jones), *An Economic History of Italy* (New York, 1961), 138–146.

7 See Léopold Genicot, in *The Cambridge Economic History of Europe*, (Cambridge, 1966; 2d ed.), I, 688–694. On Venetian economic fortunes in the fifteenth century in general, see Luzzatto, *An Economic History*, 150–155; in greater detail, *idem, Storia economica di Venezia dall' XI al XVI secolo* (Venice, 1961), 146–179; *idem*, "Il costo della vita," 290. For the monetary conversion, see Papadopoli, *Le monete*, I, 383–385. The equivalence of the *staio* is in Lane, *Venetian Ships*, 246. In 1390 the estate of Simone Morosini sold nine *staia* of wheat to the grain office for 1 lira, 10 soldi *di grossi* (one lira *di grossi* equalled 10 ducats) (PSM Miste, B. 128, Simone Morosini, Register, fol. 5r). The 1432 figure comes from Lane, *Andrea Barbarigo*, 67–68.

8 On wheat prices as general index, see Heers, *L'Occident*, 295; Luzzatto, "Il costo della vita," 286. See the regional variations in grain prices in Genicot, *Cambridge Economic History*, I (2d ed.), 683. On dowries see Francesco Ercole, "L'istituto dotale nella pratica e nella legislazione statutaria dell'Italia superiore," *Rivista italiana per le scienze giuridiche*, XLV (1908), 191–302; XLVI (1910), 167–257. These two parts shall be referred to as "Istituto dotale," I, and "Istituto dotale," II. The present reference is in "Istituto dotale," I, 280–284.

dealt with in detail here (studies by Luzzatto and others have treated it thoroughly), but its bearing on the rise in dowries can be stated briefly.[9]

Military expenses throughout the third quarter of the fourteenth century put a mammoth burden on the nobles and citizens of Venice—the assessable part of the population. At their worst, during the years of the desperate War of Chioggia with the Genoese, the fisc's levies in two years, 1379–81, drained away about one quarter of the private wealth in Venice.[10] It is true that the impost-paying public gained interest-bearing shares of the state debt (*Monte*) for most of these exactions. It is also true that *Monte* shares could be negotiated for various purposes, including dowry transactions. But by this time the government had given up its former practice of making amortization payments in addition to interest payments; moreover, after 1382 interest payments effectively dropped from 5 to 4 (and for some even 3) percent—considerably lower than the return on commercial or real estate investments; and the market price of *Monte* shares, at its low point of 18 percent of face value in 1382, had risen only to 63 percent of face value by 1400, despite governmental efforts to shore up the *Monte* by buying shares through a sinking fund.[11] So dowry payments in *Monte* shares, whether computed at the market price or at face value, were not a one-for-one solution to the squeeze on private wealth that endless *prestiti* levies had effected.

Considering the effect of these fiscal burdens on private wealth, the growth of dowry standards must have been particularly painful for Venetian patricians—"insupportable" in the words of the Senate act of 1420.[12] It is probable that dowries came to demand a much

9   The main study of *prestiti* and their economic impact is Gino Luzzatto (ed.), *I prestiti della Repubblica di Venezia (sec. XIII–XV)* (Padua, 1929), esp. clx–clxxv of Luzzatto's "Introduzione storica." See also Frederic C. Lane, "The Funded Debt of the Venetian Republic," in *idem, Venice and History* (Baltimore, 1966), 87–98; Roberto Cessi, "La finanza veneziana al tempo della guerra di Chioggia," in *idem, Politica ed economia di Venezia nel Trecento. Saggi* (Rome, 1952), 172–248. The fruits of Luzzatto's researches on this question are presented briefly in his *Storia economica di Venezia*, 140–145.

10   A measure authorizing a revision of the fisc's estimate of private wealth, passed after the War of Chioggia, indicated that the total could be as much as 1.5 million lire less than the total of 6 million lire reached in the previous estimate of 1379, at the beginning of the war (*ibid.*, 145). But see the cautionary comments of Cessi, "La finanza veneziana," 192–198.

11   Luzzatto, *Storia economica*, 147–148; Lane, "Funded Debt," 87–89.

12   ". . . propter importabilem sumptum dotium" (Barbaro, "Libro di nozze," fol. a). Especially noteworthy in this act are the suggestions that this practice is of relatively recent origin ("orta sit") and the clear indication that high dowries damaged a man's other heirs—presumably the male ones.

larger chunk of the family patrimony than had been the case earlier. For these reasons, the rise in dowries had important ramifications for Venetian economic life. However, we are primarily concerned here with effects rather than with causes. Specifically, we shall deal with the way in which these ever-larger dowries were assembled. It happens that, at least in Venice, at the same time that dowry inflation was straining the resources of Dante's frightened fathers, the fathers were in fact getting a good deal of help to meet the challenge. This non-paternal involvement in the raising of dowries is a little-known fact of Venetian social history during the early Renaissance. Yet it has importance not just for the dowry as an institution, but for the family and kinship system of Venice's ruling class. Stated briefly, a widening circle of dowry contributors encouraged a patrician social orientation in which the traditional emphasis on lineage was increasingly complemented by non-lineage ties of affection and interest.

According to Roman dowry practice, the main purpose of the dowry was to help the groom bear the burden of matrimony (*sustinere onera matrimonii*).[13] In its medieval Italian version, however, the Roman *dos* had a special twist. Unlike original Roman practice, the medieval Italian dowry came to be regarded as the girl's share of the patrimony. From this principle flowed several important effects. One was that girls were excluded from a share in the patrimony (the *exclusio propter dotem*). The *fraterna*, or enduring joint inheritance, was for brothers alone: Sisters, provided with dowries, had no further legal part to play in their paternal family's economic life. Another effect was that dowries were supposed to be "congruent"—to equal a full share in the patrimony. It was, Pertile observes, to guarantee that dowries would not *exceed* an equal share under the pressure of dowry inflation, that Venice and other cities legislated against excessive dowries.[14] Finally, and most fundamentally, the view that a girl's dowry represented her rightful share of the patrimony meant that she had an indisputable right to a dowry. This was the source of the fathers' fright.[15]

13 Ercole, "Istituto dotale," I, 197–198. See also Enrico Besta, *La famiglia nella storia del diritto italiano* (Milan, 1962), 143–151.
14 Ercole, "Istituto dotale," I, 212–213, 218–232. The main study of the *fraterna* is Camillo Fumagalli, *Il diritto di fraterna nella giurisprudenza da Accursio alla codificazione* (Turin, 1912). Among more general literature, see Besta, *La famiglia*, 207–209; Antonio Pertile, *Storia del diritto italiano* (Turin, 1894), III, 282, 322. On the *fraterna* in Venetian practice, cf. Marco Ferro, *Dizionario del diritto comune e veneto* (Venice, 1779), V, 276–278.
15 "... la dote è un diritto della figlia, cui il padre non può mai sottrarsi" (Ercole, "Istituto dotale," I, 334).

Of course not all girls received marriage portions, no matter what the legal principles demanded. Closeting them in convents was a regular practice, and at its worst led to the scandalous situation in which convents, it was said, were little better than brothels. The 1342 will of the patrician Leone Morosini illustrates why the practice was widespread.[16] He bequeathed to his daughter Lucia a dowry of 576 ducats, along with a *corredum* (in effect, a trousseau of movable goods— personal effects, household items, etc.) of 346 ducats. But his wife was then pregnant and might give birth to another daughter. Rather than divide Lucia's portion between two girls—which would have led to two undistinguished marriages—Leone simply instructed that the second daughter be placed in a convent and given an annuity of ten ducats—quite a saving over Lucia's marriage portion.

Leone proposed the convent for his unborn daughter—in fact, the child turned out to be a son—because it was cheaper than an adequate dowry. But his motive was not simply to rid himself of the burdens of daughters. If two girls were too much to deal with, Leone, like other fathers, still viewed a well-dowered daughter as a social asset. In the same will he provided that if the unborn child was a boy, then Lucia was still to have a dowry "of the right amount for a patrician girl." It was the fathers' interest in effecting favorable matrimonial alliances that kept the marriage market booming and contributed to the rise in dowries—and operated to give concrete application to the legal principles governing families' responsibilities for their daughters' dowries.

But if, according to law, fathers bore primary responsibility for their girls' marriage portions, the responsibility did not stop with them. Contemporary commentators on Roman law and the Venetian statutes asserted that when a man died or became feeble-minded (*mentecaptus*) without providing for his daughters' dowries, his sons, the girls' brothers, took on the charge. This was consistent with the principle of the *fraterna*: The sons who assumed joint proprietorship of their deceased father's estate also assumed his obligations. The same principle further dictated that when male descendants were lacking, dowry responsibility went to the deceased father's male ascendants.[17]

16 Felix Gilbert, "Venice in the Crisis of the League of Cambrai," in J. R. Hale (ed.), *Renaissance Venice* (London, 1973), 275; PSM Miste, B. 127, Leone Morosini, parchment no. 2.

17 *Volumen statutorum, legum ac iurium D. Venetorum* (Venice, 1564), Bk. II, ch. 8, p. 17v. See also Ercole, "Istituto dotale," I, 238–246; Ferro, *Dizionario*, IV, 385–386.

Even more interesting, and usually unremarked in discussions of the early Renaissance dowry, is the principle that mothers were sometimes obliged to provide dowries, specifically when the father was too poor to do the girl justice. Since mothers were not part of the lineage (they had no membership in their husbands' and sons' patrimonial group), this responsibility signifies that dowries were not exclusively the concern of the patriline. But this slight hint of economic matriliny in a society usually regarded as stoutly patrilineal may have gone even further. If an unmarried and undowered girl lacked parents, brothers, and paternal ascendants, then according to one authority, responsibility passed to her maternal grandfather and other maternal ascendants.[18]

What this indicates is that the jurists considered dowry provision important enough to commit a fairly wide kinship web to participation in it. And even though in medieval practice the dowry took on the appearance of a share in the patrimony, which was the classic patrilineal institution, the maternal line also figured in this central fact of the family's social and economic life. But though the confluence of paternal and maternal kin around dowry-raising seems by itself to caution against overemphasizing the patriarchal character of Venetian upper-class society, what we have seen so far is only legal prescription. Did it correspond to actual practice? More specifically, did hard-pressed Venetian fathers receive the help in dowering their daughters that these legal prescriptions promised?

The evidence indicates that they did, and more. In the fourteenth and fifteenth centuries, patricians showed a strong and increasing disposition to contribute to the dowries of their young kinswomen. These conclusions are based on the testimony of 305 patrician wills, all but seven from the period 1300–1450. The wills were written by members of the sprawling Morosini clan or by wives of Morosini. Although one clan cannot be regarded as representative of the entire patriciate, the Morosini wills do offer something of a cross-section. This clan was a large one, spread over the city; there were at least fifty property-owning Morosini males in 1379, at all levels of wealth; and nearly half of the wills, 140, were written by women from other

---

18 Pertile, *Storia del diritto italiano* (Turin, 1893), IV, 93–94; Ercole, "Istituto dotale," I, 237. "L'avo ed ascendenti materni sussidiariamente sono tenuti a costituire la dote alla nipote in mancanza degli ascendenti paterni, e della madre" (Ferro, *Dizionario*, IV, 386). It should be noted, however, that we have not seen this principle mentioned in any other source.

families who married into the Morosini clan.[19] It should be acknowl-
edged at the outset that testamentary bequests for dowries are not the
same as actual contributions; Venetians frequently rewrote their wills,
thus cancelling their original bequests. However, each bequest indicates an intention valid at the time made, even though later revised.
So the evidence of these wills can provide some indication of Venetian
patricians' involvement with young girls' dowries.

.There are in the wills many bequests to unmarried girls, and in
view of the principle that a girl's dowry represented her share of the
patrimony, most of them probably amounted to contributions to the
legatees' dowries.[20] Nevertheless, to avoid ambiguity the analysis is
limited to 125 bequests, in 79 wills, that the testators destined explicitly
for the dowry purpose. Forty-two of the wills were drawn up by men,
the remaining thirty-seven by women. Table I gives the distribution
of the bequests among the various recipients.

Table I shows that though they were about equally generous to
granddaughters and nieces, men outdid women in bequests to daughters

Table I Dowry Bequests

BENEFICIARIES	MALE TESTATORS	FEMALE TESTATORS	TOTALS
Daughters	50 (61.7%)	31 (38.3%)	81 (100%)
Granddaughters	7 (46.7%)	8 (53.3%)	15 (100%)
Nieces	11 (52.4%)	10 (47.6%)	21 (100%)
Sisters	4ᵃ (80%)	1 (20%)	5 (100%)
Cousins	—	3 (100%)	3 (100%)
	72	53	125 (100%)

a   Includes one sister-in-law.

19   In a fiscal census (*estimo*) conducted in 1379, the Morosini estimates ranged from
500 to 38,000 lire *a grossi* (equal to 192–14,615 ducats). The basis of the estimate was
real property. The Morosini in the *estimo* dwelt in twenty-four different parishes
(*contrade*), in five of Venice's six *sestieri*, or administrative zones (Luzzatto, *I prestiti*,
doc. 165, 141–186, *passim*). For a full-length study of patrician kinship, based on the
experience of the Morosini, we have isolated more than twenty different lineages
within the clan. In our use of the terms "clan" and "lineage" we follow Robin Fox,
Kinship and Marriage (Harmondsworth, 1967), 49–50. For a fuller discussion, see George
Peter Murdock, *Social Structure* (New York, 1949), 46–78. The 140 women's wills are,
of course, distinct from 62 wills of Morosini daughters, twelve of whom married
Morosini males.
20   See *Volumen statutorum*, Bk. IV, ch. 25–26, p. 73v. For the principle that dowries
were women's only claim on their fathers' estates, see Nino Tamassia, *La famiglia
italiana nei secoli decimoquinto e decimosesto* (Milan, 1910), 292–295.

by a ratio of 5:3. In fact, that ratio is only slightly larger than that of about 3:2 between the total number of children named in the forty-two men's wills and those in the thirty-seven women's wills.[21] Thus, part of the reason that men gave more in dowry bequests lies in the apparent fact that they had more children than women when they wrote their wills. How can this be explained? For one thing, women had a tendency, as we shall see below, to draw up wills during their first pregnancies, when, of course, their only children were *in utero*. Men generally testated after their families were already born. However, we should not make too much of this difference; only four of the thirty-seven wills in the present sample were written by women apparently in their first pregnancies, and more generally, women—like men—wrote wills at all points throughout their adult lives, and at all points in their families' developmental cycles.[22]

A better explanation is that men on the whole named their children individually and made specific provision for their respective legacies. Women, by contrast, tended to make blanket bequests to their offspring, with equal shares to boys and girls alike. In this connection it is worth noting that young married women in their first pregnancies, like other female testators in later pregnancies, did make generalized bequests for their daughters' dowries. All four of the women in their first pregnancies mentioned above provided for the dowries of their unborn children, should they be girls.[23] Thus, the appearance—to judge from dowry bequests—that men had more children may be illusory, a result of different habits of testation by men and by women.

21 Thirty-six of the forty-two men mentioned children, totalling 129. Thirty-four of the thirty-seven women mentioned children, a total of ninety-one. Included in these figures are unborn children of pregnant wives—whether mentioned in the wives' or in the husbands' wills.

22 Thus, of the eighteen mothers whose husbands were still living when the women wrote their wills, four were pregnant with their first child, four mentioned one child, three mentioned two children, one mentioned four, one mentioned seven, and the remaining five made general reference to their children without specifying their names or numbers. Taking another perspective, five of the thirty-seven female testators mentioned grandchildren, against six of the forty-two men; and ten of the women mentioned living parents, against eight of the men.

23 The four are: Elena, wife of Andrea Morosini (ASV, Notarile, Testamenti [all henceforth abbreviated NT and followed by the bundle number and the notary's name] 466, Benedetto Gibellino, no. 5, 12 July 1417); Fresca, wife of Roberto Morosini (NT 1230, Federico Stefani, no. 207, 22 Dec. 1433); Franceschina, wife of Berto Morosini (NT 721, Andrea Marevidi, no. 145, 3 Dec. 1444); Maria, wife of Nicolò Morosini (NT 746, Marciliano de'Naresi, no. 83, 27 Nov. 1426).

In fact, the primacy of paternal involvement in dowry raising that the figures in Table I reveal—50 percent of the total—is even more clearly reflected in the amounts of dowry bequests.[24] Table II shows that throughout the period fathers continued to discharge their patrimonial responsibilities as leading contributors to their daughters' dowries, and that the size of the contributions rose with the inflationary trend in dowries. But the table also shows that though non-paternal bequests did not increase in size to the same extent, they did increase in numbers—to the point that in the fifteenth century, they outstripped bequests of fathers. The effect was to give non-paternal bequests, small in average, considerable aggregate importance in the total amounts bequeathed for dowry purposes, as indicated in the bottom row of the table.

This substantial, and growing, involvement of kin other than fathers in the accumulation of dowries, coinciding as it did with an alarming rise in dowry levels, must have been welcome to hard-pressed fathers of daughters. But it raises an important question in the general context of family and kinship relations. The compensation that fathers and brothers traditionally had received for dowry expenditures was the acquisition of economic, social, and even political allies in the persons of their new sons- and brothers-in-law.[25] Did the growing involvement in dowry raising of kin from outside the patrimonial group—or, in its identity over time, the lineage—now attenuate the lineage's expectations from the marriage alliance? The answer to the question requires a closer look at the kinsmen who contributed to girls' dowries.

Since we want to discover whether the patrimonial group's concern in girls' marriages diminished as the pool of dowry contributors increased, it makes sense to divide contributors into those who belonged to the endowed girl's lineage, and those who did not. What this means in practice, since we are concerned with dowry bequests from kinsmen, is a division between the legatee's paternal and maternal kin. With that in mind, a nice parallel emerges with Table I: Just as fathers dominated among contributors within the lineage, mothers were the foremost

---

24 Based on 102 bequests in specific amounts; the remaining 23 dowry bequests did not specify amounts.
25 For examples of economic and political returns on dowry investments, see, respectively, Lane, *Andrea Barbarigo*, 28–29; *idem*, "Family Partnerships and Joint Ventures in the Venetian Republic," in *idem*, *Venice and History*, 38–39.

Table II Paternal and Non-Paternal Dowry Bequests

	TO 1330	1331–1370	1371–1410	1411–1450
Largest bequest	p[a]-769[b] (1)[c]	p-1,000 (5)	p-2,300 (22)	p-4,500 (9)
	n[a]- 4[b] (1)[c]	n- 769 (6)	n-2,000 (27)	n-2,000 (26)
Smallest bequest	p-269	p-382	p-1,000	p-1,000
	n- 4	n- 4	n- 1	n- 10
Median bequest	p-509	p-576	p-1,350	p-2,000
	n- 4	n-634.5	n- 200	n- 500
Average bequest	p-535	p-606.4	p-1,340.9	p-2,244.4
	n- 4	n-500	n- 589.6	n- 569.2
Total amounts bequeathed	p-3,214 (99.9%)	p-3,032 (50.3%)	p-29,500 (65.7%)	p-20,200 (57.7%)
	n- 4 (0.1%)	n-3,000 (49.7%)	n-15,379 (34.3%)	n-14,800 (42.3%)
	3,218 (100%)	6,032 (100%)	44,879 (100%)	35,000 (100%)

a p = paternal; n = non-paternal.
b All amounts are in ducats.
c The number of bequests in this category, during this period.

contributors from outside the lineage, accounting for nearly one quarter (24.8 percent) of all dowry bequests.

It is something of a moot point whether a married woman belonged to her husband's lineage.[26] For our purposes, however, differences on the one hand between statutory regulations governing succession to intestate fathers and those governing succession to intestate mothers, and on the other hand between men's and women's general bequest patterns, indicate that married women did not demonstrate the same patrimonial and patrilineal concern that characterized their menfolk.[27] So their participation in the dowry-raising process lay outside of the interests of the lineage. Why then did women contribute to their daughters' dowries? There was an obligation attached to dowries that required wives to benefit their children with them; some jurists even held that a woman enjoyed only the usufruct of her dowry, its real proprietors being her children. Venetian law seems to have stopped short of that view, but statutory provision for succession to the estates of intestate women was completely in favor of their children.[28] These maternal bequests are interesting less because they were made (there are, after all, cultural as well as legal reasons for that), than because of their size and importance, and the timing of their appearance as an important element in the assembling of dowries.

26 In Roman law during the Republic, a wife might be absorbed into her husband's family or not; by the Empire, the tendency was for her not to be so—to remain, rather, either under her natal *paterfamilias* or, if none existed, to be *sui iuris*. In either of the latter two cases, she was not considered agnatically related to her husband's family. See J. A. Crook, *Law and Life of Rome* (London, 1967), 103–104; Barry Nicholas, *An Introduction to Roman Law* (Oxford, 1962), 80–83. In Lombard law, wives passed over to their husbands' families by reason of the husbands' purchase of the *mundium*—roughly, protective domination—from the wives' fathers; by the time of the restoration of Roman law, however, this practice no longer prevailed in the Veneto, if indeed it ever had. See Pertile, *Storia del diritto*, III, 234–240. In practice, women retained ties both to their natal and to their marital families and lineages.

27 Succession to an intestate father excluded married daughters, whose share of the patrimony had already been advanced in the form of dowries. Married daughters were, however, admitted to equal shares in the succession to their intestate mothers' property since this property did not have the patrimonial character. See *Volumen statutorum*, Bk. IV, ch. 25, p. 73v, ch. 28, p. 74v. The same relationship holds true regarding emancipated and unemancipated sons (Roberto Cessi [ed.], *Gli statuti veneziani di Jacopo Tiepolo del 1242 e le loro glosse* [Venice, 1938], p. 207, gloss 173). On general bequest patterns, see below, note 40.

28 Besta, *La famiglia*, 149–150; Tamassia, *La famiglia italiana*, 289. Already in A.D. 1060 Venetian women were regarded as the proprietors of their dowries (Pier Silverio Leicht, "Documenti dotali dell' alto medioevo," in *idem, Scritti vari di storia del diritto italiano* [Milan, 1943–48], II, pt. 2, 294). The statute governing inheritance from intestate mothers is in *Volumen statutorum*, Bk. IV, ch. 28, p. 74v.

Table III Men's and Women's Wills

	TO 1330			1331–1370			1371–1410			1411–1450		
	NO.	%	RATIO	NO.	%	RATIO	NO.	%	RATIO	NO.	%	RATIO
Men	8	57.1	$\frac{1.3}{1}$	22	44.0	$\frac{1}{1.3}$	40	33.1	$\frac{1}{2}$	34	28.3	$\frac{1}{2.5}$
Women	6	42.9		28	56.0		81	66.9		86	71.7	
	14	100.0		50	100.0		121	100.0		120	100.0	

Women, in general, were at first slow in contributing to dowries, but in the course of our period they came gradually to represent an increasingly important source of dowry money. In part this can be attributed to a constant rise in the ratio of women's wills to men's (see Table III). The relative stabilization in the number of men's wills is curious. It could be simply an accident of documentary survival, although why should women's wills have survived more than men's? There is, however, another explanation. The most dramatic increase in the number of wills of both sexes occurred in the decades after the Black Death.[29] It is probable that the experience of the great mortality that accompanied the plague in 1348 induced survivors, and especially their descendants, to look to their own estates with greater attention. One result would be more will-making. Another would be more will-making by younger people, with the specific effects of 1) more multiple wills—i.e., several wills written by the same individual over a number of years; and 2) more women's wills, as pregnant wives, concerned over intestacy, drew up their first wills during first pregnancies, modifying the intentions contained therein in later wills, also written during pregnancy.

The evidence of the 305 wills examined here documents both these effects. Eighty-seven, or 28.5 percent, were written by thirty-six individuals. Moreover, seventy-seven of these multiple wills were bunched between 1371 and 1450, constituting 32 percent of *all* wills written during those years. In fact, among the Morosini no series of wills by a single individual was begun before 1360—close enough to 1348 to suggest the influence of that year's events, and long enough after it for an institutionalized reaction to have taken hold.

Women dominated among the multiple testators. Twenty-eight of the thirty-six individuals who wrote more than one will were women. This fact adds credibility to the hypothesis about increased will-making following the Black Death. Women in Venice had a greater opportunity to write multiple wills than did men, by reason of their earlier entry into adulthood. In the fourteenth and fifteenth centuries, the preferred nuptial age for patrician girls was 13–15, and, as far as their elders were concerned, marriage meant that they became

29 There was a momentary decline in the period 1351–1370, from which twenty-two wills survive, as compared with twenty-eight for 1331–1350, sixty-five for 1371–1390, and fifty-six for 1391–1410. However, this relative decline can be attributed to the mortality itself; moreover, the great leap in the period 1371–1390 strengthens the argument advanced below.

mistresses of their own affairs.[30] A young wife's first occasion to exercise this mastery would present itself during her first pregnancy; if she survived that and subsequent pregnancies, she would have occasion to write a number of wills as her intentions regarding her bequests changed with changes in the life cycles of her kin.[31] As it happens, twenty-eight of the 202 women's wills in our group were written, by the testatresses' own explicit affirmation, during pregnancy; and another thirty-one were written by wives who may well have been pregnant but did not say so in their wills.[32]

This statistic is even more impressive in view of the fact that only 120 of the women's wills were written by wives; of the rest, 76 were by widows and 6 by single women or nuns. One of the pregnant testatresses was, in fact, a widow, but her example seems unique in our sample.[33] So the representation of pregnant women among married testatresses was at least 23.3 percent (28 out of 120) and, considering also those possibly pregnant, may have been as high as 49.2 percent. Moreover, this pronounced tendency to draw up wills during pregnancy was a development of the later fourteenth century; in the period 1331–70, pregnant women wrote one of twenty-eight women's wills (3.6 percent); in 1371–1410, thirteen of eighty-one (16.4 percent); and in 1411–50, fourteen of eighty-six (16.3 percent).[34] There are

30 This is consistently apparent in the wills. For example, Marco di Gentile Morosini in 1359 instructed that his daughter Beriola come i o her inheritance at age 11 (NT 1023, Ariano Passamonte, no. 23). Moisè di Piero Morosini specifically instructed that his daughters marry at age 12 (NT 572, Giorgio Gibellino, no. 23). One exception was Silvestro di Marco Morosini, who in 1432 instructed that his daughters were not to marry until age 16; he increased their dowry legacies by 250 ducats for every year that they waited after that. This may suggest a changing attitude in the fifteenth century. (NT 486, Francesco Gibellino, no. 45. See also Tamassia, *La famiglia italiana*, 197–198.)

31 To cite just two examples: Beruzza, wife then widow of Marco Soranzo, who was unmarried in 1374, wrote wills in 1380, 1385, 1388, and 1401 (NT 108, Giovanni Boninsegna, no. 84; NT 921, Nicolò Saiabianca, no. 519; NT 108, Giovanni Boninsegna, no. 296; NT 575, Giorgio Gibellino, no. 704). Beruzza's nubility in 1374 is indicated in the will written that year by her brother, Gasparino di Bellello Morosini (NT 1062, Lorenzo della Torre, no. 300). Another example is Cristina, wife then widow of Vettor di Lodovico Morosini, who wrote wills in 1382, 1399, 1423, and 1432 (CI 36, Giovanni Campion, 3, I, no. 71; NT 571, Giorgio Gibellino, no. 118; NT 560, Francesco Gritti, no. 346; NT 215, Giovanni Campisano, no. 34).

32 That is, the thirty-one possibilities had no children or named their parents as executors—an indication of relative youth—or both.

33 This was Agnesina, widow of Marco di Gentile Morosini (CI 143, Stefano Pianigo, no. 41), whose will is dated 7 Jan. 1360 (1359 Venetian style). That of her husband (cited above, note 30) is dated 21 Aug. 1359.

34 In the pre-1331 period there are six women's wills, including one written by a pregnant testatress.

grounds, then, for arguing that the shock of the Black Death—and each successive visitation of the plague—induced Venetians to concern themselves more regularly than before with the disposition of their property by testation. And the fact that the increase in women's wills outstripped that of men's simply reflects women's more numerous encounters with the prospect of death because of pregnancy.[35]

But a more compelling acquaintance with mortality during the plague years only partially explains the increase in women's wills. Equally important is the consideration that in the second half of the fourteenth century, and especially during its last quarter, they had more property to dispose of. Here we are brought back to dowry inflation. Most simply, once women started bringing larger dowries to their marriages, by that fact they became more economically substantial persons, with a greater capacity to influence the economic fortunes of those around them. Once begun, dowry inflation was a self-accelerating process.[36] That is, when wives who had brought large dowries to their own marriages thought of disposing their own estates (and, as we have noted, they started thinking of it sooner and more frequently in the later fourteenth century), they naturally thought of their own daughters. We shall see that they also thought of others; but their own knowledge of the importance of large dowries would incline them similarly to look after their daughters. And the existence of their dowry money, protected by law from husbandly rapacity and, often, enlarged through fruitful real estate and commercial investment, added a further impulse to well-considered testamentary disposition in favor of daughters.[37]

35 In fact, wives generally seem to have outlived their husbands. In an as yet uncompleted analysis, we found that of 110 patrician marriages terminated by the death of one of the spouses between 1366 and 1380, 77 ended with the death of the husband and only 33 with the death of the wife (CI 114, Marino, S. Tomà, prot. 1366–1391, *passim*). However, these data need to be examined carefully before the results are fully acceptable.
36 A consideration of some importance in this regard may be the effect of increased state-bond holdings (*prestiti*) on dowry amounts. From 1343 to 1381 the state's indebtedness, and thus the amount invested in it by citizens, jumped over 1100 percent; and although it oscillated thereafter, by 1438 it was nearly 16 times as much as in 1343 (F. C. Lane, "The Funded Debt," esp. 88). See above, 573–574.
37 To protect wives' dowries, the statutes required a deposit by the husband in the amount of his bride's dowry. They also assigned priority among all claims on a man's estate—including those of his children and his creditors—to dowry restitution, and made the husband's ascendants and descendants financially liable if the husband's estate was not sufficient to repay the entire dowry of his widow (*Volumen statutorum*, Bk. I, ch. 34, 56, 61, 62, pp. 17v, 26v–29v). An example of enforcement of the statutes is that of Marina, widow of Pangrazio di Benedetto da Molin. Although her late husband had

There was thus a self-reinforcing spur built into dowry inflation, derived from a woman's right to dispose of her own property, her concern for daughters, and the increased dowries that she was bringing to marriage. To illustrate the extent of this important dimension of dowry inflation—of which women were not only the objects but the effective agents as well—we can compare paternal and maternal dowry bequests in tabular form.

Table IV reveals three things with clarity. First, mothers began bequeathing money toward their daughters' dowries only after the middle of the fourteenth century; but from then on, the frequency of their contributions grew rapidly, both in absolute terms and relative to fathers' dowry bequests. Second, the size of these maternal bequests was also on the rise, in keeping with the general trend in dowries. Finally, until the middle of the fourteenth century, mothers' dowry bequests had little impact on the total amounts bequeathed for dowries; but starting in the last third of that century, they accounted for an increasing share of parental contributions—more than one third in 1411–50. So from all three standpoints, frequency, size, and relative importance, mothers' dowry bequests were enabling their daughters to meet the challenge of dowry inflation—an inflation to which the mothers, as dowry recipients themselves, were indirectly contributing.

The importance of this maternal involvement in providing relief for Dante's frightened fathers is obvious. But it has considerable social significance as well. It means that an increasingly larger role in the critical (and to some, central) social fact—marriage—was being played by individuals whose commitment to the brides' paternal lineage was much less intense that that of the brides' fathers.

It is a question of lineage orientation. In the patrilineal order of Venice, fathers never left their lineages, and they could attend materially to the interests of a wide range of kinsmen without this attention ever exceeding the realm of lineage interest.[38] Their bequests to members

---

been emancipated ("filius divisus") from his father, the latter was nevertheless forced to make up the difference when Pangrazio's own estate was inadequate to Marina's dowry claim (CI 114, Marino, S. Tomà, prot., 1366–1391, n.p., 10 May 1368). A wife was unable to invest her dowry without her husband's consent; but in compensation, he was obliged to pay her interest when he invested it (*Volumen statutorum*, Bk. I, ch. 39, p. 19v, Bk. III, ch. 28, p. 48v; NT 579, Giovanni de Comasini, no. 95: will of Goffredo di Francesco Morosini, 21 Feb. 1349 [1348 Venetian style]).

38 In strict anthropological terms, of course, a husband was just as much a member of two conjugal families as his wife. Legally, however, a man could belong to a marital conjugal family and still be under his father's *patria potestas*, with all of its economic

Table IV Paternal and Maternal Dowry Bequests

	TO 1330	1331–1370	1371–1410	1411–1450
Largest Bequest	p[a]–769[b] (6)[c]	p–1,000 (5)	p–2,300 (22)	p–4,500 (9)
	m[a]– —	m– 200 (1)	m–1,500 (8)	m–2,000 (12)
Smallest Bequest	p–269	p–382	p–1,000	p–1,000
	m– —	m–200	m– 200	m– 400
Median Bequest	p– 509	p–576	p–1,350	p–2,000
	m– —	m–200	m– 891	m– 900
Average Bequest	p– 535	p–606.4	p–1,340.9	p–2,244.4
	m– —	m–200	m– 897.8	m– 991.7
Total amounts bequeathed	p–3,214 (100%)	p–3,032 (93.8%)	p–29,500 (84.1%)	p–20,200 (62.9%)
	m– —	m– 200 (6.2%)	m– 5,582 (15.9%)	m–11,900 (37.1%)
	3,214 (100%)	3,232 (100%)	35,082 (100%)	32,100 (100%)

a p = paternal; m = maternal.
b All amounts are in ducats.
c The number of bequests in this category, during this period.

of their natal families and to those of their marital families alike remained within the lineage. As we have seen, men were tied to both by the *fraterna*, and the hereditary nature of patrician status in Venice only strengthened their commitment to the male line. In this context, a bequest to a daughter or sister was not essentially less beneficial to the interests of the lineage than one to a son or brother. In the latter case, the lineage benefited directly; in the former, it stood to benefit indirectly from the matrimonial alliance thus established.

With mothers the case was different. They were members of two conjugal families from two different lineages, and the result was a freer, less lineage-centered social orientation. The statutes, for example, did not exclude married daughters from succession to intestate women; women's property, lacking the patrimonial quality of men's, could more readily be diffused into the families of sons-in-law.[39] And women's habits themselves attest to a more flexible social attitude. The general pattern of their bequests reveals a nearly equal regard for their natal kinsmen, and, thus, for two distinct lineages.[40]

It would be valuable to know whether the increased maternal role in dowry accumulation equipped women with a greater voice in the choice of husbands for their daughters, as is the case, for example, in modern rural Greece.[41] Although there is some evidence of general motherly interest in whom their daughters married, the documentation does not reveal the extent to which mothers actually participated in matrimonial decisions. It seems reasonable to conjecture, however, that the concern that mothers demonstrated in the form of dowry bequests and the impact of their increasingly weighty contributions at a time of dowry-raising difficulty were negotiated into greater influence in the arrangements of their daughters' marriages.

More fundamentally, the contributions of mothers to their

---

effects. In any case, descent in Venice was patrilineal; to the extent that Venetian husbands remained unemancipated from their fathers, as seems to have been the rule, it seems fair to speak of extended families in the male line, even when common residence did not prevail (see Murdock, *Social Structure*, 2–10).

39 See above, note 27.

40 This conclusion arises from an examination of the bequests in the first fifty (by alphabet) wills of married women in the sample. Of 215 total bequests to first- and second-degree relatives, 107 (49.7%) went to natal kin, 96 (44.7%) to marital kin, and 12 (5.6%) to affines. These bequests are analyzed more fully in Stanley Chojnacki, "Patrician Women in Early Renaissance Venice," *Studies in the Renaissance*, XXI (1974), 18–84.

41 Ernestine Friedl, "The Position of Women: Appearance and Reality," *Anthropological Quarterly*, XL (1967), 108.

daughters' dowries may have helped to alter the social posture of the elementary conjugal family. In a widely held view, the Italian family during the twelfth and thirteenth centuries was subsumed under and, in important social matters, subordinate to the larger kinship group—clan, consortery, etc.[42] With mothers now counting for more in marriage—the most socially involving family enterprise of all—the importance of the larger kinship group, to which intermarrying women demonstrated a relatively weak allegiance, may have diminished. To see if this was the case, we can now turn to the dowry contributions of kinsmen other than parents.

Whatever long-range effects mothers' growing contributions to their daughters' dowries had in raising dowry standards, in the short run fathers must have welcomed them. But fathers had additional cause for happiness in the dowry contributions from a wide variety of other kinsmen as well. On the whole, women contributed to the dowries of girls other than their own daughters at a higher rate than did men: 41.5 percent of women's dowry bequests were external to the marital family, as against 30.6 percent of the men's. This is consistent with what we observed about wives' enduring attachment to their natal families. But, in fact, all Venetians, regardless of sex or marital status, were stimulated to help their nubile kin. Altogether 44 of the 125 dowry bequests, more than one third, were to girls other than the testators' daughters. And nowhere is the complexity of Venetian kinship patterns and of the bonds existing among kinsmen better illustrated than in the wide variety of relationships that existed between girls receiving dowry bequests and their benefactors and benefactresses.

One group of non-parental dowry bequests was consistent both with the spirit of Roman law and with general patrimonial principles: bequests from paternal grandfathers and uncles. Eighteen of the sample's twenty-two non-parental bequests from men were of this relationship. In the context of the undivided fraternal patrimony, such bequests made good sense. A father's contribution to the dowry of his son's unmarried daughter, a type of bequest encountered seven times in the sample, amounted to a far-sighted arrangement for money that would have gone to the son anyway, and would ultimately have served him

42 See Tamassia, *La famiglia italiana*, 111–114. See also the valuable discussion of David Herlihy, "Family Solidarity in Medieval Italian History," in Herlihy, et al. (eds.), *Economy, Government and Society in Medieval Italy: Essays in Memory of Robert L. Reynolds* (Kent, Ohio, 1969), 173–184.

for his daughter's dowry. But the concern that grandfathers manifested in these bequests suggests that granddaughters' dowry prospects had a more than casual importance to them. For example, Alessandro di Michele Morosini, in his will of 1331, bequeathed his entire estate, less pious and charitable bequests, to his only child, Paolo. According to the instructions in the will, Paolo was not to come into his inheritance until age 20, except for one eventuality: If he should marry and have a daughter before his twentieth birthday, he was to make a will and in it provide for the girl's dowry in the amount of 653 ducats together with a *corredum* "worthy of a noble woman"—all from Alessandro's estate. Seventy years later, Gasparino di Bellello Morosini added 800 ducats to the dowry left to his granddaughter, Franceschina, by her late father, and this at a time when Gasparino had three living sons of his own, at least one a minor.[43]

There is a clue to the reasons for such grandfatherly concern in Gasparino's will. He declared that he wanted Franceschina to marry a "Venetian gentleman worthy of her status and acceptable to my sons." Gasparino and, presumably, Alessandro and other grandfathers like them, were willing to cut into the property of the male line—the jealous preservation of which was a toughly held principle in many wills[44]—and to alienate wealth by sending it into other men's families because such expenses were investments that promoted the interest of the lineage in two ways. First, it ensured that the line would not lose status through unworthy marriages. Second, it provided the direct male heirs with affinal connections that, precisely because they were expensive to come by, promised social and economic benefits to the lineage.

This transgenerational solicitude for the well-being of the lineage, as expressed in dowry bequests to granddaughters, is even more striking in the case of men who had unmarried daughters of their own. An example of such a man is Andreasio di Michele Morosini, brother

43 NT 1189, Piero Cavazza, no. 83; NT 571, Giorgio Gibellino, "Carte Varie," dated 28 April 1401. Gasparino's bequest complemented some real estate that Franceschina had been left by her late father.
44 *Ibid.* In his will of 1348, Andreasio di Michele Morosini bequeathed all of his real estate to his four sons with the provision that if they all died without issue, the property was to be sold, at a discount of 25 percent off the assessed value, to "aliquibus vel alicui de propinquioribus, de stipite, prolis mee" (PSM Miste, B. 182a, Andreasio Morosini, account book, n.p.). For similar sentiments, see the wills of Nicolò Morosini dottor in 1379 and of Albertino di Marino Morosini in 1450 (CI 97, Francesco Gritti, no. 1; NT 986, Francesco Rogeri, no. 110).

of the Alessandro whose will we have just considered. In his will of 1348, Andreasio left his own unmarried daughters dowries of 692 and 382 ducats, respectively, at the same time he willed a dowry of 616 ducats to any of his sons' daughters who should be her father's sole heir.[45] In such cases, the testators appear to slight their own daughters in the interest of their granddaughters. That they did so indicates that Venetian patricians had a sense of lineage as a sort of superpersonal abstraction that would live on after the testator but the well-being of which was nevertheless in his interest and deserving of his efforts on its behalf. It also indicates that they viewed its well-being not only in narrow terms of retaining wealth among males, but also in a more sophisticated sense of social and economic alliances of the kind built up through marriage.[46]

The same sense is evident in the dowry bequests of uncles to nieces. There are eleven such legacies in our sample, and eight of them were given by the testators to their brothers' daughters.[47] Of these testators, five had children of their own to provide for, including, in three cases, unmarried daughters. Yet, the avuncular providence could be impressive: In 1413 Giovanni di Piero Morosini willed 1,200 ducats toward the dowry of his late brother's daughter, while bequeathing his own daughter a dowry of 2,000 ducats.[48] The reasons for such generosity were twofold. The continued existence of the *fraterna* long after the father's death meant that the dowries of all daughters of a group of brothers came, to some extent at least, from the same common estate. But along with the common dowry burden went common advantages—the second reason for men's dowry bequests to their brothers' daughters. The economic and social benefits that a bride's father might harvest from a good marriage—at the price of a large dowry—were shared by his brothers. These were the considerations underlying Gasparino Morsini's instructions that any husband of his

---

45 PSM Miste, B. 182a, Andreasio Morosini, account book, n.p.

46 In this respect the Venetian lineage, and the clan to which it belonged, contrasts with the consorteries of Lombardy and Tuscany. See Franco Niccolai, "I consorzi nobiliari ed il comune nell'alta e media Italia," *Rivista di storia del diritto italiano*, XIII (1940), 119–124, and *passim*. On the restrictions that corporate kin groups, such as the consortery, place on relations with affines, see Eric R. Wolf, "Kinship, Friendship, and Patron-Client Relations in Complex Societies," in Michael Banton (ed.), *The Social Anthropology of Complex Societies* (New York, 1966), 5.

47 Of the other three, two are unclear about the testators' relationship to the legatee and one bequest went to the daughter of the testator's brother-in-law—it is not clear whether a sister's husband or a wife's brother is meant.

48 CI 168, Marco de Rafanelli, no. 93.

granddaughter Franceschina had to be approved by his surviving sons, the girl's uncles.[49]

The mutual involvement of brothers in the marital destinies of each other's daughters was complemented by their collective involvement in the marital destinies of their sisters. Indeed, it can be argued that the ones who bore the brunt of the entire dowry system, and especially of the inflationary trend, were the brothers of endowed girls. It was the inheritance theoretically devolving upon them, as continuers of the lineage and of the patrimony, that was diminished by each dowry that accompanied a sister to her marriage. It was probably recognition of this potential clash of interests that prompted the legislators to guarantee the inheritance rights of daughters *vis-à-vis* their brothers. On the other hand, Pertile observed that it was to protect brothers from the effects of dowry inflation that governments, such as that of Venice, attempted to put restraints on dowry amounts.[50] Yet despite the grounds for brother-sister rivalry, there are instances of brothers helping their sisters' marriage prospects from what seems to be a view of family advantage that extended beyond a narrow, and self-serving, emphasis on male inheritance. In the 1374 will in which he bequeathed 1,500 ducats to his newborn daughter, Gasparino Morosini gave 100 ducats to each of his nubile sisters.[51] In 1416, Nicolò di Giovanni Morosini, with no children of his own but with two living brothers and a sister, wrote in his will some instructions that testify to the broad view that Venetian men could hold of the interests of the lineage. After making some pious bequests, he willed the rest of his estate to his two living brothers, under two conditions. One was that from that inheritance the two brothers were to add enough to the 1,400 ducats which their father had left their sister to enable her to

49 Legally, the *fraterna* lasted for two generations of the male line (Lane, "Family Partnerships," 37; Pertile, *Storia del diritto*, III, 282). The principle of grandfatherly bequests was prescribed in the statutes. *Volumen statutorum* (Bk. IV, ch. 25, p. 72v), stated that the unmarried and orphaned granddaughters, through the male line, of intestate men possessed a right to shares of their grandfathers' estates for dowry purposes (in effect parts of the shares that their deceased fathers would have inherited had they been alive). The principle was important enough to have been included in the additions and amendments to the statutes carried out under the Doge Andrea Dandolo in 1343 (*ibid.*, Bk. VI, ch. 53, p. 110v).
50 The statute-makers devised a long and complex set of principles to guarantee that the son of an intestate father made a sufficient amount available to his unmarried sister for her dowry (*ibid.*, Bk. IV, ch. 25, p. 71v; Ercole, "Istituto dotale," I, 241–246). Pertile, *Storia del diritto*, III, 322.
51 NT 1062, Lorenzo della Torre, no. 300.

marry "in a way that befits the condition of my house and brings honor to it."[52] The other condition was that some of the money was to augment the dowries that their late brother had left to his daughters, who were Nicolò's and his brothers' nieces.

The case of solicitous brothers, like that of grandfathers and uncles, demonstrates a commitment to the continuing interests of the patrilineage. That much is consistent with the patrilineal traditions of medieval European society.[53] Even if Venetian patricians extended the range of lineage-promoting tactics to include investment in good marriages for social and economic reasons, the orientation was toward the lineage. If an occasional patrician bequeathed something toward the dowry of his wife's sister, as Fantin di Giovanni Morosini did in 1413, that was a remarkable exception.[54] The dominant impulse among males making dowry bequests, whether to daughters, granddaughters, nieces, or sisters, was to bring honor and profit to the male line to which they belonged and which they regarded as their duty to preserve. When hard-pressed fathers were helped in meeting the challenge of dowry inflation by their own fathers, brothers, or sons, this help had its roots in a long tradition of male kinship solidarity.

But among women the pattern was different. And in the context of women's increasing prominence in dowry raising, the differences are important for an understanding not only of how this major aspect of the familial experience developed, but of changes in the family's place in the larger kinship system, and in society. In certain respects, of course, women did resemble men in their dowry bequests. We have already seen the priority that they gave to their daughters. But they also resembled men in some of their express motivations in making such bequests. Like men, they regarded social suitability, marrying according to one's station, as a major desideratum for their daughters. Lucia, wife of Roberto Contarini, made a forthright statement of this sentiment in her will of 1413. If at her death her daughters did not have

52 "... cum honore et prout congruit conditionem domus mee honorificientius maritetur" (NT 1234, Francesco Sorio, no. 509).
53 On the patrilineal traditions, however, see the debate between Leyser and Bullough: K. Leyser, "The German Aristocracy from the Ninth to the Early Twelfth Century: A Historical and Cultural Sketch," *Past & Present*, 41 (1968), 25–53; D. A. Bullough, "Early Medieval Social Groupings: The Terminology of Kinship," *ibid.*, 45 (1969), 3–18; K. Leyser, "Debate. Maternal Kin in Early Medieval Germany. A Reply," *ibid.*, 49 (1970), 126–134.
54 He bequeathed 100 ducats to his "madona" for her daughter's dowry (NT 1233, Francesco Sorio, no. 257). The source for the meaning of *madona* as mother-in-law is Giuseppe Boerio, *Dizionario del dialetto veneziano* (Venice, 1856), 381.

dowries adequate to permit them "to marry well, according to their station," then they were to get more from her estate, "in order to marry better."[55] Superficially, women also resembled men in their dowry bequests to girls other than their own daughters. Against seven bequests to granddaughters by men, there were eight by women; against eleven bequests to nieces by men, there were ten by women.

It is among these non-filial bequests, however, that some interesting differences occur. A closer look at the bequests to grandchildren reveals that both women and men divided their bequests evenly between sons' daughters and daughters' daughters. But the three men who made bequests to their daughters' daughters had no sons,[56] whereas in three of the four cases of male bequests to sons' daughters, the testators also had daughters of their own (in two instances, married daughters) for whose living and prospective female offspring no dowry provision was made in the wills. The eight women's bequests to granddaughters make an interesting contrast. In three cases, the testatress had only one child. But of the remaining five, only one made a bequest to the granddaughter by one child without also remembering the granddaughters by her other children of both sexes. To illustrate this difference more clearly we can glance at the wills of Giovanni, son of the Doge Michele Morosini, and of his widow, Novella, who wrote hers in 1420. Giovanni bequeathed 2,000 ducats to any of his sons' daughters who might be her father's only child. Novella also made a bequest to a son's daughters: She willed 500 ducats toward the dowries of her son Marino's daughters. But at the same time, and unlike her husband, she bequeathed the same amount to the daughter of her daughter.[57]

The indication is clear: In their non-filial bequests men showed a

55 "E in caxo che si al maridar de mie fie le mon avesse tanto che le podesse ben maridar segondo la so condition voio che lo i se possa azonzar la parte che i tocasse de questo mio residuo in la so impromesse per maridarle meio" (NT 1255, Pietro Zane, fol. 194r).

56 However, one of them, Giovanni di Marino Morosini, in 1397, was very generous to his brothers' sons (CI 242, Giacomo Ziera, 5. prot., c. iv).

57 Maria, widow of Matteo Morosini, in her will of 1431 bequeathed 500 ducats toward the dowry of her son's daughter without reference to either her own daughter or that daughter's children, although the daughter, who was married, was to act as executor. However, the daughter was living with her husband in Negroponte (Euboea), and distance may have weakened contacts; the daughter was to be an executor only if she returned to Venice (CI 24, Rolandino Bernardi, 16. c. 41, no. 99). Novella's will is in *ibid.*, 16. c. 67, no. 184. For Giovanni's, see PSM Miste, B. 2, Giovanni Morosini, account book.

prejudice in favor of the interests of lineage, which benefited from dowry assistance given to the daughters of its male members. Where male testators helped their daughters' daughters—and thus, indirectly, the lineages to which their sons-in-law belonged—they did so only when they had no sons to carry on their own lineages. Women, however, demonstrated no such prejudice. Their contributions to their granddaughters' dowries were not governed by consideration either of lineage or of the sex of the child whose daughter was benefiting.

But does that mean that married women substituted loyalty to their natal families' lineages, for that of their husbands'? Certainly they maintained close ties to their natal families. The wills reveal that nearly half of the testamentary executors chosen by married women were primary natal kin (parents and siblings); and this was true both of women with living husbands and of widows.[58] But such continued rapport makes sense in the context which we are considering. A family investing a substantial dowry in a socially and economically desirable marital alliance could be expected to keep in touch with its son- and brother-in-law; *a fortiori*, contact would be maintained with his wife. Moreover, the wife herself, as a propertied person with the capacity to make testamentary disposition of and, provided her husband consented, to invest her property, could be expected to maintain economic ties to the family that had been the source of her property.[59]

However, women's social and economic contact with their natal families is not the same as identification with the continued interests of the natal family's lineage. In this connection, a comparison between men's dowry bequests to their nieces, already discussed, and those of women to their nieces discloses a significant difference. We noted that of eleven male bequests to nieces, eight specified the girls' precise rela-

58 Based on examination of primary-kin executors in ninety-seven wives' and widows' wills—those whose first names begin with the letters A–E. The results can be seen most clearly in tabular form:

EXECUTOR	67 WIVES'	30 WIDOWS'	ALL WOMEN'S EXECUTORS
Parents and siblings	91 (52.2%)	32 (42.7%)	123 (49.5%)
Husbands	53 (30.5%)	— —	53 (21.3%)
Children	30 (17.3%)	43 (57.3%)	73 (29.2%)
	174 (100%)	75 (100%)	249 (100%)

It is noteworthy that one out of every five wives (14 of 67) failed to name her husband among her executors.

59 For example, Tomasina, widow of Albano Zane, made business loans to her father, Andrea di Dardi Morosini, at least twice in the 1380s (CI 20, Giovanni Bon, fasc. 4, n.p. 21 March 1380; fasc. 5, n.p., 27 April 1382).

tionship to their benefactors, and in each of these eight cases she was the daughter of the benefactor's brother. By contrast, only two of the ten women's dowry bequests to nieces went to daughters of brothers; three are unclear about the relationship, and five went to daughters of the testatresses' *sisters*. If we regard a bequest of this kind as helping a lineage, the lineage to benefit was neither that of the benefactress nor her husband, but that of her sister's husband. So although women were relatively more active than men in making dowry bequests to consanguines other than their own daughters, their motives were different from those of men. Although men emphasized their own lineages, women did not share this priority. For them, considerations of the lineage, whether natal or marital, seem to have been relatively unimportant. But family ties, whether male or female, natal or marital, represented an important imperative.

What conclusions can we draw from these differences between men's and women's dowry bequests? The most important is that a distinctive, feminine, social impulse was coming to have considerable influence in patrician social relations. The aspect of this feminine orientation that set it apart from that of men was a comparatively weaker sense of lineage. Women's relative lack of concern for the interests of the lineage did not mean indifference to kinsmen. It did mean, however, that the principle of selection governing their testamentary beneficence—in the context of our discussion, their dowry beneficence —was different from the commitment to kin-group interest that characterized men. It was the principles of "religion, morality, conscience and sentiment"—the sanctions that govern relations not of the kin group, but of the family.[60] And of these, in the case of Venetian patrician women, personal regard—affection—seems to have been critical.

It can be seen in a special bond that existed among women. This point must not be exaggerated. Women did demonstrate concern and responsibility for their male kin, sometimes even attaching greater importance to them than to the females.[61] But the attachment between

60   Meyer Fortes, "The Structure of Unilineal Descent Groups," *American Anthropologist*, LV (1953), 34. He contrasts these principles governing the family, the nucleus of the "complementary line of filiation" which ties husband and wife together, with the principles that govern the descent group's interests—law and public institutions.
61   Making provision for her unborn child in her will of 1385, Cristina, wife of Antonio Querini, bequeathed it 300 ducats if a boy, but only 200 if a girl (CI 22, Miscellanea Testamenti, Notai Diversi, no. 747).

women was both different from and, in important ways, stronger than the attachment between a woman and her male kin. We can see this by taking another look at the wills, this time focusing on bequests in general. A group of ninety-seven wills of wives and widows contains a total of 415 individual bequests to primary and secondary kin.[62] Of these, 218, or 52.5 percent, went to woman and only slightly fewer, 197 (47.5 percent), to men. There does not seem to be a great difference. But if they are divided into bequests to primary and to secondary kin, the results indicate more clearly the special relationship among women. In the 302 bequests to primary kin (parents, siblings, husbands, and children), males and females benefited almost equally, receiving 154 and 148 bequests, respectively. But among the secondary-kin bene-ficiaries (aunts and uncles, nieces and nephews, cousins, grandparents, grandchildren, and first-degree affinal kin: children-, siblings-, and parents-in-law), females outnumbered males by a considerable margin, receiving seventy bequests compared with forty-three to males, or 61.9 percent to 38.1 percent.

The discrepancy between the sex ratio in women's primary-kin bequests and that in their secondary-kin bequests is revealing of the motives behind women's choices of beneficiaries. When they bestowed equal testamentary largesse on the men and women of their primary kin, they were acting under the natural impulses of loyalty and affection that domestic proximity stimulated. Young wives, married at age 13 or 14, would naturally hold tightly to the reassuring ties to their parents and siblings regardless of sex.[63] Mothers would naturally feel affection for both sons and daughters. But though the preferences for females among more distant kin also reflects affection, it is of a more discriminating kind, resulting from association by choice, not by biological chance. These preferences are in keeping with the indications of women's relative indifference to considerations of lineage. Women left property to their female relatives not to advance the interests of the lineage, but because they felt affection for these relatives. There may have been a sense of kinship responsibility at work, for example, toward aged grandmothers; and the apparent tendency of women to outlive their husbands may have provided testatresses with a number of

62 This is the same group as that used above, note 58. Excluded from consideration are unborn children and generalized bequests to groups unspecified as to number, e.g., bequests "to all my children."
63 Evidence is the tendency in wives' choices of executors, indicated above, note 58, and the patterns of their bequests, analyzed above, note 40.

elderly widowed kin toward whom they could discharge that responsibility. But such gestures are still not sufficient to account for the five-
to-three ratio of females to males among women's secondary-kin
beneficiaries. Moreover, even the type of motivation in bequests to
aged female relatives is different from lineage allegiance, because it has
a personal rather than institutional object.

In the context of the growing importance of women's property,
organized in wills and, particularly, directed toward dowries, the impulse of personal affection that is apparent in the pattern of their
bequests has a special significance. It means that a richer and more
complex set of social forces was at work within the Venetian patriciate
in the later fourteenth and especially the fifteenth century than had
been the case earlier. The male commitment to the lineage still persisted, as indeed the endurance of the patrimonial system and the
hereditary nature of Venice's ruling class dictated that it would. But
alongside the lineage orientation of males, and complementary to it,
there was appearing—in a position of considerable social influence—
the more personal attitude of women. This may have bearing on the
old but recently rekindled discussion of the emergence of a more
intense family consciousness on the part of fifteenth-century Italians.[64]
The heightened personal affection that, as some writers have argued,
constituted the hallmark of the resurgent elementary family may have
its origin in the enlarged role of women. Yet, in Venice at least, this
greater influence commanded by women and by their distinctive social
orientation did not replace attention to lineage; it simply blended with
it another set of concerns.

In the light of these considerations, the dowry inflation that caused
Venetian and other Italian fathers such anxiety can be seen leading to a
number of developments that together contributed to a reordering and
an enrichment of the social relationships within the Venetian patriciate.[65] It strengthened the traditional kinship bonds by inducing

64 See Herlihy, "Family Solidarity," *passim*; Richard A. Goldthwaite, *Private Wealth
in Renaissance Florence: A Study of Four Families* (Princeton, 1968), esp. 255–258; Randolph
Starn, "Francesco Guicciardini and His Brothers," in Anthony Molho and John A.
Tedeschi (eds.), *Renaissance: Studies in Honor of Hans Baron* (DeKalb, Ill., 1971), 411–
444.
65 For reasons of space, we have not discussed the growing practice, engaged in by
both men and women, of allotting a certain amount of money to the dowries of poor
girls, both patrician and plebeian. We have found thirty-four such generalized bequests
in the Morosini wills, or almost one for every ten wills. The impulse behind these and
the bequests to kinswomen that we have been considering were doubtless encouraged
by the dowry inflation of the time. However, there is a difference between general

kinsmen to aid beleaguered fathers of marriageable daughters. It created stronger interlineage ties by increasing the expectations that families of effortfully endowed girls entertained *vis-à-vis* the girls' husbands. And by encouraging women themselves to take a substantial part in the accumulation of their daughters' and other kinswomen's dowries, it created a condition in which impulses of personal regard, both within and between families—and lineages—assumed a larger place among the principles governing patrician social relations.

charitable bequests, usually made in the category of bequests *ad pias causas*, and those to kinswomen made among the other specific bequests to family and friends. The former fall into the category of generalized charity that was growing in importance at this time. See Brian Pullan, *Rich and Poor in Renaissance Venice: The Social Institutions of a Catholic State, to 1620* (Cambridge, Mass., 1971), 183, and *passim*.

Journal of Interdisciplinary History, v:4 (Spring 1975), 655–667.

Robert V. Schnucker

Elizabethan Birth Control and Puritan Attitudes

The eighteen-year-old Mary Fitton, second daughter of Sir Edward Fitton, was sent to Queen Elizabeth's court in 1595 with the hope that as a lady-in-waiting, she would not only receive proper training but, at a propitious time, would be able to secure a fine husband. Since she had reached the full bloom of youth, she was attracted to and became attractive to some of the young men at court. In the course of events, Mary and the Earl of Pembroke became very close friends. What probably began as a casual relationship quickly developed into a scandal that embarrassed Mary, the Earl of Pembroke, and the court. According to a letter of Robert Cecil to Sir George Carew, Mary Fitton ". . . was proved with child, and the Earl of Pembroke being examined confesseth a fact but utterly renounceth all marriage." [1] Queen Elizabeth's reaction to the situation was to place both Mary and the Earl in the Tower. As the pregnancy progressed, a number of letters were exchanged between Mary and her father. It was apparent that the unwanted pregnancy had not only stymied the paternal hopes for a good marriage but also had ruined Mary's future at court. In one of the letters that Mary received, her mother added a postscript in which she warned her daughter against harsh physics, for their use could induce abortion. Is it possible that this supposed warning was really a suggestion for curtailing the unwanted pregnancy? The pregnancy went full term and when Mary was delivered, the child was reported as dead. Some of the questions raised by this episode concern what Mary Fitton could have done to avoid conception or to abort the pregnancy, and the broader issue of the knowledge of birth control of that time.

A rather common contemporary assumption is that only recently has birth control been a matter of concern. It is often further assumed that even when there was concern in the past, very little was known about the theories needed for effectual birth control, and a limited number of techniques were available. Three scholars who have dealt with the

Robert V. Schnucker is Professor of History and Religion and Chairman of the Department of Philosophy and Religion at Northeast Missouri State University. He is the author of *Modular Learning Program for World Civilization* (St. Charles, Mo., 1973).

1 Anne (Lady) Newdigate-Newdegate, *Gossip From a Muniment Room Being Passages in The Lives of Anne and Mary Fitton, 1574–1618* (London, 1898), 42.

problem of birth control among the English of the time of Mary Fitton have argued for limited knowledge of effective birth control techniques. Ashley has asserted that the techniques used were continence and *coitus interruptus*. Stone in his masterful work on the English aristocracy has taken a position basically the same as that of Ashley. Wrigley, in studying the population trends of Colyton in the sixteenth century, stated that, as far as is known, the English limited their families ". . . by practising *coitus interruptus* . . . and no doubt procuring many abortions, possibly also infanticide."[2]

The attempts to create a successful contraceptive date back to the ancient Egyptians when alligator dung in suspension was prescribed as a spermicide. The physicians of the Greek world wrote about contraceptives and the Romans borrowed the Greek knowledge and disseminated it throughout their empire. According to Hopkins, the bulk of ancient Greek and Roman medical knowledge was contained in twenty-six writers, twenty-three of whom mentioned various techniques and formulas for birth control. One basic source of information used in the Middle Ages came partly from this core of ancient medical knowledge.[3] Another source of birth control information for the Middle Ages came from the Islamic world, particularly the writings of Al Rāzī and Ibn Sīnā. Both men devoted some of their work to a discussion of various birth control methods. A summary of the techniques that they advocated included potions to be taken orally, magical means, pessaries, penis ointments, *coitus interruptus*, violant action by the female after coitus, and avoidance of simultaneous orgasms.[4]

In addition to these techniques, there was a considerable body of folklore knowledge in Elizabethan cook books, herbals, and medical manuals concerning birth control. The two methods most frequently presented to the reading public during the Elizabethan age were oral and mechanical contraceptives, and abortion. The concept underlying oral contraceptives (which took the form of vomits and laxatives),

2 Maurice Ashley, *The Stuarts in Love, with Some Reflection on Love and Marriage in the Sixteenth and Seventeenth Centuries* (New York, 1964), 10; Lawrence Stone, *The Crises of the Aristocracy 1558–1641* (Oxford, 1965), 633ff.; E. A. Wrigley, "Family Limitation in Pre-Industrial England," *Economic History Review*, XIX (1966), 104.

3 Norman E. Himes, *Medical History of Contraception* (New York, 1963), 71; Keith Hopkins, "Contraception in the Roman Empire," *Comparative Studies in Society and History*, VIII (1965), 128–130, 132. Hopkins gives a convenient chart listing the medical authorities and whether or not they discussed abortifacients and contraceptives.

4 Himes, *Medical History*, 148. Some of the substances to be used in anointing the penis include rock salt, tar, balm, oil with white lead, sweet oil, juice of onion, balsam, and sesame oil.

was to dampen or purge the desire for coitus—a method advocated earlier by Islamic physicians. Some of the ingredients used in oral contraceptives were pepper, rue calamine, castor oil, endive, sallow flowers, woodbine, cucumbers, purslane, sorrell, succory, conserves of red roses, mint, melons, cherries, plums, apples, pears, hemp seed, rue, cummin, corriander seeds, poplar leaves, and lettuce. One emetic designed to purge the desire for intercourse consisted of radish root, agarick, and saram boiled in barley water, to be taken when cool.[5]

The mechanical contraceptives were pessaries, genital baths, and bloodletting. A typical pessary to be inserted into the vagina was composed of bitter almonds blanched and ground. Another pessary used castoreum mixed with rue and the ground roots of lilies and nenufar. The pessary supposedly would provoke the menstrual flow and thus either prevent or possibly stop a pregnancy. A variation of the pessary was the uterine clyster which today would probably be called a douche. A clyster suggested by Ferrand was made of cold herbs, camphor, and castor oil or rue. That such clysters were used or at least known is shown by the papal bull of Sixtus V, *Effraenatam*, in which he spoke against poisons in douche form used for contraceptive purposes.[6] The theory supporting genital baths was that cooling the genitals would in effect dampen desire for coitus or benumb the genitals and thus reduce the possibility of erection or orgasm. All kinds of materials were suggested to accomplish this. Langham's herbal recommended ginger and vinegar, or juice from nightshade, leek, henbane, or the great morrill. The use of such juices, oils, and ointments probably were effective to some extent, for it would be difficult to maintain an erection while the penis was bathed in a cool liquid, particularly, a slightly anesthetic one.[7]

5 This list can be found in John XXI (trans. Humfre Lloyd), *The Treasuri of Helth* (London, 1550), fols, O v v-r. William Langham, *The Garden of Health* (London, 1633), 224, 585, 681. Andrew Borde, *A Compendyous Regyment or a Dyetary of Healthe* (London, 1547), fols. G iii r, H i r. James Ferrand, *Erotomania* (Oxford, 1640), 242, 244–245. See also *ibid.*, 348.

6 John XXI, *Treasuri of Helth*, fol. O viii r; Ferrand, *Erotomania*, 348, 355–356; John T. Noonan, *Contraception: A History of Its Treatment by the Catholic Theologians and Canonists* (Cambridge, Mass., 1966), 349. The bull was issued in 1558.

7 Langham, *Garden of Health*, 332. Langham also prescribed the use of willow leaves. His directions were to crush the leaves into a pulp and apply them to the privy parts to remove the desire for coitus. A similar suggestion is found in Ferrand, *Erotomania*, 266–267. *Ibid.*, 356, suggests that one ought to rub the genitals with the gall of Cramp-fish ". . . which is a marveilous Narcotiche, or Stupefactive vertue. . . ." But Ferrand warned that such practice could cause sterility in men and upset the menstrual cycle of women.

The theory behind bloodletting as a contraceptive was related to their notion of how sperm was produced. Sperm was thought to be blood made white by the heat humor and according to Ferrand, "... an Excrement of the third Digestion, which provokes Nature either by its quantity, or quality to evacuate it...." If either the quantity or quality of the blood could be decreased, then the necessary ingredient for sperm would be missing and the desire for coitus would diminish. Thus, it seemed reasonable that a sound technique to help control sexual passion was this minor form of surgery. Some parts of the body were better suited for this surgery than others. For example, the liver vein in the arm was thought to be a prime vein for venting the heated passions of love. However, if the male suffered from Satyriasis or the female from uterine fury, the vein to be opened was not to be near the privy parts for such an opening would bring the blood to the affected areas and cause the sexual passions to increase. If all of the bloodletting techniques failed, then, in desperation, Ferrand recommended that an arm vein be opened and the patient bleed until he "... is ready to fall downe for faintnesse, and losse of blood...."[8] The effectiveness of these oral and mechanical contraceptives is not known, but the number described in the literature of that time, plus the research of Stone, Ashley and Wright, provide a *prima facie* argument that contraceptives were recommended, available, and probably used.

The second basic form of birth control to be considered here is abortion. This form of limiting family size or avoiding an unwanted pregnancy has a long, interesting, and often tragic history. It is not surprising to find that during the Elizabethan age there were works available that described the symptoms and causes of abortion, some preventatives, and some abortifacients. The preventatives listed by the medical men indicate that they had no efficacious cure for the undesired abortion. Their inability to stop non-induced or induced abortion is seen in this "cure": Apply "... vpon their Nauell a tost dipt in good red wine, strowing vpon it the powder of Roses ... and a little cinamon."[9] The literature of that day, when discussing the causes of abortion, included such excessive exercise as leaping, dancing, riding in a coach, and lifting or carrying heavy weights, falls, blows, violent vomiting or bowel movements, and immoderate sexual intercourse. There was one report of women who sought to induce abortion by lacing themselves so tightly that the foetus would either be squeezed

8 *Ibid.*, 261, 262, 339.
9 James Guillimeau, *Child-birth or, The Happy Deliverie of Women* (London, 1612), 73.

to death or expelled.[10] However, if one could read and had access to various herbals, cook books, and household medical manuals, one would discover that the books contained suggestions that could be tried in secrecy and might induce an abortion. Most of the abortifacients were in some form of pessary or suppository. These were apparently to induce enough vaginal bleeding so that the foetus would be flushed out of the womb. Some of the suggestions offered were: the dregs of oil put in the vagina would cleanse it as would holwort; the flower of *nigelia romana* when mixed with honey and placed in the vagina would cause all of the contents of the vagina to come out violently; the same result would occur when a pessary made of the root of gladyn soaked in oil de bay with the powder of worlwort shaken over it was placed in the vagina overnight. A rather fierce irritant that was recommended for use as a pessary was made from nettle leaves. Langham's herbal prescribed ". . . i dram or ii drams of the powder (of flower de luce) with . . . broth or whey, and it prouoketh the terms and causeth abortion.[11]

Oral abortifacients were relied upon to cause either violent bowel movements or violent vomiting. The idea seems to have been that the violence would loosen the foetus or weaken it so that abortion would occur. Bankes claimed that apium would function as a physic which induced abortion, while Langham stated that the seed of water cress when used orally in a preparation would function as a vomit with the final result being abortion.[12]

There were complaints and warnings about pregnancy and childbirth. The physican Boaistuau declared that there was no one more subject to miseries and infirmities than the female, especially those who were fertile, ". . . for they haue scant a monethes rest in a whole yeere, but that they are continually ouercome wyth sorow and feare. . . ." The sensitive Copland early in the sixteenth century penned a similar concern. The young bride in his poem, realizing on her wedding night that married life held nothing but a continual succession of pregnancies, child-births, and deaths, forbid her husband any access to his conjugal rights. The woman's desire to stop the monotonous existence of

---

10 Jacob Rueff, *The Expert Midwife, Or an Excellent and most necessary Treatise of the generation and birth of Man* (London, 1637), 163ff., 60. See also Guillimeau, *Child-birth,* 70.

11 John XXI, *Treasuri of Helth,* fols. O vvi v; O viii r. The use of *negilia romana* was given by Langham, *Garden of Health,* 3–4. For flower de luce, see *ibid.,* 254–255.

12 Robert Bankes, *Here begynneth a newe marer ye whiche sheweth and treateth of the vertues & properties of herbes the which is callyed an Herball* (London, 1526), fol. A ii r; Langham, *Garden of Health,* 172.

bearing children was expressed, for example, by Frances Clarke in a letter to her father. She informed him that she had just given birth to her tenth child ". . . and I pray God, if it be his blessed will, it may be my last." The husband's frustration with frequent pregnancy was given in a letter of William Blundell to one of his older children after his wife had given birth to her tenth child: ". . . you have had three sisters in the space of thirty two months. You may well think this is not the way to grow rich." [13]

With this interest in birth control on the part of the Puritans, how can one determine the incidence of contraception among them? The method of family reconstitution used by Fleury and Henry, which might have proved productive, was inapplicable since we did not have access to the necessary parish records.[14] Instead, we have tried to determine the attitudes of the Puritans toward birth control and have assumed that there was a relatively high correlation between their attitudes and their actions. We then used some readily accessible demographic data to arrive at tentative but confirmatory results that might show whether or not some Puritans practiced birth control.

Birth control was rejected by the Puritans as running counter to the purpose for marriage. In general, most of the Puritan authors of marriage manuals and the scriptual commentators accepted a threefold purpose for marriage. The Puritans were divided over placing procreation or mutual solace as the primary purpose for marriage. Cleaver, Smith, Perkins, Niccholes, and Gouge stressed procreation, while Becon, Rogers, Pritchard, Cartwright, Gataker, and Willet, although accepting the same three-fold purpose, placed mutual solace and comfort first.[15]

13 Peter Boaistuau (trans. John Alday), *The theatre of Rule of the World* (London, 1574), 62; Robert Copland, *A Complaint of Them that be to soone mayred* (London, 1535), fols. B i v – B ii r; Ashley, *Stuarts in Love*, 10. Ashley quotes from Cecil Aspingall-Oglander, *Nunwell Symphony* (London, 1945), 115.

14 T. H. Hollingsworth, *Historical Demography* (London, 1969), 181.

15 Robert Cleaver, *A Godly Forme of Household Government* (London, 1603), 157–158; Henry Smith, *The Sermons of Henry Smith* (London, 1628), 13, 14, 16; William Perkins, *Christian Oeconomie* (Cambridge, 1618), 671; Alexander Niccholes, *A Discourse of Marriage and Wiving* (London, 1615), 29; William Gouge, *Of Domesticall Duties* (London 1622), 209–210; Thomas Becon, *Booke of Matrimonye* (London, 1564), fols. DCxlviii r, DCli v–r, DClv v; John Rogers (ed. F. J. Furnivall), *The Glasse of godly Loue* (London, 1898), 179; Thomas Pritchard, *The Schoole of honest and vertuous lyfe* (London, 1579), 50; Donald Joseph McGinn, *The Admonition Controversy* (New Brunswick, N.J., 1949), 181–182; Thomas Gataker, *A Good Wife Gods Gift* (London, 1623), 39–40; Andrew Willet, *Hexapla* (London, 1608), 401.

Johnson and Epton have variously argued that the Puritans began a new ordering of the three-fold purpose of marriage in which mutual solace and comfort gained primacy.[16] But there is ample evidence that what Johnson and Epton conceive as new was in fact part of a cultural change rather than a new emphasis spawned by Puritanism. For example, one of the first statements in English to place procreation second was William Tyndale's *On the Obedience of a Christian* (1528). Schücking has argued that this idea was not original to Tyndale but came from his teacher, Martin Luther. Six years after Tyndale's publication, Agrippa's *The Commendation of Matrimony* was translated into English and published. In this work, Agrippa also pressed the argument that the primary purpose for marriage was solace and comfort. Noonan has recently claimed that among some Catholic theologians in the early sixteenth century there was a shift from the Augustinian and medieval view that intercourse was only to be used for procreative purposes. This movement was led by Thomas de Vio, Cardinal Cajetan, Dom Dominic Soto, and Sylvester da Prierio.[17] Thus, there is evidence for a movement away from the time-honored priority of procreation as the first purpose in marriage during the sixteenth century and some of the Puritans were part of this movement or at least reflected it.

Although the Puritans were divided on the primacy of procreation or mutual solace and comfort in marriage, they were united in the idea that procreation, whether primary or secondary, was not to be taken lightly nor to be frustrated through the use of contraceptives or abortifacients. In short, although knowledge of birth control techniques was available to Puritans, they rejected the practice.

There were five fundamental beliefs that prevented their approval of birth control. First, by observing the Biblical injunction to be fruitful and multiply, parents were creating the basic cell of existence upon which was constructed all of the edifices of society, whether religious or secular. This was part of the order established by God at the beginning of creation. Heywood expressed this belief by writing that "Matrimony is therefore to be esteemed and honoured, as being first

16   James T. Johnson, "English Puritan Thought on the Ends of Marriage," *Church History*, XXXVIII (1969), 429; Nina Epton, *Love and the English* (London, 1960), 143.
17   Levin L. Schücking, *Die Familie im Puritanismus* (Leipzig, 1929), 32; Henry Cornelius Agrippa (trans. David Clapham), *The Commendation of Marriage* (London, 1534), fol. B vii v; Noonan, *Contraception*, 312–313.

ordained in Paradise, and since continued upon earth, and in a pious gratitude returnes us many pious and gratious children, to be made Citizens and Saints in Heaven."[18] The importance of procreation meant more than the human establishment of the basic cell of society: It meant that man cooperated in the divine work of creation.[19] This human cooperation, wrote Heywood, ". . . purchaseth man the name of father here below, as a type of that great and Almighty Father above: here generating, as he there creating. God made nature, man here maintaines her." The Puritan divine Thomas Gataker reminded his readers that the greatest honor and dignity that God could bestow upon man was to include him as an instrument in procreation by pro-creating others as himself, ". . . producing one in all respects like him-selfe, the chiefe of God's works; of giuing being to a creature with Gods Image, wherein himselfe had beene created. . . ." Niccholes held the same belief.[20] Further, since God had become man in Jesus Christ by being born of Mary, to prevent birth was also to attack the nature of man which God took upon Himself. Birth control was degrading to humanity; it meant the prevention of the creation of a being which God had blessed and honored through the incarnation. "Be fruitful and multiply" meant more than reproduction as among beasts. It meant the reproduction of those who bore the image of God; it meant the reproduction of the species through which the deity had chosen to reveal Himself.

The second aspect of the Puritan rejection of birth control con-cerned the belief that children were a blessing from God. The Puritan physician Christopher Hooke attempted to answer two complaints of women who did not recognize the breeding and bearing of children as a blessing, but who claimed, on the contrary, that pregnancy was without any divine control, that children were a burdensome charge, and, thus, that they would rather not bear them. These complaints Hooke declared to be wretched and unprofitable, for they robbed God of the honor and thanks due Him in the procreative process. The fruit

---

18 Thomas Heywood, *A Cvrtaine Lecture: As it is read by a Countrey Farmers wife to her Good man* (London, 1638), 82.

19 Smith, *Sermons*, 13; Gataker, *Good Wife*, 34. In the second sermon, with its own pagination, Gataker makes almost the identical comments as Smith.

20 Heywood, *Cvrtaine Lecture*, 82; Gataker, *Good Wife*, 34 (second set of pagination). Niccholes made the same allusion to the divine-human cooperation in the procreative process when he stated that the world must be populated with that which is the crown and glory of God's workmanship, that which is ". . . the last and best and perfectest peece of his handi-worke . . ." (*Discourse of Marriage and Wiving*, 1).

of the womb was a divine reward, a mercy, and a blessing bestowed by God.[21] Hooke and other Puritans made it clear that fecundity was not a bane but a blessing; even if the child was illegitimate. This idea had been declared earlier in the translated works of Bullinger and was continued in the writings of Gataker, Gouge, Hieron, and Perkins. Hieron, for example, pointed to the large families mentioned in the Old Testament and declared that the larger the family, the more the parents had been blessed by God. Whately told parents of numerous progeny that they must see God's hand in their fertility, while those who were barren must seek from God the ability successfully to reproduce.[22] It was the observation of Perkins that the divine blessing of marriage was partly visible in its fruit, i.e., children. Perkins also reminded his reader that the conception and birth of any child is an act wholly dependent upon God's providence and design.[23] Thus the female could not claim any merit in her fecundity, for the ability to conceive and bear children was solely the act of God's grace and mercy.[24] The practice of birth control meant that man pitted his will against the design and mercy of God and rejected fecundity as God's special mark of grace upon the union of male and female.

We turn now to the third of the Puritan objections to birth control. Those who attempted to limit the frequency of conception or birth could bring about a reduction in the number of the elect of the body of Christ and the number of the commonwealth. The increase of the number of the elect was emphasized by Hieron in his prayer for "Some Barren Hannah, or childless Elizabeth. . . ." Here it was made clear that the chief motive for procreation was to increase the elect:

> And, good Lord, bee pleased so to order and to direct my desire herein, as that I may not in this seeke some outward contentment onely, but that my chiefe respect may be, that by mee, thy Church may bee

21 Christopher Hooke, *The Childbirth or Woman's Lecture* (London, 1590), fols. D 2 v, C i v; Samuel Hieron, *All the Sermons of Samuel Hieron* (Cambridge, 1614), 149.

22 Heinrich Bullinger (trans. Miles Couerdale), *The Christian State of Matrimonye* (London, 1541), fol. C viii v; Gataker, *Good Wife*, 36; Gouge, *Domesticall Duties*, 506; Hieron, *Sermons*, 159, 409; Perkins, *Christian Oeconomie*, 690; William Whately, *Prototypes, or the Primarie Precedent. Presidents Out of the Booke of Genesis* (London, 1640), 120a, 132.

23 Perkins, *Christian Oeconomie*, 689–690. Other Puritans who subscribed to this belief were Rogers (*Glasse of godly Loue*, 186); Robert Croftes (*The Lover, Or Nuptiall Loue* [London, 1639], fol. A 8 r).

24 Hooke, *Childbirth*, fol. D 2 r. See also Hieron, *Sermons*, 159.

increase, and that out of me, may proceede such an one by whom thy glorie may bee furthered, and the honour of thy Name aduanced amongst men.[25]

Becon and Gouge both subscribed to this belief in the purpose of procreation. Becon argued that men ought to realize that they were to be fruitful not only to continue the race, but also to fill the number of the elect so that men would become heirs of everlasting glory and dwell in the Kingdom of Heaven. Gouge emphasized this by suggesting to husbands and wives that when they prayed alone, they ought to pray for children who would become the heirs of salvation. Still other Puritans who saw procreation as a means to increase the number of the elect were Perkins, Hieron, Willet, Stubbes, and Cartwright.[26] Again, the assumption supporting this belief was that of the family as the basic societal unit, whether religious or secular. To prevent the husband and wife from increasing the family was not only a serious blow against society, but also against the body of Christ.

As a corollary to the above, the fourth belief that led the Puritans to reject birth control was the necessity for a legitimate succession within the commonwealth and within the body of Christ. Gouge's observation was typical of the Puritan concern; he favored population increase ". . . but with a legitimate brood, and distinct families which are the seminaries of cities and commonwealths."[27] There was a three-fold fear that a bastard brood might ruin both the commonwealth and the body of Christ. First, bastards might inherit that which belonged to the legitimate heirs and disrupt individual families and ultimately the commonwealth. Second, bastards might inherit the kingdom of God, which was contrary to scriptural injunction. Third, bastards might overrun the parishes causing a burden on the welfare capabilities

25 Samuel Hieron, *A Helpe unto Deuotion* (London, 1611), 159.
26 Becon, *Booke of Matrimonye*, fols. DCLi v–4; Gouge, *Domesticall Duties*, 209, 236; Perkins, *Christian Oeconomie*, 671; Hieron, *Sermons*, 409; Philip Stubbes, *The Anatomie of Abuses* (London, 1595), 60; Willet, *Hexapla*, 401; McGinn, *Admonition Controversy*, 182, 192.
27 Gouge, *Domesticall Duties*, 209. Earlier examples of this sentiment can be found in Cleaver, *Godly Forme*, 671; Perkins, *Christian Oeconomie*, 671; Bullinger, *Christian State of Matrimonye*, fol. F v r. The statement in Cleaver is almost identical to the phrase found in Bullinger. The stress on the legitimate brood was given by Thomas Carter, *Carters Christian Common Wealth* (London, 1627), 3: "See heere my bretheren, God reiecteth your seed of bastardie, begotten in your filthy fornication and abominable adultery, he chuseth none of these, it is the seed of lawfull wedlocke, whereof he maketh his choyse to inherite his Kingdome, and reaigne in glory with his beloued Sonne."

of the population.[28] Yet greater than this fear of bastards was the fear directed against birth control, for the latter would result in a decrease in the number of the elect.

There was a final element in the Puritan rejection of birth control: their conviction that as the woman bred and bore children who would become heirs of Christ, she was then most free to serve God and most preserved from sin.[29] The conception, gestation, and delivery of children were the consequence of God's judgment and grace, and a sign of His blessing. The labor pains were part of the punishment connected with original sin. The female was gladly to suffer these steps of procreation and put her trust in God.[30] Many Puritans, in discussing this, quoted I Timothy 2:25 and observed that since sin came into the world through the female, she could recover her honor by bearing children. Smith, in commenting upon the passage from I Timothy, contended that if a woman had defects (as Leah possessed, for example), she could compensate for them by bearing children of her husband, an act which Smith claimed was ". . . the right wedding Ring, that sealeth and maketh vp the marriage."[31] Implied in this gloss is a fascinating element of Puritan theology in which the female by breeding and bearing children cooperated not only in her own salvation, but to some extent in the total schema of salvation.[32] The maternal function, when accepted in faith, liberated the female from the curse which weighted upon her since the time of Eve. To use any kind of birth control would have been a sign of her rejection of the necessity of the role of motherhood, a sign of her unwillingness to free herself from Eve's curse, and a sign of her failure to cooperate in the schema of salvation.

Thus, the literary evidence seems overwhelmingly to indicate a rejection by Puritans of birth control. Does some readily accessible

28 See Robert Burton, *Anatomy of Melancholy* (Cambridge, 1621), 658.
29 Gataker, *Good Wife*, 18. See also Richard Capel, *Tentations: Their Nature, Danger, Cure* (London, 1633), 379.
30 Smith, *Sermons*, 11. Smith later made the observation that marriage was called matrimony since it ". . . signified Motherage, because it maketh them mothers, which were virgins before; and is the seminary of the world, without which all things should be in vaine, for want of men to sue them . . ." (*ibid.*, 13). Gataker quoted St. Paul as declaring that women were to marry, breed, bear, and bring up children for "That is the end of their Marriage: and to doe that, is to be a Wife" (*Good Wife*, 18-19).
31 Smith, *Sermons*, 41-42. See Rogers, *Glasse of godly Loue*, 186; Croftes, *The Lover*, fol. A 8 v.
32 Bullinger, *Christian State of Matrimonye*, fol. B vii r. See also Smith, *Sermons*, 11.

demographic data confirm this?[33] It needs to be stressed that the
following is not proof of the results of opposition to birth control
on the part of the Puritan clergy but is merely an indication of the
impact of their opposition to birth control. In a random sample of
Puritan clergy, the average number of children born per family was
6.8. This is considerably larger than the current average American
family and higher than the average among the English nobility of the
same period.[34] The sample of 6.8 is also larger than the average family
of 4.75 in Ealing in 1599 as reported by Laslett. Wrigley reported that
at Colyton between 1560–1629, 55 percent of the marriages had six or
more children.[35] If one may assume that the current United States
medical estimate for the number of non-induced abortions per pregnancy is a conservative estimate for the Puritans, it means that the
wives of the men included in the sample experienced at least 300
pregnancies—a much higher number than experienced by the same
number of wives today. Over one fourth of the sample had fewer than
two children, and of this fourth, close to half did not father children
with their wives. The percent of sterile marriages among the sample
of Puritan clergy was less than one percent below that given by
Stone for the English aristocracy living contemporaneously with the
clergy.[36] The highest number of children born was in the family of
Andrew Willet, whose only wife gave birth to eighteen children.
Twenty-nine of the sample fathered close to 250 children for an
average of 8.6, a considerably larger family size than reported by demographers studying England during this period. The significantly
larger families of the Puritan clergy seem to suggest that they took
seriously their teachings on birth control.

To conclude, the Puritans who were aware of birth control techniques,
were against them since they violated the God-given plan for marriage,
to be fruitful and multiply; birth control prevented man from creating

33   To arrive at these tentative results, we selected a random sample of forty Puritan
clergy who lived between 1560 and 1640 from the *Dictionary of National Biography*
(DNB). By checking the articles in the DNB and other biographical articles, we learned
that these men had fathered 272 children. Eleven of the men fathered fewer than two
children, and included in the eleven were five who fathered no children. The validity
of the number in the sample is based upon a model given by Wilfrid J. Dixon and Frank
J. Massey, Jr., *Introduction to Statistical Analysis* (New York, 1969), 550.
34   Stone, *Crises of the Aristocracy*, 169.
35   Peter Laslett, *The World We Have Lost* (New York, 1965), 68; Wrigley, "Family
Limitation," 97.
36   Stone, *Crises of the Aristocracy*, 168–169.

that which was in the image of God; it denied the biblical testimony that fecundity was a blessing from God and a sign of His grace; it frustrated the peopling of the commonwealth with a legitimate brood as well as completing the number of the elect; and it frustrated woman's chances to compensate for her faults through the process of procreation. Puritan attitudes toward birth control, which were apparently put into practice by their preachers, can be summed up in this statement from Thomas Becon:

> ... whosoeuer goeth about to lette or destroye thys appoyntment of GOD eyther by voew, order, profession or otherwise, the same person is an enneyme to GOD, ad aduersarye to nature, and a verye plague and a sore pestilence to mankynde. . . .[37]

37 Becon, *Booke of Matrimonye*, fol. DCli r.

Edward Shorter

Illegitimacy, Sexual Revolution, and Social Change in Modern Europe

Sexuality in traditional society may be thoûght of as a great iceberg, frozen by the command of custom, by the need of the surrounding community for stability at the cost of individuality, and by the dismal grind of daily life. Its thawing in England and Western Europe occurred roughly between the middle of the eighteenth and the end of the nineteenth centuries, when a revolution in eroticism took place, specifically among the lower classes, in the direction of libertine sexual behavior. One by one, great chunks—such as premarital sexuality, extra- and intra-marital sexual styles, and the realm of the choice of partners—began falling away from the mass and melting into the swift streams of modern sexuality.

This article considers the crumbling of only a small chunk of the ice: premarital sexuality among young people, studied from the evidence of illegitimacy. However, in other realms of sexuality, a liberalization was simultaneously in progress. There is evidence that masturbation was increasing in those years. The first transvestite appears in Berlin police blotters in 1823. Prostitution in Paris tripled in the first half of the nineteenth century. And, between 1830 and 1855, reported rapes in France and England climbed by over 50 per cent.[1] It is not the concern of this paper, however, to pin down qualitatively these other developments. This is a task reserved for future research based upon a

Edward Shorter is Associate Professor of History at the University of Toronto. He is the author of *The Historian and the Computer* (Englewood Cliffs, N.J., 1971) and is working on the large-scale transformation in popular patterns of family life and intimate relationships in modern Europe.

An earlier version of this paper was presented at the 1970 annual meeting of the American Historical Association. The Institute for Advanced Study gave the author the time to write it, and John Gillis, Joan Scott, Charles Tilly, Fred Weinstein, and E. A. Wrigley were kind enough to read it critically. Carolyn Connor and Ann Shorter prepared the graphs at the end.

1   E. H. Hare, "Masturbatory Insanity: The History of an Idea," *Journal of Menta Science*, CVIII (1962), 12 (Hare's explanation for the phenomenon—a sexual outlet imposed by Puritan restrictions on intercourse—strikes me as unlikely); Hans Haustein, "Transvestitismus und Staat am Ende des 18. und im 19. Jahrhundert," *Zeitschrift für Sexualwissenschaft*, XV (1928–29), 116–126 (the man had begun wearing women's clothes in 1797); A.-J.-B. Parent-Duchâtelet, *De la Prostitution dans la ville de Paris* (Paris, 1857), I, 32, 36; Alexander von Öttingen, *Die Moralstatistik in ihrer Bedeutung für eine Socialethik* (Erlangen, 1882; 3rd ed.), 235.

content analysis of pornographic literature and a statistical study of the dossiers of sexual offenders in France and Germany.

What is meant by "liberalization" or "sexual revolution"? With these terms I wish to indicate a change in either, or both, the quantity and quality of sexual activity. Quantity refers to how often people have intercourse and with whom—premarital, extramarital, and marital. By quality I mean to locate the style of activity upon a spectrum running from genital to "polymorphous" sexuality: A genital orientation is the concentration of libidinal gratifications in the genitals alone; polymorphous is the discovery of other areas of the body to be erogenous zones. Liberalization will thus be understood as an increase in the quantity of sexual activity or a shift on the quality spectrum from genital to polymorphous gratification.[2]

Premarital adolescent sexuality, basically a "quantitative" subject, is the easiest portion of the sexual revolution to deal with because reliable statistics pertaining to the behavior of common people may be found and correlated with other indicators of social and economic transformation. Before 1825 data on illegitimacy were accurately preserved in parish registers throughout Europe. And nineteenth-century government statisticians meticulously noted in their annual reports not only the movement of the population, but also the number of illegitimate children born in the various districts of their lands. New insights into the intimate realms of popular life may be gained from these statistics.

Starting around the mid-eighteenth century a dramatic increase in the percentage of illegitimate births commenced all over Europe;[3] illegitimacy further accelerated around the time of the French Revolution, and continued to increase until approximately the mid-nineteenth century. This illegitimacy explosion clearly indicates that a greater number of young people—adults in their early twenties, to go by the statistics on the age of women at the birth of their first illegitimate child—were engaging in premarital sex more often than before.[4] There were slip-ups, and the birth of illegitimate children resulted.

---

2 This definition permits us to utilize the distinctions Herbert Marcuse first elaborated in *Eros and Civilization: A Philosophical Inquiry into Freud* (Boston, 1955). Paul Robinson has recently reviewed the question in *The Freudian Left: Wilhelm Reich, Gaza Roheim and Herbert Marcuse* (New York, 1969).

3 See the note on the measurement of illegitimacy in the Appendix (259–260).

4 Louis Henry agrees that illegitimacy data are a valid indicator of premarital sexual morality. "L'apport des témoignages et de la statistique," in Institut national d'études démographiques (INED), *La prévention des naissances dans la famille: ses origines dans les temps modernes* (Paris, 1960), 368. When we speak of a sexual revolution, we are not talking

The alternate constructions one might place upon the statistical increase in illegitimacy are, in my view, incorrect. It is impossible to dismiss such a rise as a result of improved procedures for reporting illegitimate births. By all accounts, few bastard children slipped through the net of the baptismal register. In the 1700s, some village pastors of stern morality were inclined to enter all children conceived premaritally as illegitimate, whether born in wedlock or not. To the extent that this practice was abandoned the real proportions of the increase would be masked, but in no event enhanced.[5]

It is also untenable to argue that the illegitimacy explosion stemmed from a "compositional" effect: that, for whatever reason, late in the 1700s more unmarried young women were around than ever before, and so these unmarried women just naturally produced more bastards. To be sure, the percentage of single women in the population did increase all over the continent, but the mentalities of these women, as well as their proportion in the population, were shifting, for the rise in illegitimate fertility, measured by the number of illegitimate births per 1,000 single women, shows that they were behaving more "immorally" than in the past.[6] We are unquestionably confronting a genuine change in popular sexual behavior, not a statistical artifact.

Nor should the illegitimacy explosion be dismissed as the sudden lengthening of the gap between conception and marriage, and as nothing more than that. Some might argue that an increase in illegitimacy was a sign not of changing mentalities but merely of a pregnant girl's increasing difficulty in forcing her seducer to marry her. Or increasing illegitimacy may have stemmed from a couple's greater

---

primarily of teenagers, as may be seen from data on unwed mothers' ages presented by P. E. H. Hair, "Bridal Pregnancy in Earlier Rural England Further Examined," *Population Studies*, XXIV (1970), 65; and by Alain Lottin, "Naissances illégitimes et filles-mères à Lille au XVIIIe siècle," *Revue d'histoire moderne et contemporaine*, XVII (1970), 306. The average age of unwed mothers probably decreased somewhat in the course of the sexual revolution; on nineteenth-century Sweden, see Gustav Sundbärg, *Bevölkerungsstatistik Schwedens, 1750–1900: Einige Hauptresultate* (Stockholm, 1923; 2nd ed.), 126, table 46.

5 See the note on the measurement of illegitimacy in the Appendix (259–260).
6 In few places are time series data available on the number of single unmarried women in the population, the standard denominator for the illegitimate fertility rate. Eighteenth-century Swedish data, presented in the Appendix (264), show that illegitimate fertility was rising at the same time as the illegitimacy ratio, and shorter series found elsewhere confirm this trend. For a sophisticated measurement of illegitimacy, see Joginder Kumar, "Demographic Analysis of Data on Illegitimate Births," *Social Biology*, XVI (1969), 92–107.

willingness to see their first child born out of wedlock. Both arguments account for rising illegitimacy in terms of technical shifts in courtship practices, ignoring changes in attitudes toward sexuality among young people as a whole. Neither argument would demand that the percentage of young people sleeping together before the sealing of a formal engagement had increased.

One piece of evidence forces us to reject both of these arguments: the number of children born within eight months of their parents' marriage. In virtually every community we know about, prenuptial conceptions rose along with illegitimate births. This indicator is charted, where available, in the Appendix (260). The simultaneous upward march of illegitimacy and prenuptial pregnancy means that the rise in illegitimacy itself was *not* merely the result of increasing delay in marriage, with the level of intercourse remaining stable. Rather, if both bastardy and prebridal pregnancy rose, there is an almost complete certainty that the total volume of premarital intercourse was rising.[7] This demonstrates that engaged couples were copulating before marriage more often than before, and that many more casual sexual alliances were being constituted than in the past.

Finally, we should inspect the rough outlines of traditional sexuality. By "traditional" I refer to European rural and small-town society between 1500 and 1700. It was a period of cultural homogeneity in which all popular strata behaved more or less the same, having similar social and sexual values, the same concepts of authority and hierarchy, and an identical appreciation of custom and tradition in their primary social goal, the maintenance of static community life. We have numerous testimonies to the quality of peasant and burgher sex life, but almost none to that of the lower classes (domestic servants, laborers, journeymen, and the industrious poor). But I think it is safe to assume that the comportment of the two strata was similar. Möller has portrayed sex life among the *Kleinbürgertum* in the 1700s: man on top, no foreplay, quick ejaculation, and indifference to partner's orgasm. The gamut seems paper-thin, and the more exotic perversities which delighted the upper classes were doubtless unheard of and unimagined in provincial backwaters. More importantly, people were either chaste before marriage, or began sleeping together only after the

---

7 The certainty is not quite total because a rise in both of these indicators could be due to a drop in infanticide and abortion, or to an increase in fecundity. Yet there is no evidence that the first two lessened at all, to say nothing of decreasing on a scale sufficient to cause the illegitimacy explosion. Nor is there evidence of a change in fecundity.

engagement was sealed.[8] This is the situation from which the great liberalization emerged.

A TYPOLOGY OF ILLEGITIMACY   In order to understand why an increasing number of illegitimate children were born, two questions must be asked: (1) Why did the level of intercourse outside of marriage rise, thereby increasing the incidence of premarital conceptions? (2) Why did a greater percentage of conceptions fail to lead to marriage—why did more of this increased sexual activity result specifically in illegitimacy? To answer the first question one must distinguish, in a general way, among the reasons for having sex; to answer the second requires an understanding of the social situation in which a couple found themselves—for the stability and durability of their own relationship, and the firmness of their integration into the social order about them, would determine whether they would marry before the child was born.

The reader must be warned of the speculative character of my answers to these two questions. The explanations of shifts in sexual mentalities and the typologies of interpersonal relationships from one period to the next are preliminary efforts to make sense of badly fragmented and scattered information on intimate life. The arguments that follow thus are not to be understood as hard statements of fact, but rather as informed guesses about the likely course of events. Only the hope of spurring further research justifies this kind of speculative enterprise, for we are unable to determine what kinds of evidence to seek out until we have arguments that specify exactly what is to be sought.

As a first imprudent step, let us assume that people have intercourse for one of two reasons. They may wish to use their sexuality as a tool for achieving some ulterior external objective, such as obtaining a suitable marriage partner and setting up a home, or avoiding trouble with a superior. If they have such motives in mind as they climb into bed, they are using sex in a *manipulative* fashion. Alternatively, they may be intent upon developing their personalities as fully as possible, upon acquiring self-insight and self-awareness, and, accordingly, think

---

8 An extensive popular literature on peasant sex practices exists for the nineteenth and twentieth centuries, of which Grassl's "Bäuerliche Liebe," *Zeitschrift für Sexualwissenschaft*, XIII (1926–27), 369–380 is typical. The only scholarly works I have been able to rely on for this picture of premodern sexuality are K. Rob. V. Wikman, *Die Einleitung der Ehe: Eine vergleichend ethno-soziologische Untersuchung über die Vorstufe der Ehe in den Sitten des Schwedischen Volkstums* (Turkü [Finland], 1937), 350–355; Helmut Möller, *Die kleinbürgerliche Familie im 18. Jahrhundert: Verhalten und Gruppenkultur* (Berlin, 1969), 282–301; Peter Laslett, *The World We Have Lost* (New York, 1965), 128–149.

of sex an an integral component of their humanity. For such people, sex is a way of expressing the wish to be free, for the egoism of unconstrained sexuality is a direct assault upon the inhibiting community authority structures about them. I call this *expressive* sexuality. This level of intercourse is higher than that for the manipulative variety because self-expression is an ongoing objective, whereas once the object is attained to which manipulative sexuality was employed, the person may lapse into the unerotic torpor society has ordained as proper. Expressiveness means a lot of sex; manipulativeness means little.

But what about the sex drive? It is always with us, a dark motor of human biology moving men and women to intercourse in all times and all places. Yet its position in the hierarchy of *conscious* needs and impulses is by no means constant, but is rather a function of social and cultural variables which change from one time and place to another. Gagnon and Simon have shown for twentieth-century America that social structure and cultural stances interpose themselves between the steady thrust of the libido and the act of intercourse.[9] My point is that such factors constituted "reasons for intercourse" in nineteenth-century Europe as well. Specifically, there are two: the conscious wish to use sex as a means of manipulating other people to perform non-sexual acts, and the conscious wish to use sex as a spotlight in the introspective search for identity. Changes in these reasons for intercourse suggest that the history of the sexual revolution in Europe may be written as the transformation of lower-class eroticism from manipulation to expression.[10]

But if the social order about the expressive couple remains the same, they will doubtless get married and appear in the records of the statisticians only as contributors to the legitimate birth rate. In order to see why the child whom they conceive is born a bastard, we must look at the stability of their relationship. Instability may result when one of the partners in a relationship (normally the male) is using his social or

---

9 They summarize their thinking in "Psychosexual Development," reprinted in John Gagnon and William Simon (eds.), *The Sexual Scene* (Chicago, 1970), 23–41.

10 A case study linking romantic love and self-awareness in the eighteenth century is Rudolf Braun, *Industrialisierung und Volksleben: Die Veränderungen der Lebensformen in einem ländlichen Industriegebiet vor 1800 (Zürcher Oberland)* (Erlenbach-Zurich, 1960), 65–72. On the eighteenth-century diffusion of romantic love, see also Jean-Louis Flandrin, "Contraception, mariage et relations amoureuses dans l'Occident chrétien," *Annales,* XXIV (1969), 1370–1390; Philippe Ariès, "Interprétation pour une histoire des mentalités," in *Prévention des naissances,* 311–327, esp. 323.

economic authority to exploit the other sexually (usually the female). In such a case, marriage is unlikely to follow pregnancy. The likelihood of a subsequent marriage is also reduced when the partners are caught up in a society undergoing rapid flux, so that either the establishment of a family household is impossible, or the male can easily escape the consequences of impregnation by fleeing. The notion of stability in the social situation of the couple therefore incorporates several possibilities.

These two variables—the nature of sexuality (expressive vs. manipulative) and the nature of the couple's social situation (stable vs. unstable)—are strategic in accounting for the illegitimacy explosion in Europe. Because each has its own history (although both must be considered together) we may construct a table which cross-classifies and derives four different situations resulting in the birth of an illegitimate child:

Table 1:   The Types of Illegitimacy

	EXPRESSIVE SEXUALITY	MANIPULATIVE SEXUALITY
Stable social situation	True love	Peasant-bundling
Unstable social situation	Hit-and-run	Master–servant exploitation

"Peasant-bundling" illegitimacy lies at the intersection of instrumental sexuality and a stable social situation: persons with things on their mind other than sex whose cohabitation is sanctioned by custom. "Master–servant exploitation" denotes the coercion of women into bed by men who use their power as employers or social superiors to wrest sexual favors from them. Less than rape, the woman consents to being exploited in order to exist in peace with her superiors. There is little question of marriage when pregnancy ensues, a sign of the instability inherent both in the relationship and in the society which permits this kind of illicit exercise of authority. "Hit-and-run" illegitimacy identifies temporary liaisons where the partners articulate romantic sentiments and substantial ego awareness, and thereby are sexually expressive, yet are not inclined to remain together after a conception has taken place, or are prohibited by the force of events from doing so. Finally, in "true love" illegitimacy the psychological orientation of the partners is roughly the same as with the hit-and-run situation (although the couple may come more quickly to think of itself as a domestic unit), yet both their intent and their social environment conspire to permit a swift subsequent wedding and the establishment of a household. The child is technically illegitimate, but, like the offspring of peasant bundlers, is soon enmeshed in orderly family life. Children born of master–servant and of hit-and-run unions are more enduringly illegitimate.

All four types of illegitimacy were present in European society at all stages of historical development, but, in some epochs, some types were more prevalent than others. The explosion of bastardy may be written as the supplanting of peasant-bundling and master–servant exploitation by hit-and-run and true-love illegitimacy as the predominant types. This transition came about because popular premarital sexuality shifted from manipulative to expressive, thus elevating the number of conceptions, and because inconstancy crept into the couples' intentions toward each other, and instability into the structure of the social order in which they found themselves. The result was to make more premarital conceptions into illegitimate births.

These four types represent, in fact, four distinct historical stages in the unfolding of illegitimacy, one giving way to the next in a neat chronological progression.

Stage I Peasant-bundling was the paramount form of illegitimacy in Europe before the eighteenth century. England and Europe had always known some bastardy, on the order of 1 or 2 per cent of all births, and most parish registers turned up an isolated illegitimate child or two in the course of a decade. But these children, when not the offspring of the poor servant girl raped by the village half-wit, stemmed normally from engaged peasant couples who commenced sleeping together before marriage, as was customary, yet delayed the marriage too long. Social authorities in these village and small-town communities put enormous pressure upon hesitant males to wed their swollen fiancées, being persuasive only because the seducer had been, and would continue to be, resident locally and dependent upon the good will of his social betters.

I have not seen data on the legitimation of illegitimate children before 1800, so the characterization cannot be made exactly. Yet excellent information on prenuptial conception and illegitimacy convince me that this portrait must be essentially accurate.[11]

11 The standard work on bundling (*Kiltgang, Freierei*) is Wikman, *Die Einleitung der Ehe*. Parish register investigations now in progress have turned up in most places lots of

Stage II Master–servant exploitation became an even brighter thread in illegitimacy as the seventeenth century gave way to the eighteenth. Manipulativeness continued paramount in lower-class eroticism; the change seems to have been that people in positions of influence and authority were able, as they had not been before, to take advantage of their exalted stations. We must keep in mind that these little dramas of exploitation happened mostly within the context of lower-class life. At that humble level, the authority of the oldest journeyman of the master tanner, for example, may have been minimal in absolute terms, yet to the girl who swept out of the shop it must have appeared commanding. The abuse of social and economic power to sexual ends doubtless was more difficult in the good old days, with the rest of the community watching vigilantly for disfunctions in the smooth mechanisms of prerogatives and obligations,[12] but the stirrings of social change weakened traditional control over such goings on.

Among the evidence for this characterization is Solé's work on the city of Grenoble in the late seventeenth century. He noted that around half of the illegitimate births (illegitimacy was around 3 per cent of all births) were the work of men who held the mothers of the bastards in some kind of thralldom, as masters of domestic servants or employers of female wage labor. And many of the cases of "rapt" coming before the judiciary of Angoulême in 1643–44 involved the

---

premarital conceptions among traditional peasant populations. In addition to the graphs in the Appendix (265–272), see E. A. Wrigley, *Population and History* (New York, 1969), 88 (a third of all first children in Colyton were baptized within eight months of marriage); P. E. H. Hair, "Bridal Pregnancy in Rural England in Earlier Centuries," *Population Studies*, XX (1966–67), 233–243; Michael Drake, *Population and Society in Norway, 1735–1865* (Cambridge, 1969), 138–144 (especially good on the stability of sexual relations among the cottager class); J.-C. Giacchetti and M. Tyvaert, "Argenteuil (1740–1790)," *Annales de Démographie Historique, 1969*, 40–61. The last say that even where illegitimacy was 1 per cent, 11 per cent of all first births were premaritally conceived. Intercourse during engagement was not everywhere the rule in traditional peasant society, as is pointed out in Emmanuel Le Roy Ladurie, *Les Paysans de Languedoc* (Paris, 1966), 644. See also Patrice Robert, "Rumont (1720–1790)," *Annales de Démographie Historique, 1969*, 32–40. Oscar Helmuth Werner, *The Unmarried Mother in German Literature with Special Reference to the Period 1770–1800* (New York, 1917), describes the violence of the traditional response to libertine behavior.

12 Chaunu has speculated that in open-field communities, where communal interaction was frequent and controls omnipresent, illegitimacy came from premarital intercourse among youths of the same age. In "bocage" communities, where relative isolation weakened social controls upon the superordinates, illegitimacy came from the masters' sexual exploitation of servants. Open-field morality was, however, more strict. See Pierre Chaunu, *La civilisation de l'Europe classique* (Paris, 1970), 196–197.

master's sexual violation of the servant. "The most common case is that of the farmers (*laboureurs à bœufs*) or village officials who, upon becoming widowers, take as servants a young girl from the parish. They speak to her vaguely of marriage, then when a birth approaches chase her from the house...."[13] In the early 1700s, the illegitimacy ratio in numerous urban communities had just begun to rise, as may be seen from the Appendix (270), whereas that in small rural communities continued at an infinitesimal level, a statistical demonstration of a rise in Stage II illegitimacy. But a detailed study of fathership in parish register data is needed to confirm our picture of master–servant exploitation.

A number of large-scale social changes intervened between Stages II and III, running roughly from 1750, which had the end effect of giving lower-class people a new conception of self and thus an expressive notion of sexuality. The fabric of lower-class life was thus shaken in a way that substantially decreased a pregnant girl's chances of getting married.

Stage III Hit-and-run illegitimacy typified a period when young people swooned romantically through a social landscape of disorder and flux. There was much intercourse, but people were stepping out of their old places en route to new ones, and temporary cohabitations often failed to turn into permanent concubinages. This combination of circumstances raised illegitimacy to historic heights, for the years 1790–1860 were, in virtually every society or community we know about, the peak period of illegitimacy. The graphs in the Appendix (265–272) reveal this conclusion unmistakably.

Time-series data on legitimation demonstrate that only a quarter to a third of all illegitimate children were subsequently legitimated by the *inter*marriage of their parents.[14] The other two-thirds either died, typically a consequence of indifferent care and the lack of a secure home, or remained unlegitimated—by definition outside of a glowing familial

13 Yves-Marie Bercé, "Aspects de la criminalité au XVIIe siècle," *Revue historique*, CCXXXIX (1968), 33–42; Angoulême evidence, 38; Jacques Solé, "Passion charnelle et société urbaine d'Ancien régime: Amour vénal, amour libre et amour fou à Grenoble au milieu du règne de Louis XIV," *Villes de l'Europe méditerranéenne et de l'Europe occidentale du Moyen Age au XIXe siècle: Actes du Colloque de Nice (27–28 Mars 1969)* (Paris, 1970), IX–X (1969), 211–232. In the Norman village of Troarn, Michel Bouvet identified master–servant exploitation as a common source of illegitimacy during the 1700s. "Troarn: Etude de démographie historique (XVIIe–XVIIIe siècles)," *Cahiers des Annales de Normandie*, VI (1968), 53.
14 See the time series on the legitimation of children in the Appendix (260–261).

hearth. Some mothers eventually found husbands other than the fathers of their children; their bastards would then be raised in a domestic atmosphere, but rarely would their new stepfathers adopt them.[15] Legitimation statistics point to an unsettledness in the sexual relations between men and women, hence the sobriquet "hit-and-run."

Stage IV From about 1875, the reintegration of the lower classes into the structure of civil society appears to have removed the transient quality from romantic relationships, leaving their expressive nature unimpaired. Stable communities developed in the sprawling worker quarters of industrial cities; a cohesive lower-class subculture with distinctive values and symbols became elaborated in distinction to the bourgeois society. Outside society accepted placidly the idea of early worker marriage, and, within premarital liaisons themselves, thoughts of subsequent marriage were present at the beginning.[16]

During this stage illegitimacy ratios declined somewhat from their Stage III heights, although they did not return to the low levels of traditional society. And legitimation rates rose steadily during the last third of the century, a sign that couples who coalesced briefly for intercourse were staying together with connubial intent. The modern pattern of cohabitation is between social and economic equals, not between unequals, as in Stage II. The only survey I have been able to find of illegitimate fatherhood late in the century demonstrates that the seducers came from similar social stations as the seduced, which implies a growth of romantic, expressive sexuality in place of the manipulative, instrumental sort.[17]

These portraits of the four stages are meant as ideal types suggesting the sequence of events most places would experience. I do not intend to argue that the infinitely disparate cities and regions of Western

15 In Frankfurt am Main around 1900, only one-fifth of the illegitimate children whose mothers had married another man were actually adopted by their stepfathers (*Namensgebung*). Othmar Spann, *Untersuchungen über die uneheliche Bevölkerung in Frankfurt am Main* (Dresden, 1905), 26.

16 The resiliency of social networks in lower-class neighborhoods around this time has not been a subject of monographic investigation. One occasionally finds in the secondary literature relevant observations, such as Michel Collinet's view that the skilled workers of Paris become "sedentary" after the turn of the twentieth century (*L'Ouvrier français: Essai sur la condition ouvrière* [*1900–1950*] [Paris, 1951], 114).

17 Theodor Geiger, "Zur Statistik der Unehelichen," *Allgemeines Statistisches Archiv*, XI (1918–19), 212–220. Geiger presents some Norwegian data (1897–98) which show that in 76 per cent of the illegitimate births, both parents were from the same social class; in a further 18 per cent of the cases, a lower-class female had slept with a middle-class male; and, in a final 7 per cent, a middle-class women and a lower-class man (216–218).

Europe marched in lockstep, for the timing of each of these stages would vary from one place to another, depending on events. But the illegitimacy explosion sooner or later came to Breslau and Liverpool, to the Scottish lowlands and the Zurich highlands. Exactly when depended upon the pace of modernization.

SOCIAL CHANGE AND THE WISH TO BE FREE   What touched off the wish to be free—the great drift toward individual innovation and autonomy at the cost of community custom and hierarchy—is one of the most vexing problems of modern scholarship, and a solution to it does not lie within the scope of this paper. Weinstein and Platt state that at the psychoanalytic level, the separation of home and workplace was responsible, for as the father exchanged his continuing presence within the family circle for workaday employment outside, certain emotional connections caused sons to rebel against their fathers' authority. With fathers no longer emotionally nurturant, male children no longer had to obey them.[18] Classical sociology provides other answers: Marx with his insistence upon the capitalist economy as the generator of proletarian rebellion, de Tocqueville with his assertion that equality had proven too much of a good thing. The matter is still unclarified, and my puzzlement is as great as anyone's. But the pattern of takeoff in illegitimacy ratios, and the correlates of illegitimacy with other socioeconomic variables, suggest a partial answer to the question.

It is in the area of changes which enhanced the individual's sense of self and which correspondingly broke down allegiances to custom and to the community that we must seek the motor of the wish to be free. At many levels of social relations and of psychodynamics, sexual freedom threatens the maintenance of community life because of the radical privatism and "egoism" it instills in individuals. (The classic European tradition of conservatism was intensely aware of the nature of this threat, and often damned libertine sexual behavior as "Egois-

---

18 I have borrowed the phrase from the title of the book by Fred Weinstein and Gerald M. Platt, *The Wish to be Free: Society, Psyche, and Value Change* (Berkeley, 1969). Although I think that the overall argument in Weinstein and Platt is substantially correct, I disagree with their views on the timing of the development of autonomy: (1) The search for autonomy from the family (not just from politics) probably began late in the 1700s, not in the late 1800s, when Freud was writing; (2) Weinstein and Platt argue that women were to acquire a sense of autonomy only in the 1900s, whereas men had liberated themselves from their fathers' authority much earlier. My view is that the shift from manipulative to expressive sexuality happened as much (if not more) among women as among men, and that it occurred late in the 1700s.

mus.") Following accepted practice in the study of modernization, I shall call those areas of the economy and society effecting such changes in individual mentalities the "modern" sector. A case can be made that exposure to the modern sector at least sensitizes the population to the values of individual self-development and precipitates a readiness to experiment with new life styles and personality configurations, which then leads to action, *should all other things be equal*.

Most corrosive of the traditional communitarian order was the modern marketplace economy. This insight into the individualizing impact of capitalism upon the *local* arena is almost as old as the free marketplace itself, and Nisbet, Polanyi, and Wolf have recently reminded us of it again.[19] The notion of the individual as an isolated actor in the economy hell-bent upon maximizing his own profit was the diametric opposite of concepts binding together the traditional local corporation, be it a small-town guild or open-field village. The reality, of course, was quite different from the classical *laissez-faire* model, yet it is likely that the concept was constantly in the thoughts of those involved in wage negotiations, for example, or those who offered their services in a competitive labor market. To be sure, Western Europe had known *export* capitalism, the fabrication of goods for non-local sale, since the Middle Ages, but free markets within the *local* economy date from the eighteenth century in France and England, and from the early nineteenth in Germany.[20]

In the context of sexual history, however, a free market economy meant something a little more precise than the general exchange of goods and services regulated only by the price mechanism. In the countryside it meant agricultural capitalism and the rationalization of husbandry. The laborers and live-in hired hands who worked for improving farmers all over Europe were highly prone to illegitimacy. This is no less true of such English areas of agricultural modernization as Norfolk, Surrey, and Sussex, as it is of French departments—the

19 Robert Nisbet, *Community and Power* (formerly *The Quest for Community*) (New York, 1962), *passim*; Karl Polanyi, *The Great Transformation* (New York, 1944), Chs. 1–4; Eric R. Wolf, *Peasant Wars of the Twentieth Century* (New York, 1969), 276–302.
20 On England see E. A. Wrigley, "A Simple Model of London's Importance in Changing English Society and Economy, 1650–1750," *Past and Present*, XXXVII (1967), 44–70; on France, Louise A. Tilly, "The History of the Grain Riot as a Form of Political Conflict in France," *The Journal of Interdisciplinary History*, II (1971), 23–57. On Germany, Gustav Schmoller, "Die Epochen der Getreidehandelsverfassung und -politik," *Schmollers Jahrbuch*, XX (1896), 695–744, as well as his *Zur Geschichte der deutschen Kleingewerbe* (Halle, 1870) for local markets in non-agricultural goods.

Somme, the Eure, and the Pas-de-Calais—employing numerous rural wage laborers. In Germany, the great farms of Mecklenburg and Niederbayern employed workers among whom illegitimacy flourished.[21] Parish data from the late eighteenth century are still not abundant enough to tell if the accumulation of an agricultural proletariat produced a corresponding initial increase in bastardy, but I suspect that this finding will turn up in the work that E. A. Wrigley and Louis Henry are now directing for England and France.

In towns, a free market economy meant capitalism in the form of factory industry. A distinctive feature of factory worker life in the 1800s was staggering rates of illegitimacy. In France, local studies of industrial towns have established that female factory workers were substantially over-represented among unwed mothers in proportion to the population. In Dresden and Munich, an illegitimate child often accompanied worker parents to the altar.[22] Yet these are only examples; the systematic statistical analysis required to demonstrate such hypotheses is inordinately difficult to obtain because: (1) as noted, we simply do not know about the development of illegitimacy over time in a sufficient number of municipalities to permit us to isolate the impact of factory industrialization; and (2) what appears to be the effect of factory industry may, in fact, be the effect of residence in a city.

The fact that the single group most prone to illegitimacy was urban domestic servants gives pause to attaching too much importance to factories and to the modern economy.[23] I have argued elsewhere that urbanity itself constitutes an important independent variable in

21 A glance at maps of illegitimacy in any of these countries shows that counties, departments, or *Regierungsbezirke* with a high concentration of landownership in the hands of a few have, by and large, high levels of bastardy. I examined the statistical relationship between engrossment and illegitimacy in Bavaria in "Sexual Change and Illegitimacy: The European Experience," in Robert Bezucha (ed.), *New Directions in European Social History* (forthcoming).

22 Jules Michelet suggested that factory workers sought out sex as a compensation for the ghastliness of shop floor life. Cited in Georges Duveau, *La Vie ouvrière en France sous le Second Empire* (Paris, 1946), 423. See Ernest Bertrand, "Essai sur la moralité des classes ouvrières dans leur vie privée," *Journal de la Société de Statistique de Paris*, XIII (1872), 86–95 for occupations of illegitimate mothers in Châlons-sur-Marne, Troyes, and Reims.

23 Othmar Spann was preoccupied with this problem. See his "Die geschlechtlich-sittlichen Verhältnisse in Dienstboten- und Arbeiterinnenstande, gemessen an der Erscheinung der unehelichen Geburten," *Zeitschrift für Socialwissenschaft*, VII (1904), 287–303, and his *Uneheliche Bevölkerung*, 170–171. Illegitimacy rates of factory women and domestic servants in Berlin in 1907 were twice as high as for those groups in Prussia as the whole (measured as the number of illegitimate births per 1,000 single women of

accounting for the distribution of illegitimacy, but I was unable then, and still cannot now, fit the impact of the city into a neat theoretical structure. We can see the city accelerating illegitimacy by reducing the chances that an impregnation will eventuate in marriage. But does urban residence by itself shift lower-class mentalities from manipulativeness to expressiveness? What difference the city makes is one of the big questions in modern social science, and another unresolved puzzle in this paper.

Among the empirical evidence I can offer on this subject is that illegitimacy began to turn upward in the cities first, spreading to the villages only later. In every city in England and the continent for which data are available, the upsurge in illegitimacy commenced around 1750 or before, as may be seen from the Appendix (267–268). Second, except in England cities had much higher illegitimacy ratios than surrounding rural areas. Yet such illegitimacy may have been solely due to the fact that there were more single women in the cities than in the countryside. And, because of all of these urban maidservants, seamstresses, and the like, a higher proportion of all urban births were illegitimate than in the countryside. But that does not mean that the typical urban girl would be more likely than the typical country girl to behave immorally and produce illegitimate children. Maybe no differences existed in the morality of young women in the city and the country. Further research will clarify this question.[24]

---

childbearing age), even though overall illegitimate fertility in Berlin was only fractionally higher than in Prussia as a whole. L. Berger, "Untersuchungen über den Zusammenhang zwischen Beruf und Fruchtbarkeit unter besonderer Berücksichtigung des Königreichs Preussen," *Zeitschrift des königlich preussischen statistischen Landesamts*, LII (1912), 231–232. I am grateful to John Knodel for calling this article to my attention.

Robert Michels wrote about illegitimacy among "isolated" groups within the population, such as urban domestics and seamstresses, in *Sittlichkeit in Ziffern? Kritik der Moralstatistik* (Munich, 1928), 172–180. Abel Châtelain has been working on the entire question of maidservant migration. "Migrations et domesticité feminine urbaine en France, XVIIIe siècle–XXe siècle," *Revue d'histoire économique et sociale*, XLIV (1969), 506–528.

24 The urban-rural distinction is standard in illegitimacy discussions, and the interested reader may consult A. Legoyt, "Les Naissances naturelles," *Journal de la Société de Statistique de Paris*, VIII (1867), 62–77; Karl Seutemann, "Die Legitimationen unehelicher Kinder nach dem Berufe und der Berufsstellung der Eltern in Oesterreich," *Statistische Monatschrift*, V (1900), 13–68; Öttingen, *Moralstatistik*, and other works cited in the Appendix. Some, such as Möller in *Kleinbürgerliche Familie*, say the bigger the city, the greater the illegitimacy (289). F. G. Dreyfus talks of an urban "masse de population flottante, très mal enracinée et intégrée," *Sociétés et mentalités à Mayence dans la seconde moitié du XVIIIe siècle* (Paris, 1968), 254.

English cities are a puzzling case apart, for their illegitimacy *ratios* were often beneath those of the surrounding countryside. In London, for example, illegitimacy in 1859 was an unbelievably low 4 per cent of all births. (In Vienna in 1864, illegitimate births exceeded the legitimate.) Either something about English cities, such as their great prostitution, made them remarkably different from their continental counterparts, or many births were not being registered as bastards (something that could easily have happened in English vital statistics registration).[25]

The final sensitizing variable crucial in value change appears to be exposure to primary education. Formal education, if only of a rudimentary sort, is calculated precisely to give the individual a sense of self by teaching logical thought. Learning to read requires the acquisition of linear logic, which mode of thought then surely spreads to other intellectual processes and levels of perception, to say nothing of the logical capacities instilled by other kinds of formal education. Logic and rationality are just other words for ego control, the psycho-structural state of mind whence expressive sexuality flows. It is surely significant that the illegitimacy explosion coincided closely in time with the spread of primary education, and in space with the diffusion of literacy among the population.[26]

To review a provisional reconstruction of the psychodynamics of the sexual revolution: It appears that liberal sexual attitudes probably flowed from heightened ego awareness and from weakened superego controls. Traditional European society internalized anti-sexual values which commanded repression. But, when new values began to replace old ones, the superego restrictions on gratification gave way to the demands of the ego for individual self-fulfillment, and it was but a short logical step to see sexual fulfillment as integral to this larger personality objective. I do not mean that people became "sexualized" human beings; instead they became pluralized, seeing sex as an intrinsic part of

25   The English statistical service thought prostitution a likely explanation of low urban illegitimacy. Anon., "Illegitimacy in England and Wales, 1879," *Journal of the Statistical Society*, XLIV (1881), 397.

26   W. G. Lumley, "Observations upon the Statistics of Illegitimacy," *Journal of the Statistical Society of London*, XXV (1862), 219–274, raises the possibility of a positive correlation among bastardy and the level of education in Scotland, although he is uncertain about England (234, 260). There are strong theoretical reasons for suspecting a causal relationship between illegitimacy and primary education, but no evidence is available in published sources to permit verification. I am reluctant to put much faith in correlations among census data because so many other factors among a literate population could account for illegitimacy. The case history method seems most promising for checking this linkage in my model.

their humanity. This makes the sexual revolution an integrated movement of self-awareness, not a turbulent unleashing of carnality. If my argument is correct, behind this wish to be free lay the market economy, evoking ego orientation from those caught up in it, and primary education, stressing logical thought and control of the external world.

SOCIAL CHANGES DECREASE THE LIKELIHOOD THAT CONCEPTION
LEADS TO MARRIAGE   Let us imagine a young girl has just told her suitor that she is pregnant. He has three possible responses, in the event that he does not wish to propose marriage in short order:

(1) "I love you but we can't get married until I inherit the shoe shop at age 42."
(2) "I love you but the authorities won't let us get married because they're afraid we might go on welfare."
(3) "So long, honey."

Which of these responses hundreds of thousands of young men selected is the key to the second strategic variable in accounting for illegitimacy: the chances of conception resulting in marriage before the child was born. The response was determined by the presence or absence of three principal social conditions, and our understanding of the sources of illegitimacy will be incomplete without a quick glance at them.

Response (1), the need to delay marriage until the man could establish an independent livelihood, was doubtless spoken most often in areas of lagging artisanal economy and impartible agricultural inheritance, late in the eighteenth and early in the nineteenth centuries. Age-old custom in Europe stipulated that the ability to support a family was a precondition of marriage, and, customarily, young men would not take brides until a master craftsman's license was in the offing or until the parents declared themselves ready to abandon farming and let the son take over the big house. In the 1700s, however, population grew so rapidly that the vacant positions which would allow for economic independence were soon filled up. Though other jobs entailing economic dependence were always available (witness the howls over a shortage of rural wage laborers), these positions were not thought suitable for establishing a "bürgerliche Existenz." A hesitancy to subdivide the fields and the stranglehold of the guilds upon the expansion of the artisanal sector saw to it that these economic backwaters did not expand with the growth of population. Hence there were rising ages at marriage and cries of "overpopulation"—and illegitimacy.

This model of population growth, rising ages at marriage, and illegitimacy works best for the areas of Europe not permeated by cottage industry. Where the domestic system was found, people married earlier, yet *also* produced more illegitimate children. (I do not wish to argue a direct positive correlation between age at marriage and illegitimacy. Too many other variables intervened: such as strength of familial controls and the mentalities of the population.) But in a cottage industrial area the delay in marriage was more likely due to abandonment of the mother by her seducer (response 3), rather than to a need for patience arising from economic exigencies (response 1).[27]

Response (2) is a special Central European variant of response (1), for in most German-speaking areas from Austria to Pomerania legal restrictions on marriage were reinforced in the nineteenth century. These laws were the bureaucratic elaboration of traditional community bars upon the marriage of the indigent, and were promulgated in the first half of the century at the behest of municipal governments. Town councils all over Germany feared that permitting the lower classes to marry freely would result in the swamping of local poor-relief funds by the children of the poor. Had things been as before, with no value changes underway among the lower classes, this calculation might have proved rewarding. Yet the lower classes had by now (as we have seen) abandoned their traditional chastity before marriage, and proceeded to saddle these anxious municipalities with hordes of illegitimate children. This is why Central European illegitimacy ratios in the first two-thirds of the century were so strikingly high. In the late 1860s these laws were repealed, and, in the space of a year or two, illegitimacy ratios all over Germany sagged.[28] It must be borne in mind that these laws were not

27 For population dynamics in a society with ossified guilds and nonpartible farms, I have drawn on the case most familiar to me: the state of Bavaria. See Edward Shorter, "Social Policy and Social Change in Bavaria, 1800–1860" unpub. Ph.D. thesis (Harvard, 1968). On long-term trends in the distribution of property in rural areas, see Günther Franz, *Geschichte des deutschen Bauernstandes vom frühen Mittelalter bis zum 19. Jahrhundert* (Stuttgart, 1970), 210–227.

28 On these marriage and settlement laws, see Karl Braun, "Das ZwangsZölibat für Mittellose in Deutschland," *Vierteljahrschrift für Volkswirtschaft und Kulturgeschichte*, XX (1867), 1–80; Eduard Schübler, *Die Gesetze über Niederlassung und Verehelichung in den verschiedenen deutschen Staaten* (Stuttgart, 1855); John Knodel, "Law, Marriage and Illegitimacy in Nineteenth-Century Germany," *Population Studies*, XX (1966–67), 279–294; Mack Walker, "Home Towns and State Administrators: South German Politics, 1815–30," *Political Science Quarterly*, LXXXII (1967), 35–60. Illegitimacy *rates*, however, were much less affected by the abolition of marriage laws.

responsible for the initial take off of illegitimacy, postdating that explosion by several decades. Other factors were behind central European
illegitimacy as well, for even in the absence of such legislation several
German states experienced the highest incidence of bastardy on the
continent.

Under different circumstances than in responses (1) and (2), the man
might refuse to marry the girl altogether (response 3), and, after oblig-
ing her by "recognizing" the child at its birth, he would disassociate
himself entirely from his foundering family.[29] Chronologically, the
period of most frequent absconding was the first half of the nineteenth
century (when the other two responses were also most often heard),
yet refusals to stay by the fallen woman probably happened most in the
modern sector—factory industry and the city—rather than in the small
towns of traditional society. All statistics point to the city as a place
where conception out of wedlock meant abandonment by one's lover,
as seen by the numbers of foundlings, of single women in lying-in
hospitals (a sign, in the eyes of some, that the unwed mother was alone),
and of single women on relief. In Austria, a negative correlation turns
up in communes larger than 2,000 between the percentage of bastard
children legitimated and the size of place, indicating the relative im-
permanence of sexual liaisons in the metropolis. Some of this dismal
showing of urban places was due to the pregnant country girls who
would come to the city to bear their illegitimate children, and then return home. But, even after they have been discounted, the mid-
nineteenth century city remained a place of dislocation.[30]

29 Recognition in French and Belgian law meant that the father conceded to the child
some inheritance rights and support obligations, but this did not constitute either a
legitimation or an adoption of the bastard. In Paris during 1880–84, more children were
recognized (20.5 per cent) than legitimated (18.6 per cent), a sign of great instability in
relationships between the sexes. Keep in mind that some of those recognized also turn
up in the legitimation statistics, which means that we cannot add the two figures together
to determine the total proportion of illegitimate children brought into the charmed
circle of family life.

30 Seutemann, "Legitimation unehelicher Kinder," 42, for Austrian urban legitimation. The Dresden illegitimacy ratio in 1873–79 was around 20 per cent with non-local
mothers included, 16 per cent with them excluded, indicating that urban ratios were high
for reasons other than the "fleeing pregnant peasant" effect. Öttingen, *Moralstatistik*, 317.

A sad little literature on child mortality, foundlings, and unwed mothers on relief
shows in a way that most cold demographic statistics do not the human cost of illegitimacy. The historian must span a long emotional distance between all of this expressive
sexuality and the thousands of small tragedies behind the astonishingly high rate of
illegitimate infant mortality. See William Acton, "Observations on Illegitimacy in the
London Parishes of St. Marylebone, St. Pancras . . . during the Year 1857," *Journal of
the Statistical Society of London*, XXII (1859), 491–505; Ed. Ducpetiaux, "Du sort des

Illegitimacy reached its absolute height during the first half of the nineteenth century simply because these three kinds of responses to the announcement of a pregnancy happened to coincide. Illegitimacy declined when such social conditions ceased to obtain.

SEXUAL BEHAVIOR AND FAMILY PATTERNS   At the end, we must resolve a paradox which has emerged from the uneven distribution among the social classes of the contagion of libertine sexual behavior. The middle classes, as the lower, were exposed to marketplace mentalities and education, yet their sexual attitudes throughout the 1800s remained defiantly puritanical; indeed, the evidence of Victorianism would have it that the more one were educated, the more prudish and moralistic one became.[31] How ironical that those middle-class types who preached the gospel of autonomy—liberalism, *laissez-faire* capitalism, and universal suffrage—were the most repressive people sexually. In class terms, they were the movers and doers, the *bourgeoisie d'affaires*. Yet those who favored economic collectivism and political community were the most liberated sexually, with a high degree of personal control and autonomy. In class terms, they comprised the proletariat.[32]

If the argument about exposure to modernity and education is correct, one would expect the middle classes, rather than the lower classes, to have been in the vanguard of the sexual revolution. Other variables must have intervened to leap the gap between thinking about "the real me" and actually climbing into bed for intercourse. That is where the family enters. The lower classes were able to respond to the priming of the pump only because the family ceased for them to be an agency of social control. To go by existing evidence, it was the middle-class family which maintained the restrictive sexual taboos of traditional society, and which continued to demand chastity before marriage throughout the 1800s. For the family, sexuality and marriage went hand-in-hand. Intercourse before marriage would harm the family

enfants trouvés et abandonnés en Belgique," *Bulletin de la Commission Centrale de Statistique* (of Belgium), I (1843), 207–271; René Lafabrègue, "Des enfants trouvés à Paris," *Annales de démographie internationale*, II (1878), 226–299; Othmar Spann "Die Lage und das Schicksal der unehelichen Kinder," *Mutterschutz. Zeitschrift zur Reform der Sexuellen Ethik*, III (1907), 345–358; H. Neumann, "Die jugendlichen Berliner unehelicher Herkunft," *Jährbucher für Nationalökonomie und Statistik*, VIII (1894), 536–549.

31 See Steven Marcus, *The Other Victorians: A Study of Sexuality and Pornography in Mid-Nineteenth-Century England* (New York, 1966).

32 This paradox was pointed out to me by Fred Weinstein.

by (1) sullying the daughter and ruining her prospects of an advantageous marriage, and (2) threatening the continuation of the family name and property from generation to generation.

But even beyond this calculus of familial interest, the concept of *Ehrbarkeit* has always been a lynch pin in the ideology of the petty-bourgeois family. The quickest way to make oneself dishonorable was by sexual transgression. This notion of honor had disseminated from the master craftsmen of the guild system to all bourgeois family circles, but lower-class persons by definition were not master artisans, and, although formerly they had been willing respectfully to look on as the burghers exhorted one another to be honorable, for them this social ideology had become meaningless by the nineteenth century.[33]

One might plausibly argue that in the course of the eighteenth century population growth decapitated the authority of the lower-class family by creating so many children that parents had nothing to pass on to their extra-numerous offspring, and hence no control over their behavior. And cottage industry created alternate sources of employment to enable children to escape the authority of the family by physically removing themselves or otherwise acquiring economic independence. Once children decided to exchange the old internalized values of abstinence for new ones of self-fulfillment, parents were powerless to stop them. The petty-bourgeois family did not undergo this fate because it managed to control its fertility[34] and to preserve the sense of family tradition which said that children would follow in the footsteps of the father. To be sure, young men of middle-class origin responded to a new *Zeitgeist* of gratification by sleeping with prostitutes; but these liaisons posed no threat to the family. What we know about middle-class daughters suggests that they stayed pure before marriage. Thus the authority of the middle-class family over its offspring remained inviolate, and, as a result, middle-class youth, however sensitized by change, did not actually break out of the web of familial custom and control. But the youth of the lower classes did, which resolves the apparent paradox.

33 For this discussion of the traditional petty-bourgeois family, I rely on Möller, *Kleinbürgerliche Familie*.

34 There is now a mass of evidence, both literary and statistical, that middle-class French families had consciously adopted family limitation by about 1775. See *Prévention des naissances*; on birth control, see the most recent in a chain of local studies, Marcel Lachiver, *La Population de Meulan du XVIIe au XIXe siècle (vers 1600–1870)* (Paris, 1969), 210. The question is still unclarified for Germany.

Thus in a long chain of argumentation we get from rising illegitimacy to the emergence of class differences in family structure. The chain has a number of linkages, the solidity of which may be verified by the test of quantitative data. These may be time-series data relating the change from year to year in some possible causative factor, such as an increase in literacy, to some such index of sexual behavior as prenuptial conceptions. Or the testing may be done with "ecological" data, using census information to spot a statistical relationship between the number of factory workers in an area and the number of young people living away from home, or the number of illegitimate children in the population. I have tried to cast the argument of this paper to permit precisely this kind of verification with statistical procedures.

If the propositions presented here about sexual behavior, family structure, and social change are correct, we may expect future work to turn up the following kinds of regularities:

1. If the proposition is true that illegitimacy stemmed from a change in mentalities (rather than from some purely "compositional" effect, such as an increase in the number of single women), we should expect to find the incidence of shotgun weddings increasing in the same places and at the same times as illegitimacy. This simultaneity would indicate that the percentage of all young people practicing premarital intercourse was climbing, ruling out explanations of bastardy which fixed solely upon courtship practices.

2. If the proposition is right that exposure to primary education effected a liberalization of sexual values, we should expect parish register data to point to a higher level of illegitimacy among young women with some rudiments of education than among those without. If the hypothesis is accurate that involvement in marketplace situations brought about libertine sexual behavior, we should expect female servants within the rationalized sector of capitalist agriculture to evidence higher illegitimacy rates than servants on traditional seigneurial estates.

3. If the proposition is true that the passage from Stage III illegitimacy (hit-and-run) to Stage IV (true love) came in consequence of greater residential stability, we should expect strong areal correlations between territorial mobility and illegitimacy, taken district by district. Likewise, the notion of a transition from stage II illegitimacy (master-servant exploitation) to the subsequent romantic-love Stages may be critically inspected through parish register data: Did a tendency emerge over the years for premarital lovers to come from the same social class?

If all of the correlations turn out in the predicted direction, we may smile and use our footing on this tiny base of confidence for better leverage on other vexing questions. If the correlations turn out to be zero, or, worse yet, the reverse of what the argument had anticipated, we shall have to return to the drawing board.

Yet this is an agenda for the future. As a starting point in the unraveling of European sexual history this paper has attempted: (1) to verify with exact quantitative data the existence of a late eighteenth-century revolution in premarital sexual behavior, and (2) to speculate, with arguments about social change and psychodynamics at many removes from the actual data, why this revolution took place. Future work will doubtless modify substantially the speculative elements of this argument. Future work will probably not, however, dispute that there is something to be explained. The evidence of illegitimacy and of prebridal pregnancy point inescapably to a drastic change in the sexual experience of the European lower classes in the course of modernization.

APPENDIX

A NOTE ON THE MEASUREMENT OF ILLEGITIMACY   To avoid confusion in the terminology of measurement, I refer to the percentage of illegitimate births among all births (illegitimate births/100 total births) as the illegitimacy *ratio*; and to the number of illegitimate births per 1,000 unmarried women in the population of childbearing age as the illegitimacy *rate*. The latter measure is clearly preferable to the former as an indicator of relative illegitimacy because the ratio is dependent upon the number of legitimate births. If, for example, the number of legitimate births in a place dropped, the illegitimacy ratio would appear to rise, for fewer legitimate births in the denominator would make the illegitimate births in the numerator appear more important, even though, in fact, illegitimacy had not changed at all. Another peril one encounters in using the ratio is the possibility that differences from one place to another (or one time to another) in illegitimacy may be solely attributable to differences in the distribution of single women from one place or time to another. If there are more single women in a town, more illegitimacy may be found there, all else being equal. Yet the single women in a town with a high illegitimacy ratio may not be more immoral, or find themselves abandoned at the altar more often, than the women in another town with a lower illegitimacy ratio. The illegitimacy rate would indicate that both towns were the same.

Experienced researchers, such as the INED scholars in France, are generally convinced of the accuracy, or at least of the constancy over time, in the biases of parish register data. The only major collapse of illegitimacy reporting of which I am aware came with English civil registration of births in 1838. The Act (Statute 6 and 7 Will. IV, cap. 86) made no mention of illegitimacy, and statisticians were able to determine if a child were a bastard only if the space for the father's name were left blank. Needless to say, an unwed mother could easily invent something, or take the name of her suitor, if the man were agreeable, and no one would be the wiser. See Lumley, "Observations upon the Statistics of Illegitimacy," esp. 220–221; *Sixth Annual Report of the Registrar General of Births, Deaths, and Marriages in England* (London, 1845), xxx–xxxix. Some deficiencies also crop up in seventeenth-century English parish register data, and it is possible that an apparent early seventeenth-century peak in illegitimacy may be an artifact caused by a late seventeenth-century tendency not to register the children of common-law unions as illegitimate. I have this information from E. A. Wrigley, who says that of the genuineness of the eighteenth-century explosion there can be no doubt. For an instance of the registration of legitimate but prenuptially conceived children as *illegitimate*, see Julius Gmelin, "Bevölkerungsbewegung im Hällischen seit Mitte des 16. Jahrhunderts," *Allgemeines Statistisches Archiv*, VI (I) (1902), 248.

Hélin noted some improvement in the accuracy of illegitimacy statistics in Liège, nonetheless attributing the great rise in bastardy there to a "relâchement de contraintes sociales devenues traditionnelles depuis la Contre Réforme" (209–210). Although I an suspicious of Hélin's explanation, I think the data he reports are of excellent quality. Etienne Hélin, *La démographie de Liège aux XVIIe et XVIIIe siècles* (Brussels, 1963).

TIME SERIES ON THE LEGITIMATION OF ILLEGITIMATE CHILDREN   I have been able to obtain only two time series on legitimation: statistics for the city of Paris and for the Kingdom of Belgium. The figures represent the total number of children legitimated in a given bloc of years per 100 illegitimate children born in that time, not the illegitimate children born in a given period who were subsequently legitimated.

PARIS		BELGIUM	
Percent legitimated		Percent legitimated	
1822	7.2	1851–60	34.7
1881–84	18.6	1861–70	38.7

PARIS		BELGIUM	
Percent legitimated		Percent legitimated	
1885–89	20.1	1871–80	43.1
1890–94	23.2	1881–90	46.9
1895–99	25.6	1891–1900	57.5
1900–04	27.1	1901–10	65.2
1905–09	31.3	1911–13	61.1
1910–14	35.3		

Sources for Paris: *Recherches statistiques sur la Ville de Paris et la département de la Seine* (Paris, 1826), tables 23 and 24. *Annuaire statistique de la Ville de Paris*, yearly after 1880. Sources for Belgium: *Annuaire statistique de la Belgique et du Congo Belge*, XXXIV (1903), 109–111, and XLIV (1913), 129–131.

The standard treatments of legitimation are Moriz Ertl, "Uneheliche Geburt und Legitimation. Ein Beitrag zur Beurtheilung der 'unehelichen Geburtenziffer,'" *Statistische Monatschrift* (Austria), XIII (1887), 393–438, which reviews available statistics throughout Europe; Seutemann, "Die Legitimationen unehelicher Kinder," 13–68. Analysis of Swiss conditions may be found in yearly volumes of the *Zeitschrift für Schweizerische Statistik*, for example, XLIV (1908), 168–173, and XLIX (1913), 122–128, which yield a short time series. France is discussed in Legoyt, "Les Naissances naturelles," 71–72. Three studies trace legitimation among cohorts of illegitimate births after allowing for mortality: Eugen Würzburger, "Zur Statistik der Legitimationen unehelicher Kinder," *Jahrbücher für Nationalökonomie und Statistik*, XVIII (1899), 94–98; Othmar Spann, "Die Legitimation der unehelichen Kinder in Österreich unter Berücksichtigung der Sterblichkeit nach Gebieten," *Statistische Monatschrift*, XIV (1909), 129–138; "Legitimirung unehelicher Kinder," *Statistisches Jahrbuch der Stadt Berlin*, XXII (1895), 55–57.

SOURCES OF DATA FOR GRAPHS ON ILLEGITIMACY   The years indicated on the horizontal scale represent the endpoints of the blocs of years for which the average illegitimacy figure has been computed. The lines for prenuptial conception represent the percentage of all first births born within eight months (or thereabouts) of the wedding.

The inclusion of stillbirths in the illegitimacy statistics varies from one source to another; I have made no effort to note their presence or absence, partly because the inclusion of stillbirths elevates the illegitimacy ratios only minimally, partly because that information is missing for many places.

1. *France.* Wesley D. Camp, *Marriage and the Family in France since the Revolution* (New York, 1961), 108.

2. *Paris.* Data on *enfants trouvés* (1670–1800) and illegitimate births (1806–20) are from E. Charlot and J. Dupaquier. "Mouvement annuel de la population de la Ville de Paris de 1670 à 1821," *Annales de Démographie Historique, 1967*, 512–515. Data for 1831–1900 are from *Annuaire Statistique de la Ville de Paris*, 53–54 (1932–34), 107–108. No illegitimacy data are available for 1821–30.

3. *Brittany and Anjou (selected villages).* Yves Blayo and Louis Henry, "Données démographiques sur la Bretagne et l'Anjou de 1740 à 1829," *Annales de Démographie Historique, 1967*, 107.

4. *Lille.* Alain Lottin, "Naissances illégitimes et filles-mères à Lille," 292.

5. *Bordeaux.* Review of B. Saint-Jours, *La Population de Bordeaux depuis le XVIe siècle* (1911) in *Annales de Démographie Historique, 1968*, 182.

6. *Tamerville (Normandy).* Philippe Wiel, "Une grosse paroisse Cotentin aux XVIIe et XVIIIe siècles," *Annales de Démographie Historique, 1969*, 161.

7. *Villedieu-les-Poëles (Normandy).* Marie-Hélène Jouan, "Un bourg artisanal normand au XVIIIe siècle: Villedieu-les-Poëles, 1711–1790," *Annales de Démographie Historique, 1969*, 122.

8. *Sainghin-en-Mélantois (Nord).* Raymond Deniel and Louis Henry, "La Population d'un village du Nord de la France: Sainghin-en-Mélantois, de 1665 à 1851," *Population*, XX (1965), 582. (1) means the prenuptial conceptions of peasants and artisans, (2) those of farm laborers and weavers.

9. *Meulan (near Paris).* Lachiver, *La Population de Meulan*, 67.

10. *Boulay (Moselle).* Jacques Houdaille, "La Population de Boulay (Moselle) avant 1850," *Population*, XXII (1967), 1060.

11. *Troarn (Normandy).* Bouvet, "Troarn: Etude de démographie historique," 122–123. Bouvet's published yearly data are not convertible into ratios over blocs of time; my graph is therefore an approximate representation of the illegitimacy ratio.

12. *Leipzig.* W. Hanauer, "Historisch-statistische Untersuchungen über uneheliche Geburten," *Zeitschrift für Hygiene*, CVIII (1927–28), 663.

13. *Chemnitz. Ibid.*

14. *Frankfurt am Main. Ibid.,* 660–662.

15–18. *Freiberg, Lychen, Stroppen, Stuttgart, Durlach, Weiden, and Northeim.* Möller, *Kleinbürgerliche Familie,* 290.

19. *Hamburg.* Hanauer, "Historisch-statistische Untersuchungen," 663.

20. *Husum (Schleswig-Holstein).* Ingwer Ernst Momsen, *Die Bevölkerung der Stadt Husum von 1769 bis 1860* (Kiel, 1969), 382–383.

21. *Halle.* Hanauer, "Historisch-statistische Untersuchungen," 662.

22. *Seven parishes near Tölz (Bavaria).* Stephan Glonner, "Bevölkerungsbewegung von sieben Pfarreien im Kgl. Bayerischen Bezirksamte Tölz seit Ende des XVI. Jahrhunderts," *Allgemeines Statistisches Archiv,* IV (1896), 263–279.

23. *An Oldenburg town* (no name given). Erich Meyer, "Beiträge zum Sexualleben de Landjugend," *Zeitschrift für Sexualwissenschaft,* XVI (1929–30), 108.

24–26. *Boitin (Mecklenburg), Volkhardinghaüsen (Hesse), and Kreüth (Bavaria).* Jacques Houdaille, "Quelques résultats sur la démographie de trois villages d'Allemagne de 1750 à 1879," *Population,* XXV (1970), 649–654.

27. *Steiermark.* Otto von Zwiedineck-Südenhorst, "Die Illegitimität in Steiermark," *Statistische Monatschrift,* XXI (1895), 160.

28. *Sixteen Oberbayern villages 1760–1830,* courtesy Michael Phayer. Data for the *Kingdom of Bavaria, 1825–95* from Lindner, *Die unehelichen Geburten als Sozialphänomen,* 20. The Palatinate is included.

29. *Seventeen parishes around Hall in Württemburg.* Gmelin, "Bevölkerungsbewegung im Hällischen," 248.

30. *Göttelfingen (Württemberg).* Ilse Müller, "Bevölkerungsgeschichtliche Untersuchungen in drei Gemeinden des württembergischen Schwarzwaldes," *Archiv für Bevölkerungswissenschaft,* IX (1939), 193.

31. *Böhringen (Württemberg).* G. Heckh, "Bevölkerungsgeschichte und Bevölkerungsbewegung des Kirchspiels Böhringen auf der Uracher Alb vom 16. Jahrhundert bis zur Gegenwart," *Archiv für Rassen- und Gesellschaftshygiene,* XXXIII (1939–40), 134. I am indebted to John Knodel for the references to Böhringen und Göttelfingen.

32. *Anhausen (Bavaria).* John Knodel, "Two and a Half Centuries of Demographic History in a Bavarian Village," *Population Studies,* XXIV (1970), 367.

33. *Tirol and Vorarlberg.* Vinc. Goehlert, "Die Entwickelung der Bevölkerung von Tirol and Vorarlberg," *Statistische Monatschrift,* VI (1880), 63–64.

34. *Eibesthal (Lower Austria)*. Franz Riedling, "Bevölkerungsbewegung im Orte Eibesthal in Nieder-Oesterreich in den Jahren 1683–1890," *Statistische Monatschrift*, IV (1899), 262.

35. *Canton of Neuchâtel*. Guillaume, "Recherches sur le mouvement de la population dans le canton de Neuchâtel de 1760 à 1875," *Zeitschrift für Schweizerische Statistik*, XIII (1877), 38.

36. *Belgium*. *Annuaire Statistique de la Belgique et du Congo Belge*, XXXIV (1903), 109–111.

37. *Liège*. Hélin, *Démographie de Liège*, 256–258.

38. *Rotterdam*. A. M. Van der Woude and G. J. Mentink, "La Population de Rotterdam au XVIIe et au XVIIIe siècle," *Population*, XXI (1966), 1180.

39. *Sweden*. Gustav Sundbärg, *Bevölkerungsstatistik Schwedens*, 117, 129.

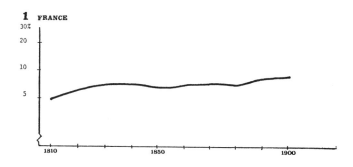

1 FRANCE

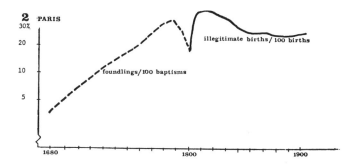

2 PARIS

illegitimate births/100 births

foundlings/100 baptisms

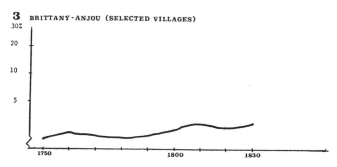

3 BRITTANY-ANJOU (SELECTED VILLAGES)

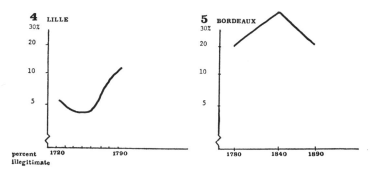

4 LILLE

5 BORDEAUX

percent illegitimate

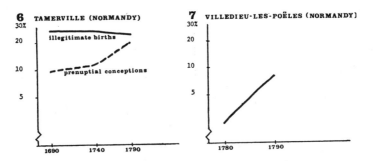

6 TAMERVILLE (NORMANDY)

7 VILLEDIEU-LES-POËLES (NORMANDY)

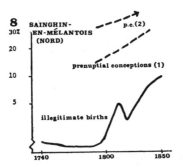

8 SAINGHIN-EN-MÉLANTOIS (NORD)

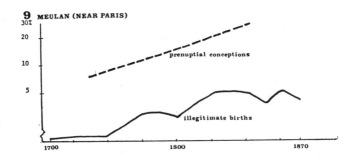

9 MEULAN (NEAR PARIS)

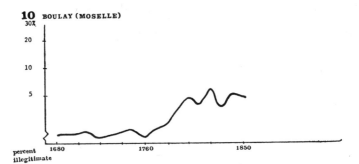

10 BOULAY (MOSELLE)

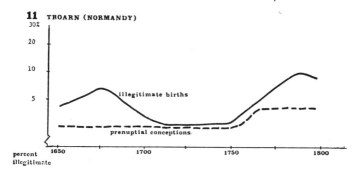

11 TROARN (NORMANDY)

illegitimate births

prenuptial conceptions

percent
illegitimate

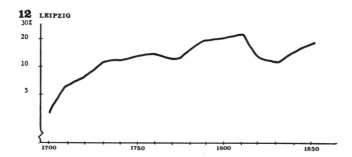

12 LEIPZIG

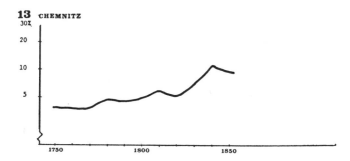

13 CHEMNITZ

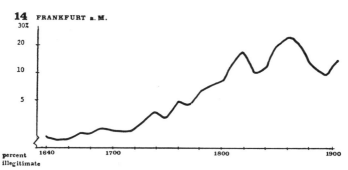

14 FRANKFURT a. M.

percent
illegitimate

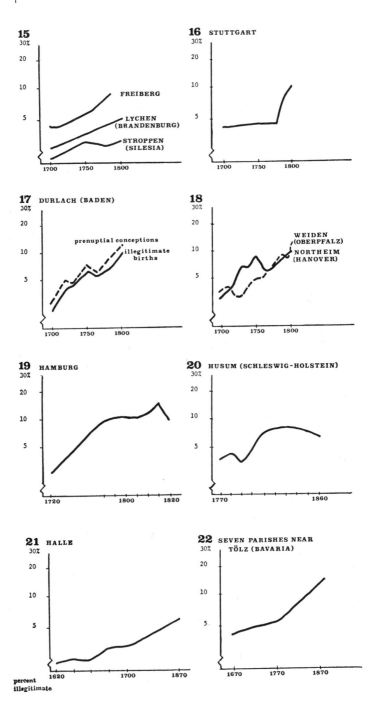

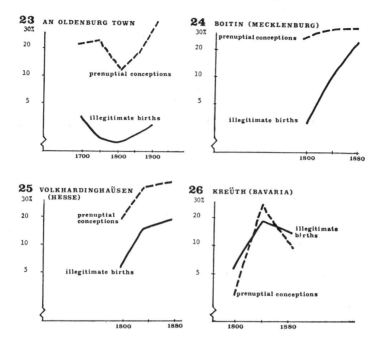

23 AN OLDENBURG TOWN

prenuptial conceptions

illegitimate births

24 BOITIN (MECKLENBURG)

prenuptial conceptions

illegitimate births

25 VOLKHARDINGHAÜSEN (HESSE)

prenuptial conceptions

illegitimate births

26 KREÜTH (BAVARIA)

illegitimate births

prenuptial conceptions

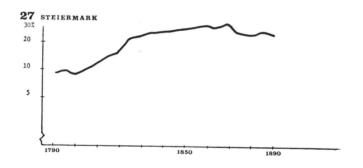

27 STEIERMARK

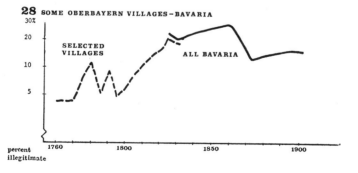

28 SOME OBERBAYERN VILLAGES—BAVARIA

SELECTED VILLAGES

ALL BAVARIA

percent illegitimate

29 SEVENTEEN PARISHES AROUND HALL (WÜRTTEMBERG)

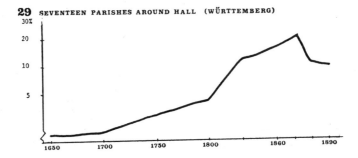

30 GÖTTELFINGEN (WÜRTTEMBERG)

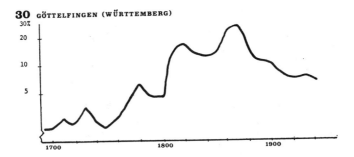

31 BÖHRINGEN (WÜRTTEMBERG)

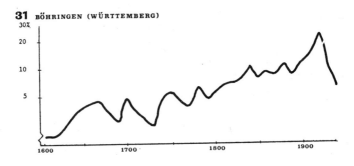

32 ANHAUSEN (BAVARIA)

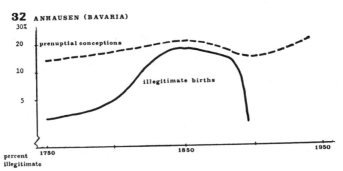

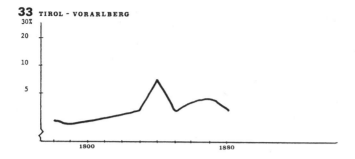

33 TIROL - VORARLBERG

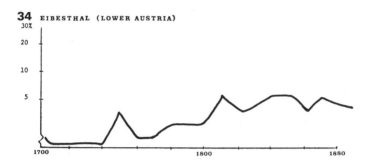

34 EIBESTHAL (LOWER AUSTRIA)

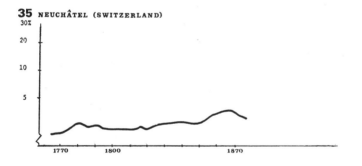

35 NEUCHÂTEL (SWITZERLAND)

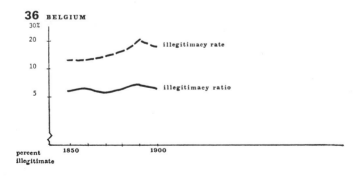

36 BELGIUM

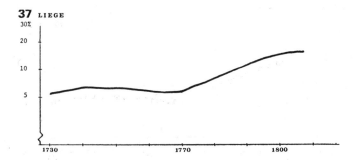

37 LIEGE

38 ROTTERDAM

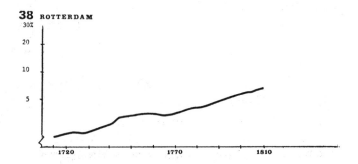

39 SWEDEN

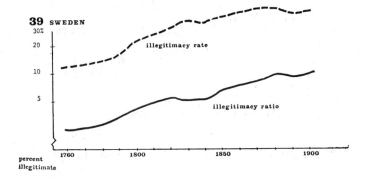

illegitimacy rate

illegitimacy ratio

percent
illegitimate

Journal of Interdisciplinary History, VII:3 (Winter 1977), 403–425.

W. R. Lee

Bastardy and the Socioeconomic
Structure of South Germany

According to Davis, the bastard ". . . is a living symbol of social irregularity, an undeniable evidence of contramoral forces."[1] Although the problem of bastardy, in its various forms (whether adulterous, incestuous, or violating caste endogamy), has traditionally faced many different types of society in which the act of marriage was an integral norm of socialization, its magnitude increased considerably in certain areas of Europe in the late eighteenth and nineteenth centuries. This development has been described as part of the thawing process of the "great iceberg" of sexuality in traditional society, culminating in a veritable "sexual revolution" and involving a growth of transvestism and prostitution, as well as rising illegitimacy rates.[2]

Certainly in Bavaria profound changes had occurred during the period from 1750 to 1850. In the late eighteenth century illegitimacy was no real social problem. By the 1820s, however, the situation was different. A priest in Ruprechtsberg claimed that few single women had not given birth to illegitimate children. "A Virgin! Rara Avis."[3] The two bulwarks of innocence, fear of God and modesty, had been breached. The seriousness of the situation cannot be doubted (Table 1). Only two other areas in Germany and Austria had higher illegitimacy rates (Table 2). Furthermore the preeminence of Bavarian bastards in the whole of Western Europe was still as severely pronounced in 1865–1870 (Table 3). Single women were conceiving five to six children each. In the parish of Gremertshausen ". . . morality and religiosity [were] . . . in such a bad condition, that deteriorations were daily visible."[4] The picture of moral decay would seem to be complete: a sexual

W. R. Lee is Lecturer in the Department of Economic History, University of Liverpool.

1 Kingsley Davis, "Illegitimacy and the Social Structure," *American Journal of Sociology,* XLIV (1939), 215.
2 Edward Shorter, "Illegitimacy, Sexual Revolution, and Social Change in Modern Europe," *Journal of Interdisciplinary History,* II (1971), 237.
3 Ordinariats-Archiv München (O.A.M.) Ruprechtsberg. Visitation 1823. Cited by Fintan Michael Phayer, *Religion und das Gewöhnliche Volk in Bayern in der Zeit von 1750–1850* (Munich, 1970), 114.
4 O.A.M. Gremertshausen. Visitation 1822.

Table 1 Illegitimacy Rates and Birth Rates in
Bavaria (1825/6–1874)

	ILLEGITIMATE BIRTHS PER 100 BIRTHS	BIRTH RATE PER 1,000 POPULATION
1825/6–29/30	19.6	
1830/1–34/5	20.4	
1835/6–39/40	20.8	36.4
1840/1–44/5	20.6	35.7
1845/6–49/50	20.5	35.1
1850/1–54/5	20.8	33.7
1855/6–59/60	22.8	35.3
1860/1–64/5	22.8	37.2
1865/6–69/70	19.4	39.6
1871 –1874	13.9	40.4

revolution had taken place, disrupting the equilibrium of traditional peasant behavior norms and replacing them with greater
freedom in sexual activity. But how viable is such a hypothesis in
the case of South Germany? To what extent were the general
causative factors found in other parts of Europe present in
Bavaria? Was there really a "sexual revolution," which could be
regarded as marking a fundamental change with preindustrial social and sexual codes?

South Germany, and specifically Bavaria, had a social and
economic factor endowment which should have militated against
a radical revolution in behavior patterns. Despite increasing acceptance of the Reformed Church, Catholicism remained a semi-
official religion to which 92 percent of the population belonged
even in 1902. Social control is often institutionalized in religion as
an adjunct to secular mechanisms and specifically in Catholicism,
which rigidly maintained the "principle of legitimacy." Significantly the Catholic Church was to take a harder and more conservative line on the "social question," with hierarchical pronouncements such as the encyclical Rerum Novarum (1891). In
Bavaria the Church's position in the late eighteenth century appeared strong. Of all peasant families, 50.5 percent were tenants of
ecclesiastical foundations. In 1776 Upper and Lower Bavaria
boasted 120 monastic foundations. A rural chaplain claimed in
1797 that ". . . no more than 10 from 1,000 parishioners failed to
attend Sunday Mass" and nineteenth-century figures reveal no
evidence of a cataclysmic change and certainly nothing compara-

Table 2 Illegitimacy in German and Austrian Territories (c. 1840)

TERRITORY	ANNUAL FREQUENCY OF ILLEGITIMATE BIRTHS	
	ILLEGITIMATE BIRTHS PER LEGITIMATE BIRTHS	ILLEGITIMATE BIRTHS PER INHABITANTS
Austria below the Ems	3.77	131.50
Steiermark	3.66	142.06
Bavaria	3.98	144.00
Baden	5.61	172.41
Saxony	6.15	184.58
Austria above the Ems	4.71	196.14
Carpathia and Krain	4.95	197.62
Bohemia	6.63	201.42
Hessen	5.71	210.03
Mecklenburg-Schwerin	6.50	222.35
Silesia and Moravia	8.02	228.49
Württemberg	7.69	242.66
Saxony-Weimar	7.10	242.67
Hanover	9.62	308.12
Mecklenburg-Strelitz	10.86	335.80
Galicia	14.06	366.26
Prussia	13.49	392.95
Tyrol and Vorarlberg	19.20	655.98
Lombardy	25.16	660.98
Oldenburg*a*	11.33	748.26
Venetian territory	31.38	832.39
Dalmatia	27.38	952.15

a without Kniphausen
SOURCE: F. Rivet, "Ueber die ausserehelichen Geburten, insbesonders in Baiern," *Archiv der politischen Oekonomie und Polizeiwissenschaft,* I (1843), 44–45.

ble to the low church attendance rates in parts of the United Kingdom revealed by the 1851 census. In Hohenkammer, average attendance rates in 1843–1848 still stood at 97.9 percent. It is against this backcloth that the "revolution" in social behavior is supposed to have taken place.[5]

5 Wolfram Fischer, "Social Tensions at Early Stages of Industrialization," *Comparative Studies in Society and History,* IX (1966), 70. Joseph Hazzi, *Statistische Aufschlüsse über das Herzogtum Baiern* (Munich, 1802), II, 123. Phayer, *Religion,* 30. K. Inglis, "Patterns of Religious Worship in 1851," *Journal of Ecclesiastical History,* XI (1960), 79. According to Horace Mann ". . . the masses of our working population . . . are never or but seldom seen in our religious congregation." H. Mann, "On the statistical position of the religious bodies in England and Wales," *Journal of the Statistical Society,* XVIII (1855), 141.

Table 3   Illegitimacy Rates per 100
births (1845/50–1865/70)

COUNTRY	1845/50	1865/70
Bavaria	20.5	19.3
Saxony	14.8	15.1
Württemberg	11.8	15.7
Denmark	11.4	10.8
Austria	11.3	14.7
Scotland	9.8	9.6
Norway	8.3	9.2
Sweden	8.8	9.3
Belgium	8.1	7.2
France	7.4	7.6
Prussia	7.5	8.3
England	6.7	6.3
Netherlands	4.8	4.0
Spain	–	5.8
Italy	–	5.0
Sardinia	2.1	–

Local kinship factors were also important throughout the period 1750–1850. Although extended families seldom existed, couples rarely had a neolocal residence completely independent of existing kinship connections. The strong identity of separate rural regions, visible in traditional costume styles, also meant that family contacts with a specific region remained strong. Godparents, for example, often came from within a radius of 5–10 km. and within individual families there was a strong element of continuity in choice. Community ties, often of crucial importance as mechanisms of social control, were reinforced by the pattern of settlement. Average population per village in Oberbayern (1808) fluctuated from 23.5 (Landgericht Miesbach) to 93.5 (Landericht Freising) and settlements of only one–two holdings were predominant near the Alps. The small, decentralized settlement pattern should have made the implementation of kinship and neighborhood sanctions more effective than in other parts of Europe, even if the result were simply to retard social change.

Demoralization in the Hegelian sense implies the loss of identity between the objective societal order and the subjective will of the individual, and both industrialization and urbanization are traditionally regarded as causative factors in this process. Certainly even prominent liberals, such as Gottfried Ludolf Camphausen and Gustav von Mevissen, stressed the power of urban life (and the development of a market economy) to weaken primal solidarities. Bavaria, however, was minimally affected by these disequilibriating macrodevelopments. The first mechanical cotton-spinning factory was not established until 1837. The question of industrial employment only became problematic after the 1850s. In the whole of the Landgericht Freising, with a total population of over 14,000 in 1830, apart from eighteen small-scale breweries there was only one factory employing one spinner and three part-time workers. Throughout the nineteenth century the agrarian sector in Bavaria remained predominant. Even as late as 1890 only 23 percent of the population lived in towns; there were only twenty-nine urban centers of more than 10,000 inhabitants. It is therefore doubtful whether the multiplier effect of urbanization on the infrastructure of rural society would have been significant. The development of a market economy was also slow and tentative, and it is difficult to see this factor as ". . . the most corrosive of the traditional communitarian order." In 1810 only 168 market centers existed in Altbayern and no additions were made until 1840. With an average population of 945, the smallest being Essing (Niederbayern) with only 317 inhabitants, it is not surprising that the economic role of these market centers in the nineteenth century was limited. In the Landgericht Freising only 28.5 percent of the annual grain crop and 0.2 percent of the region's sheep came up for sale. The development of inter-regional trade was also retarded by the fall in grain prices in the 1820s and 1830s. The whole of the Isarkreis in the early nineteenth century had only 457 registered merchants, whose turnover was officially described as not being "particularly favourable."[6]

Despite the absence of dramatic economic changes, an explosive upswing did take place in early nineteenth-century illegitimacy rates. How then is this phenomenon within a preindustrial

6 Donald G. Rohr, *The Origins of Social Liberalism in Germany* (Chicago, 1963), 9. Wolfgang Zorn, "Gesellschaft und Staat im Bayern des Vormärz," in Werner Conze (ed.), *Staat und Gesellschaft im deutschen Vormärz, 1815–1848* (Stuttgart, 1962), 119. Staatsarchiv für Oberbayern (St.A.ObB.), Regierungs Akten (R.A.) 1123/15702. Jahres-Berichte, Landgericht Freising, 1827–30. Shorter, "Illegitimacy," 249. Roman Mauerer, *Entwicklung und Funktionswandel der Märkte in Altbayern seit 1800* (Munich, 1971), *passim*. St. A.ObB. R.A. 1103/15676.

society to be explained? How valid are existing interpretations within the general European framework to the specific case of South Germany and Bavaria? Closer analysis will reveal many of their deficiencies.

It is impossible that increasing illegitimacy rates can be attributable to improved registration. Local priests were particularly assiduous in listing all illegitimate births in the eighteenth century and the maintenance of special burial plots for bastard children reinforced the need for careful differentiation.

The hypothesis relating changes in social patterns to the growth of rural industry provides a further possible explanation. Even if Bavaria had not industrialized in the period under consideration, rural industry already exercised an important role in the economy. In 1771 in the Pfleggericht Kranzberg, 21.7 percent of listed families depended to some extent on income from crafts and manufacturing. By 1788 restrictions on the spread of rural industry had been lifted and by 1809 182,216 individuals, with 70,539 apprentices and assistants were occupied in this sector.[7] Linen production was particularly noted in Upper Frankonia, shoe-making in the Palatinate, and wood-carving in Oberbayern. The disequilibrating effect on peasant society could have been considerable.

If primary social functions are normally linked to a system of occupational status, the growth of rural industry may have stimulated the emergence of new social behavior norms, as envisaged by von Benekendorf. Claims have been made of a positive correlation between the extent of rural industry and the rate of illegitimacy and it is perhaps significant that the settlement pattern associated with rural industry tended to differ slightly from that of traditional agricultural holdings, being associated with small-holdings and reduced family size. Significantly, the lowest family size located in Germany of 1.82 individuals per family related to small-holders in Calenberg-Göttingen and Grubenhagen in 1689. If it is argued that the nuclear family, despite its positive attributes in meeting the demands of primary groups, being face-to-face, permanent, effective, and noninstrumental, encountered difficulties in handling crucial tension management problems where the source of difficulty lay within the family (as in the case of illegiti-

---

7 Rudolf Braun, *Industrialisierung und Volksleben* (Zurich, 1960). St. A.ObB. General Register (G.R.) 290/1. St. A.ObB. R.A. 1103/15676.

mate offspring of family dependents), then the societal repercussions of rural industry may well have been adverse: the smaller nuclear family was even less likely to be able to cope with deviations from the norm.[8]

The applicability of this hypothesis to the case of Bavaria, however, remains doubtful. The growth of rural industry was a cumulative process which had probably reached its peak in individual sectors before the end of the eighteenth century. In many areas optimum distribution of small-holdings had been achieved by 1760 (Table 4). If this factor had been causative, why are explo-

Table 4 Percentage Distribution of Small Holdings (1/6–1/32) in Bavaria, 1760

ADMINISTRATIVE AREA	NUMBER OF HOLDINGS	NUMBER OF SMALL HOLDINGS	% OF SMALL HOLDINGS
Moosburg	2557	1359	53.1
Mering	701	550	78.9
Friedberg	1524	1078	70.7
Starnberg	1285	800	62.2
Weilheim	2217	1468	67.0
Benediktbeuren	559	302	54.0
Ettal	947	804	84.8
Mainburg	571	301	52.7
Neustadt	259	230	91.8
Vohburg	1326	872	65.7
Traunstein	1652	1026	62.1
Trostberg	804	407	50.6
Pfaffenhofen	3008	1682	56.0
Dachau	3402	2148	63.1
Kranzberg	2335	1361	58.6
Aichach	2620	1749	67.5
Landsberg (Landkreis)	3233	2349	75.7

SOURCE: P. Fried, "Historisch-statistische Beiträge zur Geschichte des Kleinbauerntums (Söldnertums) im westlichen Oberbayern," *Mitteilungen der Geographischen Gesellschaft in München,* II (1966), 19.

8 Werner Conze, "Vom 'Pöbel' zum 'Proletariat'. Socialgeschichtliche Voraussetzungen für den Sozialismus in Deutschland," in H.-U.Wehler (ed.), *Moderne Deutsche Sozialgeschichte* (Köln, 1966), 114. A. Beelitz, G. Ostermuth, H. Schlegel, and H. Pohl. "Unterschiedliche Fortpflanzung in den Fürstentumern Calenberg-Göttingen und Grubenhagen auf Grund der Kopfsteuerbeschreibung von 1689," *Archiv für Bevölkerungswissenschaft und Bevölkerungspolitik,* XI (1941), 311. Eugene Litwak and Ivan Szelenyi, "Primary Group Structures and their Functions: Kin, Neighbors and Friends," *American Sociological Review,* XXXIV (1969), 419.

sive illegitimacy rates not found prior to the nineteenth century? By 1800 other areas of Germany had extensive rural industries and a settlement distribution pattern with an equal emphasis on small-holdings, and yet this fact alone did not stimulate illegitimacy rates as dramatically as it did in South Germany and Bavaria.[9]

High illegitimacy rates have also been regarded as a consequence of the reintroduction of restrictive marriage and settlement legislation, which "narrowed the range of economic opportunities open to those wanting to establish a family."[10] In states where this type of legislation was adopted in the early nineteenth century, including Bavaria, Hannover, Wurttemberg, Baden, Hessen-Nassau, Hessen-Darmstadt, Mecklenburg-Schwerin, and Hohenzollern, influenced perhaps by such neo-Malthusians as Rau, von Mohl, and Weinheld, it is believed that a considerable number of legitimate births suppressed through marriage restrictions accounted for the large number of illegitimate conceptions. Legislation of 1818 and in particular of 1825 in Bavaria did indeed reduce marriage prospects, but certain weaknesses remain in this hypothesis.

First, the changes in Bavarian illegitimacy rates do not fit the chronological pattern of legislation. Significant changes in illegitimacy can be found in the 1780s and 1790s (Table 5), and as early as 1812–1813 the rate in Freising already stood at 19.7 per 100 births, a figure typical of other areas (Table 6).[11] Even after the lifting of marriage restrictions in the 1850s, Bavarian illegitimacy rates remained far above the average for the German Empire. In 1901 the rate for Oberbayern stood at 18.9 per 100 births and 25.3 in Munich.

Second, many of the important demographic indices connected with marriage and nuptiality remained constant for the period 1750–1850. For the constituent parishes of the Hofmark Massenhausen, for example, the overall proportion of female children eventually marrying rose from 29.5 percent in 1750–1799 to

9 Friedrich-Wilhelm Henning, "Die Betriebsgrössenstruktur der mitteleuropäischen Landwirtschaft im 18. Jahrhundert und ihr Einfluss auf die ländlichen Einkommensverhältnisse," *Zeitschrift für Agrargeschichte und Agrarsoziologie*, XVII (1969), 171–193.

10 John Knodel, "Law, Marriage and Illegitimacy in Nineteenth-Century Germany," *Population Studies*, XX (1967), 280.

11 St. A.ObB. R.A. 1105/15680.

Table 5   Decennial Illegitimacy Rates per 100 Live Births (1750–1849)

DECADE	HOFMARK MASSENHAUSEN	HOFMARK THALHAUSEN
1750–9	4.09	3.94
1760–9	3.84	3.40
1770–9	4.69	3.15
1780–9	8.55	8.77
1790–9	7.47	13.41
1800–9	7.69	11.11
1810–9	14.03	12.17
1820–9	18.04	25.53
1830–9	16.41	22.97
1840–9	15.28	55.29

34.3 percent in 1800–1849. The mean age at first marriage for women did rise, but only marginally, from 26.9 years in 1750–1799 to 27.1 in 1800–1849. On the Hofmark Thalhausen there was an equally marginal fall in this important index from 31.1 to 29.3 years. It is not surprising to find, therefore, that little change took place in the overall proportion of unmarried individuals to total

Table 6   Early 19th Century Illegitimacy Rates in Administrative Areas of Bavaria

DISTRICT	YEAR	ILLEGITIMACY RATE (PER 100 BIRTHS)
Bez. Ingolstadt	1810/11	24.0
Isarkreis	1810/11	17.0
Aichach	1811/12	12.1
Altötting	1811/12	15.5
Burghausen	1811/12	13.4
Isarkreis	1811/12	16.6
Erding	1812/13	14.5
Rosenheim	1812/13	14.5
Munchen	1812/13	18.9
Dachau	1812/13	10.1
Freising	1813/14	20.0
Rosenheim	1813/14	15.3
Starnberg	1813/14	11.3
Trostberg	1813/14	10.4
Weilheim	1813/14	7.4

population. In the Landgericht Freising 37.1 percent were listed as unmarried in 1840. If this figure is adjusted according to age-group, it corresponds closely to the late eighteenth-century figure of just over 33 percent.[12] Indeed, although the marriage rate in Bavaria in the 1820s and 1830s was lower than that pertaining to other German territories with minimal marriage restrictions, the difference only accounts for a small proportion (c. 15 percent) of the additional illegitimate births recorded.

Third, if factors affecting the ease of marriage are viewed as influencing illegitimacy rates, then an inverse correlation should be expected between the variable rates of marriage or total births and illegitimacy. This was not usually the case. In 1813–1814 both the number of solemnized marriages and illegitimate births rose. During the late 1840s a similar parallel is found, with illegitimacy rates falling at a time when total births fell at a faster rate.[13] To this extent the restrictive marriage legislation of 1825 does not appear to have had a decisive effect on relative rates of illegitimacy.

It has also been argued that the Secularization of 1803 was responsible for the dramatic increase in illegitimacy.[14] Despite the Concordat of 1817, the Church was slow to recover and the first Benedictine monastery was not reopened until 1830. The reduction in personnel was accompanied by enforced land sales and a reorganization of parish boundaries. As a result traditional moral norms, which had rested on a firm Christian basis, were displaced and the "secularization of sexual life" led directly to the illegitimacy problem. The validity of this explanation rests on an assumed effectiveness of Church control in the late eighteenth century and an accepted over-lapping of Church and peasant value patterns. Behind the impression of conformity furnished by communion attendance figures, however, there is little evidence of effective social control. The Church had ceased to take an active interest in the running of the economy and ecclesiastical foundations were inevitably landlordish in character. Many churches prior to Secularization were incorporated with monastic foundations and the priest was not locally resident.[15]

---

12 Bayerische Statistisches Landesamt. Survey of 1840. St. A.ObB. G.R. 302/42.

13 Ludwig August von Müller, *Von Riedels Commentar zum Bayerischen Gesetze über Heimat, Verehelichung und Aufenthalt* (Nördlingen, 1887), 151–152.

14 Phayer, *Religion*, III, 255.

15 Cf. Hartwig Peetz, "Der Haushalt des Klosters Polling im 18. Jahrhundert," *Jahrbuch*

Other signs of an ineffective role function in the late eighteenth century can be adduced from the following factors: first, social and linguistic barriers mitigated the significance of face-to-face contact. The majority of theological students came from the better-off sections of society. Latinized ecclesiastical ritual hardly coped with the innate superstitious nature of peasant religious belief. On Good Friday, for example, bread was rubbed on the cross, the crumbs being stored for later use in baking in the belief that doing so would prevent indigestion. The communication barrier was substantial. According to one contemporary (1786) ". . . In the sermons . . . one hears nothing but complaining . . . today over the decadent, irresponsible times, tomorrow over free-thinkers and godless books . . . and all this for an audience, among whom perhaps hardly three have ever held a book in their hands and who do not know what the sermon is about."[16]

Second, evidence is also available for a noticeable decline in peasant support for the Church in the eighteenth century. For the thirteen churches of the Hofmark Massenhausen, voluntary contributions fell from 135 Gulden (1769) to 98fl.33kr.Ih1. (1802).[17] The average decennial frequency of peasant endowments of ecclesiastical foundations also fell from 6 in 1700–1749 to 3 in 1750–1799.

Third, if the reduction in Church authority implicit in the Secularization acted in a causative role in facilitating increased illegitimacy, why did the extensive erosion of the Church's position in the late eighteenth century not produce a similar effect? Restrictions had been placed on the Mendicant orders (1749–1769); the Decimation Bull of 1757 allowed taxation of Church property and the Bull of 1798 had enabled the Kurfürst to appropriate one-

für Münchner Geschichte, IV (1890), 318; Rudolf Haderstorfer, *Die Säkularisation der oberbayerischen Klöster Baumberg und Seeon* (Stuttgart, 1967), 14–15. St. A.ObB. Amts Register (A.R.) 2359. Eleven of the 20 parishes in the Pfleggericht Kranzberg were incorporated prior to 1803.

16 Franz Xaver Freninger (ed.), *Das Matrikelbuch der Universität Ingolstadt-Landshut-München. Rectoren, Professoren, Doctoren. 1472–1872. Candidaten 1772–1872* (Munich, 1872), 79. Anita Brittinger, "Die Bayerische Verwaltung und das volksfromme Brauchtum im Zeitalter der Aufklärung," unpub. diss. (Munich, 1937), 8–9. K. Böck, *Das Bauernleben in den Werken bayrischer Barockprediger* (Munich, 1953), 28 ff.

17 On the basis of a list of voluntary contributions for all Massenhausen settlements dating from 1835–36, the average level per head had fallen from 45 kreuzer in 1769 to just over 4 kreuzer.

seventh of all ecclesiastical property. All of these measures struck at the symbolic position of the Church without affecting the "moral" behavior of parishioners or leading to dramatically high illegitimacy rates.

A further explanatory hypothesis regards formalized primary education, with its emphasis on linear logic and a sense of self, as a prime force in the disruption of social values in the nineteenth century. Undoubtedly increased literacy did promote added awareness of optional forms of social behavior. In Austria after the introduction of compulsory attendance in 1774, the increased influx of popular novels from north Germany contributed to the "anti-catholic" feeling of certain social groups. In England loss of faith in the nineteenth century could easily be associated with specific literary works. If this were equally true for Bavaria, increased literacy may have minimized the magical and superstitious elements in religious belief and thereby led to a conflict between individual and socio-religious behavior norms.[18]

There was educational reform in the early nineteenth century. School attendance was made compulsory for children between six and twelve years in 1802 and improvements were made to the curriculum in 1804, 1806, and 1811. The training of teachers was improved by the establishment of nine seminaries between 1803 1817. In 1783 probably over half of the people in Bavaria could neither read nor write.[19]

In the opinion of contemporaries, however, these attempts at educational reform achieved very little. Figures for the Hofmark Massenhausen indicate that in the period 1840–1847 only 58 percent of men and 50 percent of women from small-holdings could sign their names. In Thalhausen 60 percent were illiterate in the period 1820–1839. Given the predominance of small-holders in many rural areas, it would seem that overall levels of literacy had hardly improved from the late eighteenth century. Structural deficiencies in the educational sector still abounded. Secularization did not lead to the utilization of appropriated income for local educational needs, and the rate of foundation of new schools was

18 Shorter, "Illegitimacy," 252. Otto Brunner, "Staat und Gesellschaft im vormärzlichen Oesterreich im Spiegel von J. Beidtels Geschichte der Oesterreichischen Staatsverwaltung, 1740–1848," in W. Conze (ed.), Staat und Gesellschaft, 71. Susan Budd, "The Loss of Faith in England, 1850–1950," Past & Present, 36 (1967), 109–112.
19 Peter Anton Winkopp, Bibliothek der Denker und Männer von Geschmack. Der Zustand der Aufklärung in Bayern (Munich, 1783), I, 471.

slow. Even in 1833 the average teacher-pupil ratio in the Land-gericht Freising stood at 1:103, although in Neufahrn this rose to 1:209. According to Sendtner, Bavaria lagged behind all other German states in the promotion of education.[20] The aims of the educational system were too limited, but despite the narrow terms of reference, the schooling provided was still insufficient and had little overall effect. It seems unlikely, therefore, that the high il-legitimacy rates could have been the result of changes in this sphere.

Finally there is the possibility that social isolation and class stratification increased during this period. The gradual erosion of corporate bonds signified the change from a structured society of separated groups (Stände), differentiated even by sumptuary legislation, to a legally uniform civil society, where the inter-nalized corporative constraints no longer held. According to Franz von Baader (1765–1841) traditional German society could only be retained by greater emphasis on corporate professional organiza-tions. It is possible that corporate cohesion deteriorated in the late eighteenth century. In Austria one effect of Joseph II's "Gesinde" legislation abolishing patriarchal authority was to exclude servants from the family by a reduction in cooperative contact within the employer's household. Adolf von Knigge (1798) viewed the sweetest of all relationships between the household father and his dependents (both by kinship and contract) as a thing of the past.[21] It is therefore possible that such phenomena as increased urbaniza-tion and the acceptance of new educational theories may have ad-versely altered the control mechanisms within both the individual Stände and the monogamous patriarchal family.

Once again, however, this general hypothesis proves unsuit-able as an explanation of the high illegitimacy rates in Bavaria. The family role hardly altered. It remained, as a unit centered on a specific holding, the immediate source of social welfare, including the provision of marriage dowries, provisions for physically dis-abled children and for elderly parents. Throughout the period under consideration the legal basis of these obligations did not al-

20 St. A.ObB. R.A. 1124/15703. Otto Sendtner, *Ueber Lehre und Zucht in den Schulen* (Munich, 1826), *passim*.
21 W. Fischer, "Social Tensions," 77. Günter Brakelmann, *Die Soziale Frage des 19. Jahrhunderts* (Witten/Ruhr, 1964), 195. Rolf Engelsing, "Dienstbotenlektüre im 18. und 19. Jahrhundert in Deutschland," *International Review of Social History*, XIII (1968), 397.

ter. The retention of this role, connected with the traditional inheritance pattern, was to provide a strong element of continuity in rural society. Equally there is little evidence of an erosion of corporate bonds within the various strata of rural society. In the Gemeinde proceedings an awareness of corporate responsibility is predominant in the early nineteenth century. The Gemeinde was the highest form of organization in most rural areas, and the allocation of increased powers to this body in the course of the early nineteenth century (as in 1825, 1834, 1848, and 1850), together with the maintenance of consensus and participational action would, if anything, have tended to reinforce cohesion within rural society in Bavaria.[22]

None of the traditional explanations of the disruptive factors facilitating high illegitimacy rates appears appropriate to Bavaria. How then is this dramatic phenomenon to be explained? Basically, increased illegitimacy did not imply a dramatic change in behavioral norms. Illegitimacy did not mean exclusion from contemporary society. It did not conflict, in the opinion of the peasantry, either in the late eighteenth or early nineteenth centuries, with traditional moral norms. The increasing number of bastards is to be explained primarily in economic and legal terms and not in connection with Secularization nor a nascent "sexual revolution."

Although tradition in primitive societies often acts as a force for consolidation, social control relies essentially on the application of different pressures to ensure the continued retention of existing norms, including physical and anticipated sanctions and psychological punishment. In Bavaria illegitimacy had been accepted into the framework of rural society in a way which made social controls unnecessary. There was no inherent conflict between illegitimacy and the retention of the family as the basic unit. Illegitimate children received their due share in family settlements. It was commonly regulated that in the event of a bride's death illegitimate children from other relationships were to be accorded the same rights as legitimate issue.[23] In other spheres a similar lack

22 J. Pflaumer-Rosenberger, *Die Anerbensitte in Altbayern* (Munich, 1939), *passim.* Gesetzblatt (GBL) (Munich, 1834), 109; GBL. (Munich, 1848), 98; GBL. (Munich, 1850), 341.

23 St. A.ObB. Hofmark Thalhausen, 10, Marriage Protokoll of 1833. This provides a typical example of the procedure. In the case of the later death of the bride, her three illegitimate children from another relationship were to be granted full inheritance rights.

of ostracism is visible. Cases where illegitimate children inherited a family holding are found in the 1780s as well as in the 1840s, despite the fact that illegitimate children, being institutionally outside the family under Roman Law, would normally be outside it in the legal sense. Medical attention given to children in their first year of life remained pitifully poor (only 7 percent of those dying from weakness, atrophy, or intestinal infection received attention in 1888–1889), but bastards received equal, if not preferential, treatment. There is also no evidence of a policy of slow starvation of newly born illegitimate children, as can be found in certain areas of France in the nineteenth century.[24]

On a further level traditional concepts of social stability were essentially a function of two major variables—(a) the normative and consensual commitment of the individual of the society and (b) the integration of the norms held by these individuals.[25] It would appear in the case of peasant society in Bavaria that consensual commitment did not preclude the wider acceptance of illegitimacy. Church officials frequently complained that the Gemeinde Vorsteher, as elected representatives, were seldom active enough in combating illegitimacy. Reports from the Landgericht Freising stressed that the central courts could not act against infringements of the moral code, especially in relation to illegitimacy, if denunciations were not passed on by local authorities. The absence of sanctions imposed by the peasantry is further emphasized by the frequency of illegitimate conceptions within individual families. In Fürholzen, for example, all listed illegitimate births in the period 1750–1850 came from ten of the twenty-three holdings. Of the daughters from these tenements, 64.9 percent reaching adulthood gave birth to illegitimate children.

It would therefore seem that illegitimacy, at least within certain families, constituted a social norm rather than a threat to the existing family structure. This aspect is also reinforced by the continued practice of naming illegitimate children after their putative

24 Horace H. Robbins and Francis Deak, "The Familial Property Rights of Illegitimate Children: A Comparative Study," *Columbia Law Review*, XXX (1930), 308–329. Jacques Bergeron and Rene Marjolin, "Hygiène des Nouveau-nés," in J. Bertillon (ed.), *Bericht für den internationalen Hygiene Kongress in Paris* (1893), 111.
25 William J. Goode, "A Theory of Role Strain," *American Sociological Review*, XXV (1960), 495.

father, even after the legislation of 1825 had specifically prohibited doing so without a prior examination of the paternity claim.[26] Although the legislation had an immediate effect in urban areas, the situation in rural areas remained unchanged. It can therefore be concluded that individuals responsible for illegitimate children were not themselves subject to criticism from their neighborhood or kinship groups. Their social standing within the peasant community was not endangered by paternity claims and assertions, even if false. Rural society was apparently indifferent as to whether children listed in the parish registers were legitimate or not. It did not follow the Church's lead in the attempted imposition of social controls. One of the key elements influencing role performances—the esteem/disesteem with which peripheral social networks or important reference groups will respond to the performance—was therefore inoperative as a means of controlling rising illegitimacy rates.

There were a number of practical reasons why high illegitimacy rates could be tolerated without disrupting the continued functioning of traditional rural society in Bavaria. In the first instance, infant mortality among illegitimate children remained extremely high throughout the period under discussion.[27] For Oberbayern in the period 1815–1869 infant mortality rates for illegitimate children actually rose from 38.9 to 42.0 per 100 live births. On the Massenhausen estate over 50 percent of all illegitimate births in the decades 1800–1809 and 1840–1849 died in the first year of life. To this extent high rates of illegitimate births did not imply in concrete terms a long-term social or economic problem. Secondly it is also clear that pregnancies resulting from nonmarital unions seldom resulted in a change in work pattern. Routine employment was continued almost to the day of birth, and resumed a few hours afterwards.[28]

If no formal sanctions were imposed within the family, a psychological sanction linked with a monetary fine or corporal punishment had been retained by the state throughout the

26 Josef Klemens Stadler, "Die Familienname der unehelichen Kinder in Altbayern," *Zeitschrift für Bayerische Landesgeschichte,* IX (1936), 434.

27 Georg Mayr, "Die Sterblichkeit der Kinder während der ersten Lebensjahre in Süddeutschland insbesonders in Bayern," *Zeitschrift des kgl. Bayerischen Statistischen Bureaus,* II (1870), 210.

28 H. Küstner, *Leitfaden der Berufskrankheiten der Frau* (Stuttgart, 1919), 90. Gottfried Lammert, *Volksmedizin und medizinische Aberglaube in Bayern* (Würzburg, 1869), 103.

eighteenth century. On the basis of Roman Law draconic penalties were imposed on extramarital relationships, as in the Bavarian legislation of 1649, 1660, and 1727. Although the carrying of the so-called "stone of infamy" is only cited once in late eighteenth century criminal codes, public degradation remained a main prop in the legal system of punishment. In the course of the latter decades of the eighteenth century, however, there was a tendency toward criticism of existing punishments, and an easing in the definition of illegitimacy.[29] By mid-century it was accepted that this easing excluded children born up to one month after marriage and to women who had been promised marriage, but had been deserted later by the prospective husband. The Reichtags-Abschied of 1731 allowed illegitimate children who had been later legitimized entry into urban guilds, and the Prussian Edict of 1765 attempted to remove some of the stigma attached by certain sections of society to illegitimacy.

Although legal reforms in Bavaria had initially been discouraged by the fact that 157,000 Gulden had been collected from fines exacted between 1766–1776 and 1784–1794 under the "Law of Levity," the legislation of 1780 did produce an amelioration by substituting a fine for the first offense in place of public degradation. The edict of 1808, however, abolished all monetary fines for pregnancies arising from extramarital relationships. Illegitimate children were also able to enjoy equal rights at baptism. In stark contrast to the punitive laws of the eighteenth century, the Law Book of 1813 included no form of legal punishment for illegitimate births, and by 1827 the traditional degradation pole had disappeared from all cities and markets in Bavaria. The gradual lifting of legal sanctions undoubtedly had a significant impact on peasant attitudes towards illegitimacy. Certainly in Massenhausen and Thalhausen the initial rise in illegitimacy rates in the late eighteenth century is coincidental with the introduction of legal reforms (see Table 5). The priest in Hebertshausen claimed that the failure of the state to designate illegitimate births as infringements of the moral order had led to the acceptance of bastards as part of the way of life. In Wippenhausen one of the main reasons for the decline in morality was that illegitimacy went unpunished

29 Georg Carl von Meyr (ed.), *Sammlung der Churbaierischen Generalien und Landesverordnungen* (Munich, 1773), 111, 116. Wolfram Peitzsch, *Kriminalpolitik in Bayern unter der Geltung des Codex Juris Criminalis Bavarici von 1751* (Munich, 1968), 90 ff.

by the lay authorities.[30] The only way to cure the shamelessness which thereby arose was through the repeal of the lax civil laws and the reintroduction of stiffer church penalties. To the extent that public degradation and heavy monetary fines or corporal punishment did act as a constraint on the actual birth of illegitimate children, then it is arguable that the legal reforms of the late eighteenth and early nineteenth century would have removed an important external sanction.

From a financial point of view the propensity of single individuals to conceive children out of wedlock would also have been stimulated by economic developments in the early nineteenth century. The majority of parents of illegitimate children were normally listed as being in service. This applied, for example, to 70.6 percent of the fathers in Massenhausen and 78.7 percent of the mothers. It is important to note, therefore, that the economic standing of agricultural employees (Gesinde) underwent a definite improvement in the early nineteenth century.

Labor shortages began to be felt in the primary sector from the late eighteenth century onwards. The cumulative implementation of labor-intensive agricultural reforms, without a concomitant rise in labor productivity and in the context of population growth rates well below the European average, meant that the supply situation gradually became acute. In 1809, for example, employment regulations could not be enforced in the Landericht Erding because of acute labor shortages and the competitive bidding-up of wage levels for rural Gesinde to ensure adequate supply. By the end of the eighteenth century peasants with large, integral holdings frequently had to decide whether it was financially more profitable to engage the requisite number of servants to cultivate all available land, or to employ only those necessary to produce a marginal return on investment. Money wages for agricultural servants (both men and women) rose considerably (Table 7). In the Landgericht Tölz, for example, where a "Knecht" had been content with 40-60 Gulden in 1808, he was demanding a year later 60-80 Gulden and getting it.[31]

30 O.A.M. Wippenhausen, Visitation of 1821.
31 Alois Schlögl (ed.), *Bayerische Agrargeschichte* (Munich, 1954), 16–25. Johann Wernicke, *Das Verhältnis zwischen Geborenen und Gestorbenen in historischer Entwicklung und für die Gegenwart in Stadt und Land* (Jena, 1896), 67. St. A.ObB. R.A. 1103/15676. Lorenz von

Table 7   Wage Index for Servants in Gulden (1654–1859)

	OBERKNECHT		MITTELKNECHT		OBERDIRN	
YEAR	WAGE	INDEX	WAGE	INDEX	WAGE	INDEX
1654	15	100	10	100	6	100
1750	24	160	21	210	12	200
1776	26	173	24	240	18	300
1780	30	200	30	300		
1790	18	120	15	150		
1801	54	360				
1830	50	333	35	350	24	400
1859	90	600	60	600	44	722

In real terms, however, the purchasing power of the agricultural servants in the early nineteenth century had risen by an even greater margin. The effect of a series of good harvests in the 1820s on the Bavarian economy was considerable. By 1825 grain prices had fallen fourfold from their 1817 level. Although this had severe effects on grain producers, the serving class benefited from a further increase in relative purchasing power. The long-term extent of this trend was considerable. If the wage of an "Oberknecht" in 1623 had been equivalent to 2 Scheffel of rye, it amounted to 7½ Scheffel in 1792 and 11 Scheffel in 1895. Evidence of their increased financial security was mirrored in contemporary reports. An increased expenditure on clothing was noted in a number of quarters. Official reports from the 1830s continually refer to their indulgence in "luxury." Little attempt was made to save money despite the foundation of regional savings banks and what did remain from consumer expenditure went to support the payment of alimony for illegitimate children. Agricultural servants by the 1820s and the 1830s, as a result of general economic developments, were in a far better position to indulge their own tastes than their predecessors had been, faced, for example, by the economic difficulties of the 1770s.[32] In economic terms the price paid

Westenrieder, *Gedanken über die Bevölkerung und Landeskultur in Baiern* (Munich, 1788), 237. St. A.ObB. R.A. 1103/15677-8.

32   Gustav Heinrich Haumann, *Ueber die zur Zeit in Deutschland herrschende Noth des landwirtschaftlichen Standes* (Ilmenau, 1826). Jürgen Kuczynski, Studien zur Geschichte der zyklischen Ueber-produktionskrisen in Deutschland 1825–1866. *Die Geschichte der Lage der Arbeiter unter dem Kapitalismus* (Berlin, 1961), I/ii. Hanns Platzer, *Geschichte der ländlichen Arbeiterverhältnisse in Bayern* (Munich, 1904), 205. St. A.ObB. R.A. 1123/15704.

for illegitimate children by the 1820s could more easily be afforded.

Once the economic and legal constraints were removed, a further group of supplementary social factors also help to provide a realistic explanation of the high illegitimacy rates in Bavaria.

Although the nuclear family, based on the husband-wife relationship, was predominant, certain elements of matrifocality can be observed in the structural pattern of peasant families. The economic functioning of the family holding often depended on the role of the wife, whose responsibilities included the allocation of available jobs among the family workers. If the work of the man was relatively well-defined and bound by routine, the wife was expected to modify her labor input in step with economic circumstances. Significantly the customary "year of mourning" was seldom observed and a widower was likely to remarry very shortly after the death of the spouse. Although it would be unjustified to take this argument too far, two established patterns of matrifocality—a low rate of legal marriage and high rates of illegitimacy—were phenomena common to Bavaria, and the eighteenth century did indeed witness an increased discussion of female emancipation, signified by the publication in 1780 of von Hippel's book, *On the Civic Improvement of Women*.[33]

A further social factor affecting the propensity towards high illegitimacy rates was that lower-class illegitimacy did not constitute such a problem as similar rates among higher social groups would have done, and therefore was not faced with extensive social disapproval.[34] On Goode's scale, listing fourteen different types of illegitimacy, lower-class illegitimacy has a particularly low ranking. If it is argued that the level of disapproval is positively correlated with the amount of disruption or status discrepancy created, then once tangible constraints had been removed, little would have stood in the way of an increase in illegitimacy in Bavaria.

Finally, it is clear that children, whether legitimate or il-

33 Sidney M. Greenfield, "Industrialization and the Family in Sociological Theory," in Bernard Farber (ed.), *Kinship and Family Organization* (New York, 1966), 414. H. Scharnargl, "Straussdorf, eine sozialökonomische und soziologische Untersuchung einer oberbayerischen Landgemeinde mit starkem Flüchtlingsanteil," unpub. diss. (Erlangen, 1952), appendix, Table 9a. Klaus Epstein, *The Genesis of German Conservatism* (Princeton, 1966), 229.

34 W. J. Goode, *The Family* (New Jersey, 1964), 23.

legitimate, were not regarded as fully integrated members of society. Until the child had developed skills of one form or another his economic usefulness to the family was limited and the level of parental attention, particularly in the early years of life, was minimal. Children were seldom regarded as individuals. In Mittelfels it was stated that farmers would rather lose a child than a calf and parental attitudes noticeably deteriorated after the birth of the fourth or fifth child.[35] This negative pattern of parent-child relationships is also reflected in the stereotyped naming of children and the absence of medical attention in cases of illness. Given this background of general indifference the "principle" of legitimacy would not have been regarded as being of primary importance.

What then remains of the original concept of a "sexual revolution" in the context of Bavarian conditions? If the conception of an illegitimate child was not regarded as an infringement of existing social regulations, other criteria of morality provide no indication of a cataclysmic change equivalent to such a revolution. Cases of adultery in Massenhausen only rose from nine (1750–1799) to thirteen (1800–1849), an increase hardly indicative of a dramatic reorientation in value patterns. Only two cases of rape are listed. Provided that comments on illegitimacy are omitted, a picture of basic moral and sexual conformity emerges and there is little evidence of a substantial decline in traditional standards of behavior.

Even as an isolated phenomenon, however, the dramatic illegitimacy rates of the early nineteenth century may still be taken to indicate that a greater number of young people were engaging in premarital sex than in previous decades. And yet even this aspect of the so-called "sexual revolution" must be placed in doubt. Such an assertion appears strange, given that 60 percent of all existing and past societies examined permitted premarital sexual realtions and that in Western Europe as a whole the general pattern of courtship during the eighteenth century is known to have included premarital sexual intercourse.[36] Significantly the incidence of premarital conceptions is just as high in individual parishes on the Hofmark Massenhausen in the period 1750–1799 as in the first half of the nineteenth century, and it seems unlikely that young people in their twenties, although employed as Gesinde, would have been effectively excluded from participation on their own in-

35 Hazzi, *Statistische Aufschlüsse*, II, 137.
36 W. J. Goode, *The Family*, 21.

itiative. Various possibilities emerge (verification is a different matter), including a greater resort to foetal abortion, infant murder, and contraception. All three forms of family limitation are known to have been practiced with varying frequency in eighteenth century Bavaria.[37] It is therefore possible that the only major difference in sexual behavior between the late eighteenth and early nineteenth centuries lay in the degree to which precautions were taken to avoid unwanted pregnancy. Once the economic and legal constraints on illegitimacy had been removed, there was no reason why illegitimate conceptions should not have been allowed to run their full course.

In all human societies a high value is placed upon fertility. Human beings are socialized from early childhood to marry and beget children. Bavaria was no exception to this rule. However the phenomenon of high illegitimacy rates does pose problems in that the conception of children even in relatively permissive societies is largely limited within existing marital relationships. There can be little doubt that illegitimacy rates did rise in many parts of Europe in the period from 1750 to 1850, and that this development was particularly marked in the Catholic territories of South Germany and Austria. A great deal of groundwork remains to be undertaken before the causative factors behind this phenomenon can be established with any degree of certainty. In Bavaria, if an interconnection is posited as having existed between the economic infrastructure and changes in social and sexual behavior patterns, it is difficult, given the retarded development of a cash economy and secondary sector, to explain the phenomenon in terms of a revolutionary change. Perhaps existing views of normality in relation to preindustrial social codes, emphasizing a state of equilibrium, did not allow for an element of flexibility sufficient to accommodate considerable changes, including high illegitimacy rates, without involving any substantial reorientation in accepted social roles.

The present study does not pretend to formulate a science of moral/social behavior in preindustrial South Germany. At the most it can be said to reveal a form of agrarian society where norms of moral behavior were intrinsically indigenous, restricted

37 William Robert Lee, "Some Economic and Demographic Aspects of Peasant Society in Oberbayern from 1752 to 1855, with special reference to certain Estates in the former Landgericht Kranzberg," unpub. diss. (Oxford, 1972), 72–97.

on the one hand by the general range of experience of the peasantry, and on the other by economic and legal regulators. In relation to the problem of illegitimacy the conflict of official and indigenous role-obligations was resolved in favor of that course of action adopted by the peasants, both in the late eighteenth and early nineteenth centuries. High illegitimacy rates, once the economic and legal sanctions had been lifted, could therefore be fully accommodated on the local level without involving a "sexual revolution."

Journal of Interdisciplinary History, VIII:3 (Winter 1978), 459–469.

Edward Shorter

Bastardy in South Germany: A Comment Lee

has recently argued in these pages that the startling increase in illegitimacy which took place in Bavaria between 1750 and 1850 resulted not from a "sexual revolution" but from an increase in real
wages, which made it easier for people to support children born
out of wedlock.[1] I am certainly sympathetic to his wage arguments, and to much of the logic of the article. But no sexual revolution at all? Not even a touch of saucy rebelliousness, an angry-
young-person-against-the-*Hofbauerntum* syndrome?

His argument partly depends, of course, on what we mean by
a "sexual revolution." If we insist on a dramatic breakaway from
previous sexual styles, on homosexuality, oral intercourse, and the
bondage-and-domination scene, then *d'accord:* no "sexual revolution" in early nineteenth-century Bavaria. But if we take this
mildly sensationalist notion of a "revolution"—which I myself am
partly responsible for foisting upon the trade—to mean the sudden
rejection by a whole generation of young people of their parents'
values towards premarital intercourse, I think that such a revolution *did* occur in Bavaria, and all over Europe, between the middle
of the eighteenth and the middle of the nineteenth centuries.

Here Lee and I differ. He argues that "this illegitimacy did not
imply a dramatic change in behavioral norms. . . . It did not
conflict, in the opinion of the peasantry, either in the late
eighteenth or early nineteenth centuries, with traditional moral
norms" (416). This, I think, is simply wrong.

The mainstay of Lee's case is that the Bavarian peasantry had
always accepted illegitimate children as more or less full-fledged
family members, and that at the village level no one became very
upset about out-of-wedlock conceptions. Illegitimate and legitimate children would inherit alike, work side by side, and enjoy
roughly equal moral status in the local community. Because, according to Lee, this continued to be true in 1850 as well as in 1750,
the great upsurge in bastardy had in no way conflicted with accepted local mores. Hence, no sexual revolution.

Edward Shorter is Associate Professor of History at the University of Toronto.

1 W. R. Lee, "Bastardy and the Socioeconomic Structure of South Germany," *Journal of Interdisciplinary History*, VII (1977), 403–425.

In my view, Lee has confused two types of illegitimacy. He studied Oberbayern, one of Bavaria's seven right-bank-of-the-Rhine provinces. And his Oberbayern peasants, in this large-farm, impartible inheritance region, represent perfectly the first type of illegitimacy: betrothal license, which meant men and women who were firmly engaged to marry and so went ahead and had sex, producing out-of-wedlock children because the ceremony could not take place until the man inherited his father's farm at age 34. In southern Bavaria, Austria, and German Switzerland marriage had always been late, high proportions of the population had always remained single, and illegitimacy had always been substantial compared to other parts of Europe.[2] Because engagements could run as long as a decade, betrothal license within such a context was thoroughly "traditional." Accidents happened, but were not so serious because a secure economic place awaited the infant. Normally the only other unwed mothers were rape victims.[3]

Lee so focused upon this first type that he has missed the second, more "modern" variety of illegitimacy. The point I wish to make is that "modern" illegitimacy was mainly responsible for the great bastardy explosion on which his article concentrates. "Modern" means men and women having sex not within the ac-

2 Although no overall study of this homogenous region exists, numerous local monographs have recently become available. On Switzerland see Silvio Bucher, *Bevölkerung und Wirtschaft des Amtes Entlebuch in 18. Jahrhundert* (Lucerne, 1974); Markus Schürmann, *Bevölkerung, Wirtschaft und Gesellschaft in Appenzell Innerrhoden im 18. und frühen 19. Jahrhundert* (Appenzell, 1974). On the persistence of these features into a more recent period, see John Friedl and Walter S. Ellis, "Celibacy, Late Marriage and Potential Mates in a Swiss Isolate," *Human Biology*, XLVIII (1976), 23–35. On Austria see Klaus Arnold, "Der Umbruch des generativen Verhaltens in einem Bergbauerngebiet," in Heimold Helczmanovszki (ed.), *Beiträge zur Bevölkerungs—und Sozialgeschichte Österreichs* (Vienna, 1973); Franz Fliri, *Bevölkerungsgeographische Untersuchungen im Unterinntal* (Innsbruck, 1948); Gisela Winkler, *Bevölkerungsgeographische Untersuchungen im Martelltal* (Innsbruck, 1973). See also Inge Rohn, "Bevölkerung und Landwirtschaft in Kitzbühel," in Eduard Widmoser, *Stadtbuch Kitzbühel* (Kitzbühel, 1967), I, 197–222, for a demographic analysis which discusses both the town and the surrounding countryside. The most recent work on Bavaria seems to have been done by non-Bavarians: John Knodel, "Two and a Half Centuries of Demographic History in a Bavarian Village," *Population Studies*, XXIV (1970), 353–376; Jacques Houdaille, "Quelques résultats sur la démographie de trois villages d'Allemagne de 1750 à 1879," *Population*, XXV (1970), 649–654. (One of the three villages, Kreuth, is in Bavaria.)

3 Jacques Rossiaud's important article, "Prostitution, jeunesse et société au XVe siècle," *Annales:ESC*, XXXI (1976), 289–325, makes clear how often out-of-wedlock pregnancy in the premodern era was the result of rape. A good discussion of "traditional" illegitimacy in Upper Bavaria may be found in Hanns Platzer, *Geschichte der ländlichen Arbeitsverhältnisse in Bayern* (Munich, 1904), 186–193.

cepted context of delayed inheritance but within the context of wage labor. In the "modern" form young people have no prospects of a decent settlement, no hope of gaining an established situation as large-peasants or master craftsmen in the local community, but they go ahead and have sex anyway. The revolutionary element here is that before 1760 or so the journeymen craftsmen, agricultural laborers, and live-in hired hands who later produced the illegitimacy boom seem to have stayed continent until marriage, or at least if not, the women did not get pregnant.[4]

After 1760 or so these numerous subpeasant groups started to change their minds about waiting chastely for a marriage that might never take place. They began sexual relations in their early-to-mid-twenties—to go by statistics on the mother's age at the first illegitimate birth.[5] And because they did not practice birth control (married couples did not, at least), a tremendous increase in illegitimacy eventuated.

Contrary to Lee's theory, this boom in bastardy among the propertyless evoked loud complaints from the village elders. In no way was it accepted as "normal" by the established community, and the infants born to these furtive unions underwent fates much worse than those of their legitimate counterparts. I would therefore argue that two forms of bastardy nestled side by side in Bavaria: the "traditional," premarital births of the *Hofmark* (large farms in Oberbayern) which continued over the years at a relatively stable level, and the explosively growing *Concubinate* and *Winkelehen* (backstairs coupling) of the propertyless.

Various evidence indicates that bastardy increased most rapidly among the propertyless. Phayer, for example, who studied the illegitimacy boom in the parish of Dietramszell, which is not far from Lee's Kranzberg, found that "all illegitimate births occurred to members of the better-off working class [*gehobene Unterschicht*] and the lower class [*untere Klasse*]." The illegitimacy ratio (number of illegitimate births as a percent of all births)

4 I have elsewhere rehearsed the justification for concluding that this particular rise in illegitimacy was caused by a rise in premarital intercourse, and not—as Lee suggests—by an increase in fecundity or a decrease in abortions. See Shorter, *The Making of the Modern Family* (New York, 1975), ch. 3.

5 The Oberpfalz government, for example, reported in 1863 that "on the basis of statistical . . . surveys, illegitimate births occur on the average at the age of 24." Bavarian Hauptstaatsarchiv in Munich, Ministerium des Innern (MI) 52139, 20 June, 1863, report to Interior Ministry.

among the former was 20 percent, among the latter 28 percent. "In every instance the people involved were the young, unmarried sons and daughters of little shopkeepers, shoeing smiths, weavers, and the like."[6] Phayer concludes that by 1817 "a new orientation predominated among the rural populace," leading to sexual behavior that would have been unthinkable in the old regime.

A second way to confirm this hypothesis is to observe the social profile of illegitimacy in a more systematic way—across Bavaria as a whole. The census of 1840 lets us correlate the number of illegitimate children alive in that year (measured as a percent of all children under 14) with various other variables indicating property ownership and social status. The following table shows some of the correlations:

Table 1   Correlations Between the Number of Illegitimate Children as a Percent of all Children in the Rural Counties of Bavaria in 1840 and the Percentage of:

	CORRELATION COEFFICIENT PEARSONIAN r:
Married couples	$-.50$
Unwed couples cohabiting	.15
Agriculture sole occupation	$-.23$
Day laborers	.40
Farm servants	.33
Propertyless craftsmen	.13
Artisanal workers	.19
Paupers	Not significant
"Lower classes"[1]	.44

1 The following groups were counted as "lower class": cottagers, day laborers, domestic farmhands and servants, propertyless independent craftsmen, artisanal workers, and servants of professional people. Paupers were excluded.
SOURCE: *Beiträge zur Statistik des Königreichs Bayern,* I (1850), 30–113.
Included in the "rural" areas are a number of small towns. Data for the larger cities, however, were given separately by the census.

It is clear, then, that by 1840 illegitimacy in Bavaria as a whole was closely associated with the presence of a large lower-class population of rural craftworkers, agricultural servants, and laborers. An *inverse* association exists between illegitimacy and

6 Fintan Michael Phayer, *Religion und das Gewöhnliche Volk in Bayern in der Zeit von 1750–1850* (Munich, 1970), 98.

large-holding peasants—people with enough land to avoid having to take on supplementary work and who had been the main group associated with bastardy in the preexplosion period.

Another indication that illegitimacy was interwoven in the lives of the landless lower classes is that a goodly number of contemporary observers *said* that it was. As the Bishop of Regensburg complained in 1839, "Yet scarcely forty to fifty years ago only one or two illegitimate children were to be found in a community. . . . Now there are communes, especially around the patrimonial iron foundries [*Hammer- und Fabrikgüter*] in which one encounters 45–50 and still more illegitimate children."[7] Such laments could be pulled by the dozen from the austere administrative correspondence of the early nineteenth century. The entire corpus of social commentary in the years before 1848 hammers away at the point that illegitimacy was coterminous with misery.[8] It happened among the marginal people who were trapped on the fringes of the social order. The following list of unmarried mothers apparently living alone in 1836 in the village of Neudrossenfeld highlights precisely that group most typical of the world of bastardy:

— Agnes Kummerer, age 36, 3 children, no property, "is not able to support herself."
— A group of five people, all with different family names, two children, living in the same house, "these families live in the most needy condition and the commune must pay the school fees for the children."
— Katharina Ebert, age 53, one child, occupation spinning, no property, lives in rented room.
— Magdalene Kufner, age 44, two children, occupation knitting, no property, "is totally impoverished and the commune must pay 3 gulden, 12 kreuzer school fees for the two children."
— Three women named Hofmann, ages 26, 40, and 48, three children, occupation spinning and knitting, no property, "support themselves scantily, whereby the commune must pay the school fees for the children."

7 MI 46556, 25 April, 1839, communication to Interior Ministry.
8 See Shorter "Social Change and Social Policy in Bavaria, 1800–1860," unpub. Ph.D. diss. (Harvard University, 1968).

— Margarethe Geierin, age 36, two children, no property, occupation "Vagabunda," must be completely supported by the commune.[9]

These wretched, trapped women were leagues removed from the solid peasantry that Lee describes, tolerant of bastardy as a normal part of the social order.

It is possible that these thousands of unfortunates really were accepted at the village level, regardless of what the Bishop of Regensburg and the government bureaucrats thought. If Lee is correct, it is to the villagers themselves, not the nation's social authorities, that we must go. And here opinion is mixed. I have encountered a considerable amount of testimony to the effect that many villagers considered bastardy no great offense. Joseph Hazzi, for example, a government bureaucrat on tour of Oberbayern around 1800, observed of the population of Marquartstein County: "They are eager to marry early and produce many children, among them so many illegitimate that it is considered not so much a sin as a good deed."[10] The provincial government of Unterfranken argued in 1839 that "among the rural population, especially among the so-called middle class [Mittelstande] . . . the view has gained predominance that the natural satisfaction of the sex drive is no longer forbidden by the police and morally not terribly sinful either."[11] Judge Puchta of Erlangen County had grown so accustomed to the idea of out–of–wedlock pregnancy among his clientele that in notarizing marriage contracts he would normally ask whether illegitimate children were present.[12] Yet these were middle-class officials looking from the outside in; to them illegitimacy doubtlessly seemed acceptable because so much of it was occurring.

When we let the village fathers themselves speak, a fearful, condemnatory vision of bastardy emerges which is as different from Lee's picture of indifferent acceptance as night is from day. Many "little people" had an opportunity to express their views on the root causes of poverty in the social order when, in 1848, King Max ordered an essay contest to be held on that subject. The bun-

9   MI 53272, excerpt from report of 3 Nov., 1836. The implication of the report is that these women were unmarried.

10   Statistische Aufschlüsse über das Herzogthum Baiern (Nürnberg, 1801), III, 657.

11   MI 46556, 30 Feb., 1839, report to Interior Ministry.

12   MI 46556, 22 Feb., 1837, report from Mittelfranken government to Interior Ministry.

dles of responses are packed with illiterate, semilegible missives from what appear to be ordinary villagers. Jacob Giel, a schoolteacher in Mörlbach bei Uffenheim, described how illegitimacy happened: "Some fellow from village X buys a little house in village Z. His fiancée has a little money too, and like the man has also been for a long time in service, having now several illegitimate children." But the village administration, for complicated reasons, denied the couple permission to marry. "So their fortune runs out. They sell the dwelling again, with a loss. They produce another batch of illegitimate children. The man tries to forget his woes for a few minutes with drink. A few more years in service flow by and you have—a proletarian. No! Four or five proletarians now!"[13]

Michael Genssperger, a cottager (*Söldner*) from Ottering in Dingolfing County, had a less enlightened analysis: "As for the maintenance of illegitimate children, a very irksome matter for communities, the trouble would be easily alleviated if the father had to pay a 7 gulden penalty into the community chest and the mother were punished with open humiliation or monetary fines, as used to happen, because now the illegitimate children have become far too many, and often some light-headed young thing [*liederliche Dirne*] will have given birth to 6, 8 and 10 and still more children, heeding no warnings, not even of the clergy . . . ."[14]

What so many respondents wanted was a return to the old regime, when the village as a whole could deal ruthlessly with out-of-wedlock conception, humiliating the "whores," as one writer put it, "making them wear a blue sign for ridicule," keeping the premarital fornicators away from the maypole dances, having the local seigneur "give speeches in praise of the virtuous maidens while mocking the scoundrels and whores [*Schelmen* and *Huren*], who crept away for shame." But after 1806, when such fornication penalties were made illegal, things became different, the writer continued, "and now it's the *Schelmen* and *Huren* who are the dancing masters."[15]

In these bundles of scratched-off briefs, any hint of the "full accommodation of high illegitimacy rates on the local level" of which Lee speaks is difficult to discern (425). For these village es-

13 Hauptstaatsarchiv, Ministerium des Handels (MH) 9616, no. 491, Jan., 1849.
14 MH 9612, no. 22, n.d.
15 Letter from Johann Fink, "Bauer," in Weissenbrunn, Altdorf County, 27 Jan., 1849.

sayists, burning with fire and brimstone, bastardy was anything but a matter of "social indifference."

What happened in reality was the bifurcation of these little communities over sexual morality. Within them a sizable portion of established opinion clung to the traditional peasant notion that premarital sex was bad unless the couple could count on inheriting a farm or craftshop. Yet a growing "subculture," composed precisely of the propertyless young men and women whose sexual drives had previously been so brutally repressed, were challenging this "charter culture" view of no-sex-unless-you-have-an-establishment and proceeding to seize the options for sexuality and "happiness" that an increasingly romanticized, individualized, popular culture was holding out. That all this premarital sex might end in later wretchedness of the Neudrossenfeld variety was doubtlessly obscure to them.

Joseph Walther, a retired schoolteacher in Saal (Königshofen County), made clear how deeply this cultural rift over sexual matters divided so many villages and small towns. "A community of 94 families elects its reeve every three years," he wrote. "And each time the question comes up: should we choose someone who's strict about morality and order, who puts limits on abuses and fooling around [Ausschweifungen], and who conscientiously enforces the laws of the land? Twenty-eight would desire this fervently, but sixty-six are horrified by it, and elect one of their own. Then for entire nights the village bars are full of drinkers and the streets full of night-time roamers [Streuner], the houses full of shameless and seduced daughters . . . the villages full of illegitimate children." And what can the government do about it? asked Walther rhetorically. "Whoever wants to be re-elected has to look the other way."[16]

Lee's final argument is that, not only at the level of the village but in the family itself, illegitimate children enjoyed equal status with legitimate children. That they could inherit property and otherwise participate in family life is, according to him, one of the signs of a "matrifocal" family system. Leaving aside for the moment the question of whether Bavaria was in fact a "matrifocal" society, let us see if the assertion is true that Bavarians were "generally indifferent to the principle of legitimacy" because parents

16 MH 9614, no. 231, 16 Jan., 1849.

treated both legitimate and illegitimate alike. Lee's view is that both were treated equally *badly,* in a culture where "children were seldom regarded as individuals" (423). My view would be that, however poor the quality of marital "mothering," that of non-marital was considerably worse, reflecting a fundamental inequality in the situation of the illegitimate.

For one thing, relatively few bastards were absorbed into the circle of family life, to go by statistics on legitimation. Only about a fifth of the illegitimate babies ever ended up legitimated, 15 percent from 1835 to 1859, 20 percent from 1882 to 1884.[17] Because many of these children died before legitimation could take place, the real percentage of survivors who found themselves legitimated is probably more like a third.[18] An additional fraction of bastards doubtlessly lived in a family situation, although unlegitimated by their unmarried parents, if we may go by the sudden spurt in legitimation which took place in the mid-1860s as Bavaria's marriage legislation became liberalized.[19] But the main fact remains that, far from being a "functional" or "accepted" part of rural society, a majority of bastards remained unlegitimated social outcasts.

And they were treated as outcasts, being, for example, breastfed less often. "The highest mortality of the illegitimate Bavarian children in 1871–74 falls not in the first month of life but in the second and third, a result of the fact that already in these months the breastfeeding of the children has been terminated, and the injuriousness of worse treatment is making itself apparent."[20]

Although Lee argues that both kinds of children received equally poor treatment, in fact illegitimate infants perished considerably more frequently than legitimate ones. This discrimination started with the birth process: whereas over the years from 1835 to 1859 only 3.0 percent of legitimate infants were stillborn, 3.7 per-

17 *Beiträge zur Statistik des Königreichs Bayern,* XI (1863), 87; Friedrich Lindner, *Die unehelichen Geburten als Sozialphänomen: Ein Beitrag zur Statistik der Bevölkerungsbewegung im Königreich Bayern* (Leipzig, 1900), 188.

18 *Generalien-Sammlung der Erzdiozese München und Freising. Die oberhirtlichen Verordnungen und allgemeinen Erlässe von 1821 bis 1846,* (Munich, 1856), II, 411, an estimate of Munich's episcopal chancellery.

19 The percent legitimated rose from 15 in 1862 to 22 by 1868. Josef Kaizl, *Der Kampf um Gewerbereform un Gewerbefreiheit in Bayern von 1799 bis 1868* (Leipzig, 1879), 159.

20 L. Pfeiffer, "Die Kindersterblichkeit," in A. Jacobi *et al.* (eds.), *Hygiene des Kindesalters* (Tübingen, 1882; 2nd ed.), I, 287, 327.

cent of the illegitimate were. And in Unterfranken the figures were 2.6 percent for legitimate, 3.7 percent for illegitimate. Many more bastards died in the first year of life: 31 percent of the legitimate (in itself, a horrifying rate), and 37 percent of the illegitimate in the kingdom as a whole over the period from 1835 to 1859. Childbearing in general meant a slaughter of the innocents among these Bavarians, but with the illegitimate babies mortality had an expressly cruel edge.[21]

The surrounding community made even less tolerable the hostile start which illegitimate infants received in life. Although the Catholic Church officially deplored the practice, individual priests would often refuse to baptize bastards, because the local parish would not want to take responsibility for the infants' subsequent poor relief should their parents fall destitute. So, for example, the priest in Grunthal (Wasserburg County) denied baptism to the newborn child of Barbara Gogg, a laborer's unmarried daughter who had been in service locally. Gogg was obliged to carry the child "three hours' distance" to Mühldorf for baptism. In a similar case a Fraham mother had to carry her child to Rottenkirchen for baptism, seeing it then die on the trek home.[22]

Most illegitimate children, unlike those Lee studied in Kranzberg County, grew up poor, usually unwanted, and were prone to commit petty crimes and violent acts.[23] "If a single woman has several children, it is difficult for her to find work, and the community can only support her with alms or let her subsist on minor theft from the fields and woods [Flur-und Waldfrevel], or place her children in foster homes at its cost. The sort of upbringing the children receive in the former case is only too well known: they grow up without any fatherly discipline, and so does it happen that the girls soon follow the footsteps of their mother."[24] Illegitimate dynasties arose in this way, such as that started around 1800 in the village of Neunkirchen when an unwed mother gave birth to a son who, immediately after reaching puberty, himself

21 *Beiträge zur Statistik des Königreichs Bayern,* XI (1863), 91, 96, 97.
22 These examples are from Ordinariatsarchiv Munich, Pfarr-Matrikel, 1749–1845, letter from Magistrat Mühldorf of 1 March 1844. I am grateful to Phayer for this reference.
23 For a typical description, see the letter from the local cleric in Haag to the Oberfranken government, 12 Feb., 1834, in Kreisarchiv Bamberg K3 718.
24 MI 52137, 23 June, 1853.

impregnated two women. He had learned the weaver's trade but never settled down to regular work, earning his way instead as a sometime pack-peddlar. He went on to sire three illegitimate children with a third woman, and after she died he produced yet another by a fourth woman, who already had one bastard child herself. At the time of the report, this woman was pregnant again, she and her husband living from "deception and petty theft."[25]

Here we have the core of the illegitimacy explosion, a mushrooming lower-class population that existed from wage work and hovered on the threshold of vagrancy. Family ties were unstable and uncertain; the offspring were rejected by the established social order, and their origins were judged a blatant affront to all the values of prudence and economic security which traditional peasant society represented. It is these people, not that minority of farmers' sons born out of wedlock under betrothal license, who were behind the stunning increase of illegitimacy in Oberbayern—Lee's chosen ground—from 4 percent in 1760, to 18 percent in 1825, to 28 percent in 1860.[26]

Did this great rise in bastardy involve a "sexual revolution"? If the sexual activation of an entire generation of single, lower-class young people in the space of thirty years, the passage of tens of thousands of servants and laborers from chastity to nonvirginity, can be judged a sexual revolution, I would say that Bavaria had one. Why, exactly, remains unclear.

25   MI 46556, 3 April, 1838, Archbishop of Bamberg to Munich.
26   Data on the period 1760 to 1825 from Phayer's compilation of statistics in the manuscript Pfarrmatrikel at the Ordinariatsarchiv in Munich. The 1860 ratio is from Lindner, *Uneheliche Geburten,* 218.

Journal of Interdisciplinary History, VIII:3 (Winter 1978), 471–476.

W. R. Lee

Bastardy in South Germany: A Reply

Shorter, although accepting a great deal of the arguments presented in my original article, bases his rejoinder almost entirely on the assumption that two distinct types of bastardy coexisted in Bavaria (and by implication in most other areas affected by the "sexual revolution"). On the one hand there existed a "traditional" type of bastardy, associated with large farms (not necessarily the seigneurial estates, or *Hofmarken*), linked with existing patterns of inheritance and remaining essentially stable throughout this period. On the other hand there emerged increasingly a "modern" form of illegitimacy in the early nineteenth century associated with a radical change of attitudes on the part of the "propertyless" and the poorer sections of the community, which accounts entirely for the illegitimacy explosion. This final defensive position, however, can also be broached at a number of different points and its general assumptions placed in considerable doubt.

In the first instance, although not seeking to deny entirely the tangible repercussions of a betrothal license both in the late eighteenth and early nineteenth centuries, it would be rather incautious to attribute all cases of illegitimate conceptions in the pre-explosion period to the operation of this tacitly accepted indigenous custom. A surprisingly high proportion of illegitimacy in the period 1750 to 1799 was a result of multiple illegitimate births (children born to a single woman from a number of different illicit unions). In the seven parishes within the Massenhausen estate, 30.3 percent of illegitimate conceptions in the late eighteenth century fell into this nontraditional category, which cannot be positively related to the structural pattern of inheritance customs.

An equal element of caution is required before accepting any simplistic variation in the social pattern of illegitimacy between the pre- and post-explosion periods. Statistical evidence would seem to place in question the assumption of any radical difference in the social background of those women most prone to conceive illegitimate offspring during this crucial period (see Table 1). Although there was indeed a proportional decline in illegitimate conceptions associated with unmarried women from large integral

W. R. Lee is Lecturer in the Department of Economic History, University of Liverpool.

holdings, there was a substantial increase in this category from one-fourth and to a lesser extent one-half holdings, which can also normally be regarded as representing the better endowed sections of rural society. Significantly there was no drastic rise in the proportional level of illegitimacy from the small-holdings ($\frac{1}{16}$), and this type of distribution was almost identical in the case of the putative fathers of illegitimate children (see Table 2). Indeed on the Massenhausen estate the proportional representation of the "poorer" elements only rose from 54.34 percent (1750–1799) to 57.73 percent (1800–1850). There small-holdings in any case constituted 57.08 percent of total established holdings. On this basis, therefore, the overall distribution pattern of illegitimacy according to social class did not undergo any radical transition as a result of the illegitimacy explosion, but was subject to an interesting shift in emphasis between the different peasant groups that are traditionally placed in the upper regions of the rural social ladder.

Table 1   Social Distribution of Mothers of Illegitimate Children, according to Size of Parental Holding: Hofmark Massenhausen, 1750–1850

	HOLDING SIZE				
	I	$\frac{1}{2}$	$\frac{1}{4}$	$\frac{1}{8}$	$\frac{1}{16}$
Cases (1750–1799)	25	13	5	7	33
% (1750–1799)	30.1	15.6	6.0	8.4	39.7
Cases (1800–1849)	59	53	42	26	145
% (1800–1849)	18.1	16.1	12.9	8.0	44.6

Thirdly, if Shorter's hypothesis is to be credited with any general applicability, it would be expected that the "inheritance" element within illegitimacy as a whole would gradually be submerged during the course of the later illegitimacy explosion. If one examines the comparative incidence of premarital conceptions as a general index for the posited "traditional" component in total illegitimacy, however, this would not appear to be the case. Premarital conceptions, preceding the inheritance of holdings, whether connected entirely with the primary sector or attached to domestic industry, more than doubled in number between the late eighteenth and early nineteenth centuries, evincing a trend completely at variance with the posited hypothesis.

On the basis of these three particular facets of the pattern of illegitimacy in Bavaria, therefore, the postulated variance between the "traditional" and "modern" forms of illegitimacy can be put in some considerable doubt. Indeed such a conclusion would once again emphasize the paramount importance of placing any analysis of social patterns of behavior within the context of the underlying economic conditions. This prerequisite, however, is something that has often been ignored in the attempt to formulate general models of social change during this particular period. If the arguments in relation to the social pattern of illegitimacy are accepted, very little remains of the other ancillary defensive positions adopted by Shorter in this debate. Bavaria, in any case, was not an area of large farms. By the mid-nineteenth century average land endowment per family varied from 9.3 hectare (Upper Bavaria) to 7.9 hectare (in the Palatinate).[1]

Table 2   Social Distribution of Fathers of Illegitimate Children, according to Size of Parental Holding: Hofmark Massenhausen, 1750–1850

	HOLDING SIZE				
	I	½	¼	⅛	1/16
Cases (1750–1799)	10	4	3	4	25
% (1750–1799)	21.74	8.69	6.54	8.69	54.34
Cases (1800–1849)	23	22	26	11	112
% (1800–1849)	11.85	11.33	13.40	5.69	57.73

The process of proto-industrialization, or the "territorialisation of craft production," in the course of the late eighteenth century had in any case produced a situation in Bavaria where smallholdings even in the preexplosion period were already in a distinct majority.[2] Furthermore, the process of secularization and the subdivision of holdings in the course of the early decades of the

1   Heinrich von Haag, *Kurze Beschreibung der landwirtschaftlichen Verhältnissen in Bayern* (Munich, 1890), 10.
2   Pankraz Fried, "Historisch-statistische Beiträge zur Geschichte des Kleinbauerntums (Söldnertums) im westlichen Oberbayern," *Mitteilungen der Geographischen Gesellschaft in München*, II (1966), 19; Eckart Schremmer, "Standortausweitung der Warenproduktion im langfristigen Wirtschaftswachstum. Zur Stadt-Land-Arbeitsteilung im Gewerbe im 18. Jahrhundert," *Vierteljahrschrift für Sozial und Wirtschaftsgeschichte*, LIX (1972), 1–40.

nineteenth century contributed to a significant reinforcement of the economic position of the poorer sections of rural society. In Massenhausen, for example, 52.7 percent of all land subject to subdivision prior to 1848 went to smallholders (⅟₁₆).[3] It was precisely the broad group of "shoeing smiths, weavers," and agricultural laborers, supposedly responsible for the illegitimacy explosion, which benefited from a process of land redistribution that significantly altered their social position. Indeed, if illegitimacy during the early decades of the nineteenth century was associated with the lower class, why does the census material of 1840 produce such low levels of correlation in relation to "propertyless craftsmen," "artisanal workers," and in particular "paupers," of whom there was a substantial and growing number in early nineteenth-century Bavaria?

Equally the evidence produced to show that illegitimacy by the mid-nineteenth century was not acceptable to the majority of the rural population is once again open to criticism. The so-called "little people" who contributed to the prize essay of 1848, particularly in a society which remained largely illiterate,[4] were far more likely to be representatives of a minority view than reliable exponents of broad underlying social attitudes. Certainly the evidence of schoolmasters in this context should be viewed with some reservation, as they, together with the clergy, who of course were traditionally opposed to the maintenance of indigenous moral codes by the peasantry (including the acceptance of illegitimacy), belonged effectively to an isolated and literate minority. Indeed some of the evidence presented only serves to reinforce the original contention that illegitimacy was openly accepted by the peasantry as a whole and did not conflict with their indigenous code of morality. Both in Saal and Massenhausen the majority of the rural population was not in any sense motivated to institute restrictions on existing behavioral norms, whether they related to local dances, fashionable clothing, licensing hours, or illegitimate conceptions. Further evidence of the degree to which illegitimacy was accepted by rural society in general in Bavaria is furnished by the fact that the number of legal settlements involving illegitimate

---

3 William Robert Lee, "Some Economic and Demographic Aspects of Peasant Society in Oberbayern from 1752 to 1855, with Special Reference to Certain Estates in the Former Landgericht Kranzberg," unpub. D. Phil. diss. (Oxford, 1972), 196.

4 Jakob Sendtner, *Ueber Lehre und Zucht in den Schulen* (Munich, 1826), 18.

offspring rose dramatically during this period; in the case of the Hofmark Thalhausen, for example, from 1 (1790–1799) to 17 (1840–1849). A typical example can be seen in the terms of the marriage Protokoll of 1833 relating to a small-holding in Thalhausen. In the case of the future death of the bride, her three illegitimate children from another relationship were to be accorded the same legal rights as any legitimate issue.[5] German law in any case had traditionally viewed illegitimacy in a relatively favorable light that did not necessarily involve a loss either of social standing or of legal rights.[6] To this extent the rise in illegitimacy rates cannot be viewed as constituting a radical change in rural attitudes or the emergence of a "saucy rebelliousness" on the part of Bavarian peasants.

The traditional hypothesis is essentially far too simplistic. In terms of its conceptual base, its diagnostic assessment of social phenomena, and its attempted explanation of the causal factors behind the rise in illegitimacy rates, fundamental weaknesses are apparent. Indeed, it is significant that Shorter is now prepared to concede that his earlier attempts to explain the so-called "sexual revolution," at least in the context of the Bavarian evidence, can no longer be supported. They offer very little insight into the process of role accumulation and behavioral norms as far as the indigenous rural population was concerned. But the attempt to rehabilitate the general concept of the so-called "sexual revolution" would also seem to have failed, precisely because the initial hypothesis was based largely on secondary evidence that failed to penetrate the precise economic and social aspects of illegitimacy, either before the rise in overall illegitimacy in the late eighteenth century or during the early decades of the nineteenth century. What has now been put forward as an explanation of the illegitimacy phenomenon seeks essentially to reconcile the economic data with the observed patterns of social behavior.

In a society where illegitimacy did not infringe upon the indigenous moral codes of rural groups and where the treatment of bastards did not vary significantly from that accorded to legitimate offspring (either in legal terms or in relation to parental care and attention), the significant increase in illegitimacy during the early

5   Staatsarchiv für Oberbayern, Hofmark Thalhausen, 10.
6   Richard Schröder, *Lehrbuch der deutschen Rechtsgeschichte* (1922), 44.

decades of the nineteenth century can be seen essentially to reflect changes in the underlying pattern of peasant society. As a result the increase in illegitimacy could be accommodated within the existing social structure without leading to undue social tension. If there were a bifurcation of views, it was simply a reflection of the degree to which the class structure in preindustrial South Germany fostered an adverse reaction to this phenomenon on the part of the nonindigenous elements in rural society—in particular the Church, certain sections of government, and members of the minority literate community. For peasant society as a whole, high rates of illegitimacy did not constitute to any degree a "sexual revolution" but simply reflected behavioral norms acceptable to the majority of Bavarian peasants during this critical period.

Journal of Interdisciplinary History, VIII:4 (Spring 1978), 627–667.

Cissie Fairchilds

Female Sexual Attitudes and the Rise of Illegitimacy: A Case Study

One of the most puzzling aspects of European demographic history is the apparent rise in illegitimacy in the late eighteenth and early nineteenth centuries. Illegitimate births formed only a miniscule number of the total registered births before 1750; in France the figure is on the order of 1 or 2 percent. But by the end of the eighteenth century an illegitimacy ratio of 5 percent is common, and by the middle of the nineteenth, levels of 10 and 20 percent are the norm, and some are even higher.[1] It is estimated, for example, that fully one third of all the children born in Paris in the years between 1815 and 1848 were born to unwed mothers.[2]

Recently an interesting and provocative attempt to explain this phenomenon has been made by Shorter. In a series of articles and in his book, *The Making of the Modern Family*, Shorter ties the rise in illegitimacy to a change in the attitudes toward sex of lower-class women, a change so great as to amount to a "sexual revolution."[3] Writing very much within the framework of mod-

Cissie Fairchilds is Associate Professor of History at Syracuse University and author of *Poverty and Charity in Aix-en-Provence, 1640–1789* (Baltimore, 1976).

Funds for the research for this article were provided by a University of California Regent's Summer Fellowship for Junior Faculty. An earlier version was presented at the Third Berkshire Conference on Women's History at Bryn Mawr College, 1976. The author wishes to thank the following people for their helpful suggestions for revision: Thomas Dublin, Carolyn Lougee, David Ringrose, Robert Ritchie, Carole Shammas, and Barbara Shapiro.

1 For illegitimacy ratios see Peter Laslett, *The World We Have Lost* (New York, 1970; 2nd ed.), 142; Daniel Scott Smith and Michael S. Hindus, "Premarital Pregnancy in America, 1640–1971: An Overview and Interpretation," *Journal of Interdisciplinary History*, IV (1974), 566–567; Jean-Louis Flandrin, *Familles: parenté, maison, sexualité dans l'ancien société* (Paris, 1976), 176–184; Wesley D. Camp, *Marriage and the Family in France Since the Revolution* (New York, 1961), 108.

2 Louis Chevalier, *Labouring Classes and Dangerous Classes* (New York, 1973), 311.

3 Edward Shorter, "Illegitimacy, Sexual Revolution, and Social Change in Modern Europe," *Journal of Interdisciplinary History*, II (1971), 237–272; "Capitalism, Culture and Sexuality: Some Competing Models," *Social Science Quarterly*, LIII (1972), 338–356; "Sexual Change and Illegitimacy: The European Experience," in Robert J. Bezucha (ed.), *Modern European Social History* (Lexington, Mass., 1972), 231–269; "Female Emancipation, Birth Control, and Fertility in European History," *American Historical Review*, LXXVIII (1973), 605–640; "Differences de classe et sentiment depuis 1750: l'exemple de la France," *Annales: E.S.C.*, XXIX (1974), 1034–1057; *The Making of the Modern Family* (New York,

ernization theory, Shorter ties his attitudinal change to the urbanization and economic modernization that Europe experienced in the late eighteenth and early nineteenth centuries. Shorter asserts that as the economy modernized, more and more women sought employment in urban areas. As they left their rural communities to move to the cities, they also left behind traditional values that stressed that premarital sex was wrong, and the parents and neighbors who could enforce such values. Once in the urban workforce, women found the economic independence that helped complete their emancipation. They also found the values of the market place, emphasizing personal autonomy and self-gratification, and began to search for self-fulfillment, which, Shorter says, they found in illicit sexual encounters. Hence the rise in illegitimacy.[4]

Shorter's hypothesis of a sexual revolution has recently been challenged by Tilly, Scott, and Cohen.[5] They begin by bringing together a mass of evidence to question Shorter's notion of the emancipating effect of women's work. Women's work, they say, even during industrialization, was performed within the context of the family economy, and therefore did not necessarily emancipate women from the control of either their families or traditional values. Hence they argue that there is no evidence that women's attitudes toward sex changed significantly in this period. The only evidence Shorter has of changing sexual attitudes is, they say, the rise in illegitimacy itself, and this, they maintain, can be adequately explained as a product of the persistence of traditional sexual attitudes in the changing economic context of urbanization and modernization. Scott, Tilly, and Cohen suggest that women had traditionally entered illicit relationships largely

1975). It should be noted that Shorter's interpretation has evolved considerably over time, becoming less qualified and more dogmatic with each succeeding work. My exposition of his argument is drawn mainly from the last three articles cited above, in which his ideas about illegitimacy are most fully developed.

4 Recently (in his article in the *Annales* and in his book) Shorter has expanded his notion of a sexual revolution to encompass not only the rise in illegitimacy but also changes in lower-class marriage patterns. Shorter suggests that the new female values encouraged marriages for love rather than for prudential considerations, and maintains that women's increased thirst for sexual fulfillment pushed up the fertility rate of lower-class marriages in the nineteenth century.

5 Louise A. Tilly, Joan W. Scott, and Miriam Cohen, "Women's Work and European Fertility Patterns," *Journal of Interdisciplinary History*, VI (1976), 447–476. See also Tilly and Scott, "Women's Work in Nineteenth Century Europe," *Comparative Studies in Society and History*, XVII (1975), 55–58.

in the hope of snaring a husband and founding a family economy of their own. But they were less likely to be successful in the quest in the nineteenth century, when increased geographical and occupational mobility allowed men more easily to abandon the women they had seduced. Thus, they argue, it was not a change in women's attitudes toward sex that produced the rise in illegitimacies; instead they rose because women acted according to traditional attitudes in the altered circumstances of economic modernization.[6]

Thus there are at present two diametrically opposed interpretations of the rise in illegitimacy, one that attributes it to changes in women's attitudes toward sex and one that ties it to the persistence of traditional sexual attitudes in changing economic circumstances. It is noteworthy that both interpretations turn on the question of the sexual attitudes of lower-class women, yet both present little solid evidence about what these attitudes actually were. Almost the only evidence Shorter cites to prove the existence of his "sexual revolution" is the horrified comments of middle-class observers about the immorality of the lower classes, but such comments prove little, for throughout history elite groups have been horrified by the behavior of their social inferiors.[7] Tilly, Scott, and Cohen do somewhat better in this regard, for they try to bring together evidence from secondary sources that shows how women might have illegitimate children without having indulged in especially promiscuous behavior. But basically both interpretations tend to begin with the question of the nature of women's work, and proceed to deduce from this what sexual attitudes *must have been*. It is this that makes the debate frustrating for the historian interested in female sexual attitudes. The debate has raised many important questions, not only about the increase in illegitimacy but also about women's sexual behavior in general, but it has not gone very far in actually answering them.

Ideally suited for the task of exploring the sexual attitudes of the women who contributed to the rise in illegitimacy are the

6   As for the remainder of Shorter's sexual revolution, Scott, Tilly, and Cohen maintain that it too was largely a product of changing economic circumstances. Romantic marriage arose when economic modernization made property arrangements dependent on marriage outmoded. The birth rate increased when economic circumstances encouraged earlier marriage and larger families.

7   This was pointed out by Christopher Lasch in his fine review of Shorter's book in *The New York Review of Books* (December 11, 1975), 51–52.

déclarations de grossessen statements required by French law of women about to give birth to illegitimate children, detailing when, where, and under what circumstances they became pregnant.[8] *Déclarations* were usually, although not inevitably, taken in the seventh or eighth month of pregnancy by hospital administrators, judges in the local courts, or the mayor and consuls of peasant villages. These officials tried to find out the following information: the name, age, birthplace, residence, and (occasionally) occupation of the unwed mother; the name and social status of her father; and the name and social status of the alleged father of her child. But quite often the *déclarations* went beyond this basic minimum of information to give the woman's story of her sexual experiences in more or less her own words. Depending on the patience and/or prurience of the official recording the statement, many of the *déclarations* go on over pages and pages, full of details about when and how the couple met, what they said and did during courtship, and when, where, and how often they had intercourse. These stories make the *déclarations* unique sources not only for the study of illegitimacy but also for the exploration of the sexual behavior and attitudes of lower-class women in general, for in no other source do we find, as we do in the *déclarations,* lower-class women actually describing their sexual experiences.

The *déclarations* therefore lend themselves to two kinds of analysis. First, the information about the ages, occupation, social status etc. of the unwed mothers can be analyzed quantitatively to isolate patterns in illicit sexual behavior which might help explain the rise in illegitimacy. Second, the women's stories can be used to begin to answer the broader questions of what sex was like for lower-class women in eighteenth-century France, and how they felt about it.

---

8 *Déclarations de grossesse* were first required by an edict of Henri II in 1556. Their ostensible purpose was to protect the life of the unborn child: it was thought that official cognizance of her pregnancy would discourage an unwed mother from doing away with her child once it was born. The real purpose, however, was probably the protection of public morality. It was hoped that the humiliation involved in making a *déclaration* would discourage repetition of the sin and would so embarrass the woman that she would hide her shame from public view—something very important in a society that believed that good and bad conduct were inculcated largely by visible examples. (For the legal aspects of the *déclarations,* see Marie-Claude Phan, "Les Déclarations de grossesse en France (XVI–XVIIIᵉ siècles): Essai institutionnel," *Revue d'histoire moderne et contemporaine,* XVII (1975), 61–88.

With these two purposes in mind I examined 3,001 *déclarations* registered at the hôtel-Dieu St.-Jacques in the town of Aix-en-Provence in the years from 1727 to 1789. This sample was deliberately chosen to test the hypothesis that urbanization and economic modernization lay behind the rise in illegitimacy. Unlike the two samples of declarations already analyzed by French historians, from Lille and from Nantes,[9] the *déclarations* from Aix include cases from both urban and rural areas, for copies of *déclarations* taken elsewhere in Provence were apparently forwarded to St.-Jacques. Further, unlike the bustling industrial and commercial centers of Lille and Nantes, Aix was a city little affected by economic modernization in the last half of the eighteenth century. Aix was instead a commercial backwater which survived economically because it was an administrative center of church and state.[10] This meant that it was probably more typical of French provincial cities than either Nantes or Lille.

GLOBAL TRENDS: DID ILLEGITIMACY RISE IN PROVENCE? Ideally we would answer this question by constructing comparative illegitimacy rates or ratios for the period before and after 1750, when most authorities agree that the rise in illegitimacy began. Unfortunately the difficulties in ascertaining the legitimate birth rate (let alone the illegitimate one) for the large and amorphous area from which our sample is drawn makes this impossible. We are therefore left with the evidence of global trends in the number of *déclarations* registered each year, a less than ideal indicator since (unlike an illegitimacy ratio) a rise in the number of *déclarations* could reflect population growth, a rising birth rate, or simply more complete recording of bastard births rather than an actual increase in illegitimacy. Nevertheless it should provide a rough indicator of trends. The information on yearly averages of *déclarations*, summarized in Fig. 1, reveals a clearly rising trend until 1764. From 1727 to 1749, an average of 51.9 *déclarations* were

9 Alain Lottin, "Naissances illégitimes et filles-mères à Lille au XVIIIe siècle," *Revue d'histoire moderne et contemporaire*, XVII (1970), 278–322; Jacques Depauw, "Amour illegitime et société à Nantes au XVIIIe siècle," *Annales: E.S.C.*, XXVII (1972), 1155–1181. An English translation of the latter can be found in Robert Forster and Orest Ranum (eds.), *Family and Society: Selections from the Annales* (Baltimore, 1976).

10 For a more complete description of the economy and society of Aix and its surrounding area in this period, see Cissie C. Fairchilds, *Poverty and Charity in Aix-en-Provence, 1640–1789* (Baltimore, 1976).

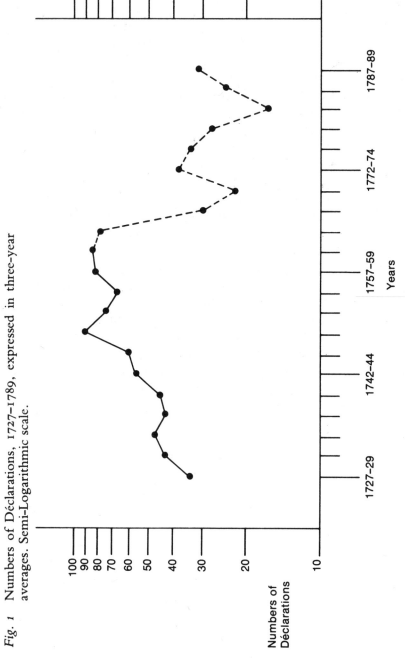

Fig. 1 Numbers of Déclarations, 1727–1789, expressed in three-year averages. Semi-Logarithmic scale.

registered at St.-Jacques each year. In the period from 1750 to 1764, the yearly average rises to 84.5. Unfortunately after 1764 our evidence becomes much more spotty because of a change in record-keeping, which was itself an important side effect of the rise in illegitimacy. Apparently so many *filles-mères* entered St.-Jacques to give birth in the early 1760s that hospital resources were severely strained. This simulated a change in the method of financing this care.[11] In turn this apparently brought a change in record-keeping. Until 1764 (the year when the new law went into effect) the hospital administrators copied the *déclarations* that they received into the hospital registers.[12] Only a few of the actual *déclarations* were preserved. But after 1764 the administrators became increasingly careless in their copying. By the 1770s the registers cease and we have only the original *déclarations*.[13] It seems that only a minority of these were preserved. Although the number of *déclarations* appears to decline in the 1770s and 1780s, it is probable that this merely reflects poor record-keeping and that the rise of illegitimacy actually continued.[14] Thus Aix would seem to provide a case where the rise in illegitimacy began in the absence of significant urbanization and economic modernization.

TYPES OF ILLICIT RELATIONSHIPS   If urbanization and economic modernization did not cause the rise in illegitimacy in Aix and its environs, what did? In order to isolate possible contributing factors, I first divided the cases into two groups, those dating from 1727 to 1749, when illegitimacy was infrequent, and those from 1750 to 1789, after the rise began. I then separated out the cases in which enough information survived to tell us something about

11 Before 1763 the supposed fathers were responsible legally for expenses. But it proved so difficult to collect from them that in 1764 responsibility was shifted to the *viguerie* in which the child was conceived. See Nicole Sabatier, *L'Hôpital St.-Jacques d'Aix-en-Provence, 1519–1789* (Aix, 1964), III, 1335–1376.
12 Archives departementales, Bouches-du-Rhône, annex in Aix-en-Provence, Series XXH, G28 to G33. Hereafter abbreviated as A.D. (Aix), XXH.
13 A.D. (Aix), XXH, IE 33–34, 40, 43–52.
14 I do not think that the gaps in the evidence for the later period will invalidate our conclusions about the rise in illegitimacy, for there is no reason to assume that those *déclarations* that happened to be preserved were in any way unrepresentative. Indeed, our picture of sexual relations is more likely to be valid for the later period than for the earlier one, since it is the original *déclarations* that usually include the women's stories and thus are more revealing about sexual practices and attitudes.

the nature of the relationship which had resulted in the woman's pregnancy. These totalled 796 of 1,142 cases for the earlier, pre-1750 period, and 1,772 of 1,859 cases for the years after 1750. I then divided these cases according to the type of relationship involved. A reading of the *déclarations* revealed that the *filles-mères* themselves showed a striking similarity of background. As the tables in Appendix I show, most were in their mid-twenties, lower-class women of rural origin who followed the occupations of textile worker, day laborer, or domestic servant. But the types of illicit relationships they were involved in and the reasons they entered into them varied widely. Three distinct patterns of relationships were discernible: those in which the man involved was superior in social and economic status to the woman, those in which the two sexual partners shared an approximate equality of status, and those in which there was, strictly speaking, no relationship at all, but instead a one-time or short-term encounter, usually involving either rape or prostitution.[15] Each of these types of relationships showed distinctive characteristics. The major variables in these relationships (the ages and geographical mobility patterns of the women involved, and the method and length of courtship) were analyzed by means of the contingency tables reproduced in Appendix II.

The frequency with which our three types of relationships occurred in the years from 1727 to 1749 has been summarized in Table 1.

RELATIONSHIPS OF INEQUALITY   As indicated, 28.7 percent of the cases in which the nature of the relationship can be identified fall

15   One other pattern of illicit relationships is visible in the *déclarations*: that involving upper-class women. Such cases were rare (28 of 1,142 cases in the years 1727–1749 and 29 of 1,859 cases from 1750–1789) and have been excluded from the discussion that follows. Why the cases involving upper-class women were so few is not clear. Perhaps standards of morality were simply more strict for women of the upper classes; noble and bourgeois families could probably keep closer watch on their daughters. But it is also possible that so few upper-class women show up in the statistics because they found it easier to obtain abortions, or at least to conceal their pregnancies and avoid making *déclarations*, a practice apparently widespread, for although the penalty for failure to make a *déclaration* was death, the municipality of Aix found it necessary to pass no fewer than seven ordinances in the years from 1659 to 1732 against midwives who connived at concealing pregnancies. (Sabatier, *L'Hôpital St.-Jacques*, III, 1147). Upper-class women could more easily afford such services. But the most likely reason why so few upper-class women are found in the *déclarations* is the simple fact that they were not as economically and physically vulnerable to seduction as their lower-class sisters.

Table 1 Patterns of Illicit Relationships, 1727–49

	NUMBER		PERCENT	
Relationships of inequality	229		28.7	
master–servant		36		4.5
other		193		24.2
Relationships of equality	529		66.5	
servant–servant		124		15.6
other–rural		142		17.8
other–rural–urban		164		20.6
other–urban		99		12.4
Short-term encounters	38		4.7	
rape highly probable		13		1.6
promiscuity highly probable		25		3.1
Total sample	796		99.9	
Total number of cases	1,142			

SOURCE: A.D. (Aix), XXH, G28–G31; XXH, E33–34.

into the category of relationships in which the man was socially and economically superior to his sexual partner. This category consists exclusively of two kinds of cases. First, there are all of the cases in which a comparison of the social status of the woman's father (used in preference to her own social status, because it was given more frequently) and that of the putative father of her child reveal the latter to be of a superior social class.[16] Second, it includes all of the cases in which the man offered some sort of economic inducement to the woman—a promise to "take care of" her, to give her a job, to give her food—to persuade her to have relations with him.[17]

16 Obviously such classifications involve great problems. First, we have only the woman's word as to who fathered her child, and, since fathers could be sued for the support of illegitimate children, it was to a woman's advantage to accuse a wealthy man. But on the other hand, upper-class men often forced their paramours to conceal their identities, suggesting that they accuse instead a lower-class type or a "person unknown." In 1770, for example, Thérèse Cavaillon, a domestic servant, stated that her mistress had secretly offered to pay her expenses if Thérèse accused an unknown in place of the true culprit, her mistress's son. (A.D. [Aix], XXH, IE 43, Déclarations de grossesse, 1770–71). I am assuming for the sake of simplicity that these two types of lies probably cancel each other out.

A second problem in this analysis arises from the immense complexity of Old Regime social structure and the ambiguities of its nomenclature. In my decisions about social status I have in general followed Adeline Daumard and François Furet, *Structures et relations sociales à Paris an milieu du XVIIIe siècle* (Paris, 1961). Ambiguous cases were omitted.

17 With these cases I have tried, doubtless not always successfully, to separate those

What made lower-class women so vulnerable to seduction by their social and economic superiors? Illicit relationships between upper-class men and lower-class women were hardly peculiar to eighteenth-century France; throughout history, wherever arranged marriages and the double standard flourished, upper-class men have used lower-class women for illicit sexual pleasure. Pomeroy mentions, for example, the sexual abuse of female slaves by Athenian citizens in ancient Greece.[18] But certain circumstances connected with the nature of women's work in eighteenth-century France made female day laborers and domestic servants especially vulnerable to such seduction.

It was customary among the rural poor for daughters to leave their homes at an early age—twelve was not uncommon—to go out to work, either because their fathers had died and left the family destitute or because their wages were needed to supplement the family income.[19] At worst such young women would join the gangs of farm laborers who wandered the countryside, drifting from harvest to harvest. At best, if they had a skill, they might find a place in the textile industry. Most typically of all, they became domestic servants. Similarly, girls with urban backgrounds, the daughters of city artisans or wage laborers, would begin working at an early age to help support their families. But unlike their country cousins, they tended to live at home while they worked, and to eschew domestic service in favor of employment as shopgirls or textile workers.

These were the only types of women's work available in a provincial town like Aix, which had little industry and lived off the patronage given to the service sector by the administrative organs of church and state. The women in our sample follow these typical employment patterns. Many of them left home to seek work because their families were destitute. Perhaps an indication of destitution is the fact that in 50.8 percent of all of the

women who were normally respectable and driven to this bartering of their favors through want from those who were habitual prostitutes. The latter are considered in a separate category. See below, 647–648.

18 Sarah B. Pomeroy, *Goddesses, Whores, Wives, and Slaves: Women in Classical Antiquity* (New York, 1975), 90–91.

19 For excellent descriptions of daughters' contributions to the family economies of the poor, see Olwen Hufton, "Women and the Family Economy in Eighteenth-Century France," *French Historical Studies*, IX (1975), 1–22; *The Poor in Eighteenth-Century France, 1750–1789* (Oxford, 1974), 25–69.

1,142 cases in our early period, either the woman's father or both of her parents were dead by the time she made her *déclaration*.fifi Others left home to help contribute to the family income, but frequently returned for visits.[21] This would suggest that Scott, Tilly, and Cohen are more nearly right than Shorter about the effect of women's work: leaving home to work did not necessarily emancipate women from family control or traditional values. Women's work *was* related to illegitimacy however, but in a much more straightforward fashion: the simple fact was that, whatever their work, women earned barely enough for subsistence. Women might do the same kinds of work as men, in the textile industry or as heavy laborers, but they were invariably paid about one-third less.[22] In the most popular form of women's work, domestic service, the wages were miniscule, although at least in theory the fringe benefits of room and board and security in old age made up for this. But many servants changed jobs frequently, and a spell of unemployment could leave a servant— or any other woman—destitute, with no alternatives but theft or prostitution.[23]

Therefore we can see how vulnerable lower-class women would have been to economic appeals and threats from men. Often the *déclarations* explicitly stated the economic motives involved in the relationships they record. Magdeleine Pilla had intercourse with Jean Joseph Bent because he paid her four *sous* each time, while Marguerite Signoret had intercourse with a baker's son who gave her bread, and Marguerite Gavauden had intercourse with a lawyer who promised to help her in a lawsuit.[24]

20 Similarly, Lottin found that in 70% of the cases recorded in Lille, the women had lost one or both parents. (Lottin, "Naissances illegitimes," 20). Death of the father is not, of course, necessarily evidence of destitution. One wishes for more information about the economic circumstances of these families; unfortunately the *déclarations* do not provide it.
21 The *déclarations* give many indications of the persistence of home and family ties. Here is one example. Marguerite Bon left her family to work as a carder in the small town of Aubagne, but returned home to visit her parents on weekends. During one of these trips home she met Jean Viderant, also an apprentice hatter. She came back every weekend after that to see him, and they decided to marry. But after surprising her one night in a "dark doorway," and taking her by force, he vanished. (A.D. [Aix], XXH, IE44, Déclarations de grossesse, 1772–73).
22 Olwen Hufton, *Bayeux in the Late Eighteenth Century: A Social Study* (Oxford, 1967), 82.
23 Hufton, *The Poor in Eighteenth Century France*, 311–313.
24 A.D. (Aix), XXH, IE44, Déclarations de grossesse, 1772–73; XXH, IE43, Déclarations de grossesse, 1770–71; XXH, E48, Déclarations de grossesse, 1780–81.

But even when the economic motive was not explicitly stated, I think that the economic vulnerability of the woman was the keynote of all of these relationships of inequality.

Another indication that the women's vulnerability drove them to these relationships is the fact that women who took part in affairs of inequality tended to be younger than those in the other two types of relationships. As a rule, women who had illegitimate children were in their mid-twenties; the average age of the women in the 771 cases in which age was given in the years from 1727 to 1749 was 24.8, while the median age was 24. But age tended to vary, albeit rather weakly, with the type of relationship, as is shown in Contingency Table 2 of Appendix II, in which the 694 cases where both the age and the type of relationship were given were cross-tabulated. This shows that women involved in relationships of inequality tended to be younger than those in the other categories. In relationships of inequality more women turn up in the younger-age categories and fewer in the older categories than we would expect if ages did not vary with the type of relationship. For example, the expected figure for women 15 to 19 is 16.4, although the actual figure is 32; the expected figure for the age 25 to 29 category is 42.2, although the actual figure is 24. Another indication that women in relationships of inequality tended to be younger is the fact that many cases of this type were long-standing liaisons that had begun when the woman was quite young. Thirty-year-old Catherine Folie, for example, stated that she had been the mistress of Josef Richaud, innkeeper at the *Cheval Blanc,* for eleven years, which implies that the relationship had begun when Catherine was nineteen.[25] Although this age pattern may reveal nothing more than the fact that upper-class men were more attracted to very young women, I think it results from the fact that younger women may have been more naive and therefore more easily seduced.

Still another sort of female vulnerability appears in a special subcategory of relationships of inequality: those between masters and servants. As Table 1 shows, 4.5 percent of our 796 cases for which the pattern of the relationship can be discerned fall into this category. In fact, there were probably many more of these cases than this figure indicates, for I have classified as master-servant

25 A.D. (Aix), XXH, G29, Expositions des femmes enceintes commencé le 28 novembre, 1729.

only those cases in which this relationship is explicitly stated. But probably many of the other relationships of inequality belong in this category as well. An indication that master-servant affairs were widespread is the fact that the second most frequent reason given by wives in eighteenth-century France when they petitioned the church for legal separations was their husbands' adultery with a servant (physical abuse was the first).[26]

In master-servant relationships the woman was doubly vulnerable, for added to economic pressures were the perils of proximity. A servant had nowhere to hide if her master were bent on her seduction. Thérèse Cavaillon, for example, stated in her *déclaration* that the son of the house had constantly pursued her. Her only refuge was her attic room. But one day he forced his way in and raped her at knife-point.[27] But such force was rarely needed; in most cases the economic power of the master sufficed. Marguerite Angellin slept with her master although, she said, he was "married and even a grandfather," because "he said that if she didn't he wouldn't pay her wages."[28] And Thérèse Roux, who had endured a long spell of unemployment before Louis Seste hired her as a servant, said that at first she had resisted Seste's advances, "but since he was her master she was obliged to consent."[29]

Thus the keynote of relationships of inequality would seem to have been the male exploitation of various types of female vulnerability. Yet this must not be overstressed. Not all of these women were innocent victims; some were clearly gold diggers out for all that they could get. One can have little sympathy for women like Marguerite Gueirand, a laundress who had an affair with M. Caillol, a master tool-maker who owned his own shop and had a sick wife. Marguerite not only got Caillol to promise to marry her when his wife finally died, but also persuaded him to give her his wife's clothes and other possessions in the meantime.[30] And if not all of the women in these relationships were innocent victims, neither were all the men heartless seducers. The fact that the man was economically superior to the woman did

26 Alain Lottin, "Vie et mort du couple: Difficultés conjugales et divorces dans le nord de la France aux XVIIe et XVIIIe siècles," *XVIIe Siècle*, 102-103 (1974), 71-72.
27 A.D. (Aix), XXH, E43, Déclarations de grossesse, 1770-71.
28 *Ibid*.
29 A.D. (Aix), XXH, E34, Déclarations de grossesse, 1747-57.
30 A.D. (Aix), XXH, IE44, Déclarations de grossesse, 1772-73.

not necessarily exclude either sexual attraction or genuine affection from their relationship. Indications of such affection abound. Some of these liaisons were quite longstanding, lasting years and even decades.[31] Often the couple had other illegitimate children besides the one for whom the *déclaration* was made.[32] Such relationships were in reality common-law marriages. Frequently the men in these liaisons expressed concern for the welfare of their paramours; this most often took the form of promising always to "take care of" them.

Despite these qualifications, however, the fact remains that the keynote of most of these relationships of inequality was exploitation. A final indication of the exploitative quality of these relationships is what happened to the two partners after their affair ended. For the man there seems to have been little social opprobrium connected with being cited in a *déclaration,* although admittedly a few of them tried to persuade their mistresses to conceal their identities. But for the woman the consequences of an illicit affair were usually disastrous. Frequently men forgot about their promises of care when they learned that their women were pregnant—Marguerite Donnat, recipient of such a promise, tells how her revelation of her pregnancy led to a quarrel, which ended when her lover "put her out of the house without giving her any money"—and maid servants discovered pregnant by their mistresses were inevitably fired.[33] Once discharged and publicly disgraced, these women found it very difficult to get another job and were often forced to turn to prostitution to support themselves and their children, if they lived.[34]

---

31 The few cases from the pre-1750 period that give some indication of the length of the liaison have been analyzed in Contingency Table 4 of Appendix II. This shows that the length tended to vary with the type of liaison, and the category of relationships of inequality tended to have proportionately more longer relationships than any other category.

32 One example, dating from 1730, is the case of Jeanne Telene, daughter of a rural agricultural laborer, then twenty-two years old. She had been the mistress of Sieur André de Chateaudouble for four years, and had borne him two other children. (A.D. [Aix], XXI, G29, Expositions des femmes enceintes commencé le 28 novembre, 1729).

33 See A.D. (Aix), XXH, E34, Déclarations de grossesse, 1747–51; A.D. (Aix), XXH, G29, Expositions des femmes enceintes commencé le 28 novembre 1729, for examples of maidservants fired for being pregnant.

34 Most illegitimate babies probably died shortly after birth. In the years from 1768 to 1775, 71% of the abandoned children cared for in St.-Jacques died during their first year. (Fairchilds, *Poverty and Charity*, 84).

RELATIONSHIPS OF EQUALITY   Despite the perils of seduction by a superior, the majority of women in our sample became pregnant as a result of relationships with men of approximately their own social class. As Table 1 shows, 66.5 percent of the identifiable relationships in the pre-1750 period were relationships of equality. The psychodynamics of such relationships varied considerably from those of relationships of inequality. Women's economic vulnerability was still a major factor, but it took a different form: it was the promise of marriage that enticed a maid to sleep with a footman, a laundress with an apprentice hatmaker, a shepherdess with an argicultural laborer. Marriage was of overwhelming importance to lower-class women. Not only did it legitimize their sexual relationships in the eyes of society, and save them from the scorn accorded to spinsters, but it also provided them with their only hope of economic security. It was only within the context of a family economy, with husband, wife, and children all working to contribute to the family income, that a lower-class woman could hope to survive.

Women therefore took promises of marriage seriously, even if the men who made them did not. And in 10.4 percent of our 529 relationships of inequality some such promise was made. This may at first sight seem a very small proportion. But we must remember that only a very few of the cases in the pre-1750 period give any details at all about the relationship—80 to be exact (see Table 3 in Appendix II). Thus, of the relationships of equality about which we have information, 55 of 68, or 80.9 percent, mention a promise of marriage. It is probable that many more promises of marriage were made—or at least implied—than were recorded.

How seriously are we to take such promises? Did women have reason to lie about the existence of a marriage proposal? Did men toss off such promises casually or were they the product of a genuine commitment? Unfortunately it is impossible to answer these questions with any certainty. Some women might have had an economic motive for lying about a promise of marriage, for if their lover promised marriage they could sue him for *rapt de seduction*. But this held true only if the woman were under twenty-five, and if the courtship had taken place without the consent of her parents.[35] Women may also have lied about marriage pro-

---

35   Sabatier, *L'Hôpital St.-Jacques*, III, 1218-1220.

posals to excuse their conduct, although in most of those cases they probably deluded themselves into really believing that the promise had been given. As for the sincerity of the man making the promise, this too is impossible to assess. Only very gullible women would take seriously the proposals occasionally given in relationships of inequality (see Table 3 of Appendix II). These were usually promises to marry their paramours after their wives died. But most promises given in relationships of equality seem to have involved a genuine commitment. Often these cases reveal a long period of acquaintanceship and courtship before the promise was made. They frequently mention formal application for the parents' consent, and occasionally note that the banns had been posted. A few cases even state that the man promised to convert from Protestantism to Catholicism in order to marry the girl.

Thus I think most promises claimed were actually made, and made with sincerity. This is important because once marriage was promised, the whole relationship took on a different complexion. Women could convince themselves that they were genuinely in love with a man whose intentions were honorable. Tulle Lemay speaks of how, "when a young man so ardently and repeatedly asked her to be his wife," she "insensibly began to feel less indifferent toward him."[36] Also, a promise of marriage apparently made sexual intercourse between the engaged couple socially acceptable, indicated by the small but nevertheless perceptible number of prebridal pregnancies found in legitimate marriages in this period.[37] Some men even used the argument that intercourse before marriage would guarantee the match. Her lover asked Marianne Gregoire to give herself to him because, he said, it would win over his parents and thus end the difficulties in the way of their marriage. Similarly, Marie Magdeleine Bellon was told that her marriage "depended on her letting herself be seduced and becoming pregnant to make his parents consent" to the union.[38]

Therefore it is probable that most of the relationships in which the sexual partners were equal in social status were, in the

36 A.D. (Aix), XXH, E35, Déclarations de grossesse, 1752–57.
37 In one Provençal village, Lourmarin, 18.4% of all legitimate first births from 1681 to 1830 were prebridal pregnancies. (Thomas F. Sheppard, *Lourmarin in the Eighteenth Century: A Study of a French Village* [Baltimore, 1974], 40.)
38 A.D. (Aix), XXH, E50, Déclarations de grossesse, 1785–86; XXH, E35, Déclarations de grossesse, 1752–1757.

minds of the women at least, prebridal pregnancies gone wrong. These women had intercourse with their lovers not primarily because of a search for sexual adventure or fulfillment, but because they hoped it would lead to marriage or, indeed, they thought that they were already as good as married. A further indication of this is the pattern of age distribution in relationships of equality. As Table 2 of Appendix II shows, if relationships of inequality tended to include more younger women than we would expect, in relationships of equality the opposite is true; we find unexpectedly large numbers of women in the upper-age brackets. In the category of "other relationships of equality" the expected number of women for the 15 to 19 age group is 36, while the observed value is 20. In the 35+ age group the expected value is 33.5, while the observed value is 53. Most women in relationships of equality were mature women who had every reason to expect that their equally mature lovers were serious about their relationship. Indeed, well over half of the women in this group were *older* than the probable median age of marriage (23.5 years) in Provence in this period.[39] This reinforces our perception that most women entered into these relationships with something permanent in mind. Anne Goivan, the twenty-five-year old daughter of a *ménager* in the small village of Grignan, probably spoke for most of the women in these relationships of equality when she stated that the only reason she had let Antoine Goiran, the son of a neighboring *travailleur*, court her for two years, let alone sleep with her, was that he seemed serious about getting married.[40]

If most relationships of equality shared this common hope for marriage on the part of the women, they were nevertheless not all alike. Relationships among the lower classes in the countryside differed from those among the urban lower classes, and certain occupational groups also showed distinctive patterns. Relationships in which both partners were servants, for example, must be singled out because of the threat to a woman's virtue when her potential lover lived under the same roof. Servant girls were as physically vulnerable to advances by their fellow servants as they were to the attentions of their masters. The story of Magdeleine Comte, a maidservant in a large household, illustrates this. Magdeleine had long been pursued by a certain Mittre, a

39 Sheppard, *Lourmarin*, 38.
40 A.D. (Aix), XXH, E40, Déclarations de grossesse, 1764–65.

footman in the same establishment. Finally he cornered her when they were alone in the kitchen, and threw her on a chair, saying that he wished to have his way with her. After that she avoided the kitchen whenever possible. But one day a guest in the house sent her there on an errand, despite her protests, and Mittre caught her again.[41] Another indication of the vulnerability of servants is the fact that they tended to be younger than the women in the other types of relationships of equality, as Table 2 of Appendix II shows.

But if the woman's vulernability seems to have played a large role in servant-servant relationships, one also suspects that maid-servants were more likely than other lower-class women to enter into illicit relationships purely for sexual pleasure. Although we know very little about the conditions of domestic service in eight-eenth-century France, it seems probable that few servants could hope to marry and continue working as servants. Places for mar-ried couples were doubtless rare. Therefore, although some serv-ant-servant relationships did have promises of marriage (see Table 3, Appendix II), one suspects that the chance of these relationships actually resulting in marriage was slight. Probably many female servants gradually came to realize that their only chance for com-panionship and sexual fulfillment lay in an illicit relationship. Many illicit relationships between servants seem to have started when the household adjourned to the country for the summer.[42] One can imagine how the pleasant weather plus the relaxation of household discipline encouraged the blossoming of romance. The sexual roundelays that playwrights such as Pierre Marivaux set in country chateaux seem to have had a basis in fact. After all, for servants, sex was probably the one available escape from the constricting discipline of their lives. Often servants made love on the beds of their masters, an easy and enjoyable protest against their lot.[43]

As for the variations between rural and urban relationships, it is usually thought that urban areas in early modern Europe had

41 A.D. (Aix), XXH, E35, Déclarations de grossesse, 1752–57.

42 The location of the sexual encounters is given in only a very few of the *déclarations*. Of the 48 servant-servant cases for which the location is recorded, 21 took place in chateaux during the summer.

43 For an example, see the case of Genevieve Gontard, A.D. (Aix), XXH, E33, Expo-sitions de grossesse, 1725–46.

a tradition of consensual unions and common-law marriages, among the lower classes.[44] There are traces of this in our sample— twenty-eight-year-old Marguerite Baudon of Hyères lived with Joseph Portonier for fourteen years before she made a *déclaration*— but they are very few.[45] An analysis of the length of liaisons given in Table 4 of Appendix II shows that there was not a disproportionate number of relationships that lasted longer than six months in urban areas. In fact, patterns of length of relationship in urban areas follow those observed for the rural lower classes.

Most of the urban cases seem to have concerned courting couples (see Table 3, Appendix II for promises of marriage) who met either at work, like Marie Agnelier and Pierre Grasson, who were both employed in the shop of a *tailleur*, or at their lodgings, like Thérèse Ferand, who became acquainted with the man who would become her lover when he moved into the house where her family lodged in the one hopes aptly named rue du Paradis.[46] The stories of these courtships give little indication of the debauchery which both contemporary upper-class observers and Shorter ascribe to those who dwelled in the "proletarian subculture" of urban areas. In only one of these cases is mention made of the cabaret, that supposed den of iniquity for the urban lower classes. Magdeleine Peleissier, who worked in a *fabrique des toiles*, was courted by Henry Feraud, a worker in the same shop. One night he took her to a cabaret, where the combination of his marriage proposal plus the *eau de vie* that he bought to celebrate led her to succumb to his advances.[47] But this is exceptional. More frequent are mentions of the problems of obtaining parental consent and the waiting and saving for marriage (Marie Chau had saved a dowry of 60 *livres* out of her earnings).[48] Given these delays, it is little wonder that many couples jumped the gun. The main problem for such courting couples seems to have been finding a place where they could be alone. If either the man or

44 Tilly, Scott, and Cohen, "Women's Work and Fertility," 468.
45 A.D. (Aix), XXH, G29, Expositions des femmes enceintes commencé le 28 novembre 1729.
46 A.D. (Aix), XXH, E46, Déclarations de grossesse, 1776–77; XXH, G32, Livre des Expositions des Femmes Enceintes Commencé le 27 mars 1752.
47 A.D. (Aix), XXH, E46, Déclarations de grossesse, 1776–77.
48 A.D. (Aix), XXH, E40, Déclarations de grossesse, 1764–65.

the woman had lodgings with a modicum of privacy, they slept together there. If not, they had intercourse out of doors.[49]

The final distinctive pattern in relationships of equality occurs among the peasants and artisans in small towns and villages. Table 1 of Appendix II shows that cases which took place in rural areas formed only 35 percent of the "other lower class" cases. Considering the enormous geographical area from which our rural cases were drawn, since cases from all over Provence were apparently forwarded to St.-Jacques, this percentage seems very small. Although there might have been a massive underreporting of rural cases, it seems permissible to conclude that this relatively low percentage was the product of extremely strict morality in the countryside. Further evidence for this conclusion can be found in an examination of the methods of courtship summarized in Table 3 of Appendix II. This shows that the overwhelming majority of the cases in which we find long courtships and promises of marriage were rural—an indication that most of these cases were legitimate courtships gone wrong. We also find that the majority of cases in which force was used *and* marriage promised occurred in rural areas. This seems to point up a characteristic of rural courtship: after the couple became engaged, it was apparently customary for the man to use force on the woman in a sort of ritual rape that probably set the tone for their future marital relations. What happened to Marguerite Girard was typical of these rural relationships of equality. Marguerite was the daughter of a shepherd, and lived with her parents in the Dauphiné. She had been courted for a year by François Noble, also a shepherd, and they planned to be married. He gave her a gold cross as a betrothal present. One evening François came to her father's house, and, finding her alone, threw her on the bed, stuck a handkerchief in her mouth, and raped her. After this they had intercourse in her father's house twice a week "like a married couple." But then François deserted her.[50] This pattern of promise of marriage, ritual rape, sexual relations approved by the family, and then desertion dominated these rural illegitimacies (and the

---

49 Of the 43 cases in this category where the location of the sexual encounter is given, 15 occurred out-of-doors, 5 in the man's lodging, 19 in the woman's rooms, and 4 in the woman's family home.

50 A.D. (Aix), XXH, IE43, Déclarations de grossesse, 1770–71.

ritual rape before marriage was probably found in legitimate marriages in the countryside as well).[51]

SHORT-TERM, CHANCE ENCOUNTERS   Mention of the use of force brings us to our final major category of cases, those in which there was no lasting relationship between the sexual partners, pregnancy instead resulting from a more or less chance encounter. In this category there are two main subdivisions: cases of rape or cases in which rape was highly probable, and cases of prostitution and generally promiscuous behavior.

As Table 1 shows, among our relationships there were only thirteen cases (1.6 percent of the identifiable total) in which rape by an unknown was either claimed by the woman or could be inferred from other information in the *déclaration*. The latter are those cases in which the women were either travelling alone (usually going from town to town looking for a job) or working as harvest-hands, and stated that their partner was a "man unknown." For inevitably it was women in such situations who turned up in the cases where rape was claimed. The physical vulnerability of the maidservant sent alone into the countryside on an errand and of the female harvest-hand forced to bed down at night with her male co-workers in a barn or hay loft should be obvious.[52] The rapists were "men unknown," but often the women identified them from their clothing as soldiers or deserters from the army.

Very different is the other subcategory of short-term encounters, those in which the woman's behavior seems to have been promiscuous. Included in this category are, first of all, all those women who could not identify the father of their child or who, like Françoise Paure, could not distinguish among two, three, or even four possible candidates.[53] Included also in this

51 As Table 7 of Appendix II shows, the ritual rape was occasionally found in relationships of equality in urban areas as well. But it seems to have been primarily a rural phenomenon.

52 A typical story of a rape is that of Françoise Forton, a thirty-year-old farm servant who lived in the village of Salenes. She was sent by her mistress to Riez to deliver a message and a basket of melons. She joined up with a woman she met on the road for protection, but they were stopped by four unknown men, who dragged them into the woods and gang-raped them. (A.D. [Aix], XXH, E50, Déclarations de grossesse, 1752–57).

53 For Françoise Paure see A.D. (Aix), XXH, G32, Livre de Expositions des Femmes Enceintes Commencé le 27 mars 1752. It should be noted that women occasionally claim

category are all inn servants, who seem to have casually slept with customers whose names they often did not know. Typical of the inn servants was twenty-four-year old Marthe Peyrig, who had been a servant at the sign of the Bras d'Or in Lambesc for two years. She said that one night an army officer staying at the inn asked her to carry his luggage to his room, and after what she described as "certain discourses," they had sex.[54] It is highly probable that most of the female servants in inns and cabarets were part-time prostitutes. At any rate, the Bras d'Or contributed at least one other case to the *déclarations*. Not surprisingly women in this category tended to show up more frequently than one would expect in the younger age groups.

These, then, were the patterns of illicit relationships in Provence in the years before 1750. Apparently very few of the cases involved permissive or promiscuous behavior. Most of the illegitimacies in this period resulted from the physical and economic vulnerability of lower-class women, which made them susceptible to seduction by their masters or to promises of marriage from their swains. Women had sex out of wedlock because they were promised money or marriage or simply because they could not avoid it. Sex was for them a means to an end rather than an end in itself.

PATTERNS OF ILLICIT RELATIONSHIPS AFTER 1750   Did the patterns of illicit relationships change significantly after 1750 in ways which might help to explain the rise in illegitimacies which began in Aix, as elsewhere in France, during that period? Table 2 summarizes the number of identifiable cases in each of our categories of relationships in the years from 1750 to 1789, with comparable percentages for the earlier period.

The first point to notice is the changes that take place in our three basic categories of relationships. We see a dramatic drop in the relative size of the category of relationships of inequality and an almost equally dramatic rise in the proportion of relationships in which the sexual partners were social equals. Cases in the category of short-term encounters also show a rise. Depauw

---

that the man was unknown to them in order to protect the identity of their lover. For an example, see the case of Marianne Perret, A.D. (Aix), E35, Déclarations de grossesse, 1752–1757. It is of course impossible to tell how many of these cases there were.

54   A.D. (Aix), XXH, IE44, Déclarations de grossesse, 1772–73.

Table 2 Patterns of Illicit Relationships, 1750–1789

	NUMBER		PERCENT	PERCENT 1727–49
Relationships of inequality	343		19.4	28.7
master–servant		63	3.6	4.5
other		280	15.8	24.2
Relationships of equality	1,263		71.2	66.5
servant–servant		107	6.0	15.6
other–rural		584	33.0	17.8
other–rural–urban		313	17.1	20.6
other–urban		259	14.6	12.4
Short-term encounters	166		9.3	4.7
rape highly probable		84	4.7	1.6
promiscuity highly probable		82	4.6	3.1
Total sample	1,772		99.9	
Total number of cases	1,859			

SOURCE: A.D. (Aix), XXH, G32–33; XXH, E40, 43–52.

found these same basic changes in the *déclarations* from Nantes for this period.[55] The decline in the relationships of inequality and the rise in the relationships of equality would at first sight seem to indicate that Shorter's sexual revolution has indeed occurred, for it suggests that in the latter half of the eighteenth century young women of the lower classes were less inclined to have sex with men of the upper classes for economic gain, and more inclined to enter into relationships with young men of their own social class for, one presumes, reasons of sexual attraction or affection. This turn toward affective rather than instrumental relationships would seem to suggest a spread of more permissive attitudes toward sex among lower-class women.[56]

55 Depauw, "Illicit Sexual Activity," in Forster and Ranum (eds.), *Family and Society*, 172.

56 It should be noted that the relative decline in the number of relationships of inequality may be a reflection of a change in the mentality of the *men* rather than the women involved in such relationships. Upper-class men may have increasingly turned away from extra-marital sex with their social inferiors. Perhaps they increasingly found partners for their sexual adventures among women of their own social class. For surely it is these women, some of whom were soon to be the feminists of the French Revolution, who were more likely to have embraced the emancipated attitudes of Shorter's sexual revolution than their lower-class sisters. On the other hand, it is also possible that as bourgeois values centering on home and family spread through the upper classes, men of superior social status were more inclined to take their marriage vows seriously and less inclined to indulge in extra-marital affairs of any sort.

But an examination of the relative changes within the sub-categories of relationships of equality throws doubt upon Shorter's hypothesis that attitudinal change contributed to the rise in illegitimacy. If Shorter were correct about the mechanisms of such change, we would expect that most of the growth in illegitimacy would be concentrated in the subcategory of women who moved from a rural to an urban area, for Shorter argued that it was the emancipation from family control which enabled women to adopt more permissive sexual attitudes. Yet in our sample we see not a rise but a slight relative decline in the number of women who fall into this category. In the earlier period women who had moved from the country to the city and had affairs with men of their own social class formed 40.4 percent of the cases in the "other lower class" category, and 20.6 percent of the cases as a whole. But in the years from 1750 to 1789, the comparable figures are 20.7 and 17.7 percent. Obviously it was not Shorter's newcomers to the city who were contributing to the rise in illegitimacy in Provence.

Similarly, if Shorter were correct about the eroticism of the "proletarian subculture" in the cities, we might expect that the cases in which the woman was born and lived in a totally urban milieu would show a substantial increase in the years after 1750. But in fact they show up in approximately the same proportion of our cases after 1750 as they did in the pre-1750 period. The most important change we find in these urban cases in the later period is the fact that the women involved in them tended to be younger than before, as a comparison of Table 6 with Table 2 in Appendix II shows. In the years before 1750, ages tended to vary moderately strongly with the type of relationship, and women in relationships of equality tended to cluster in the higher-age brackets. After 1750 the variation is much less strong, due to the fact that women were entering into relationships of equality at younger ages. This was especially true of women in the urban (and rural-to-urban) other lower-class category, as Table 6 shows. But before we conclude that this proves Shorter right, since it indicates that lower-class women in urban milieus were increasingly taking a more permissive and less marriage-oriented attitude toward premarital sex, we should note that the age of marriage itself was probably falling in Provence in this period. In the Provençal village of Lourmarin, for example, the most popular age of marriage for women was 24 to 25 in the years from 1696 to 1755, but after 1757 the figure dropped to 19.[57] Thus, even though they were younger, there is no reason to suppose that these women were less marriage-oriented than the urban lower-class women in the earlier period. The information on courtships and promises of marriage summarized in Table 7 of Appendix II bears this out. It reveals little change from earlier patterns. And Table 8 reveals that there was little change in the length of relationships among the urban lower classes, with neither a massive increase in the number of consensual unions nor a dramatic drop in the average length of the relationships, both of which we might have expected if these urban women were taking a more permissive attitude toward sex.

Again, if Shorter were correct, we might have expected that the category of servant-servant relationships would show an increase, since we have argued that these cases were probably the most permissive and least marriage-oriented of all of our relationships of equality. But instead of a rise we find not only a relative but also an absolute decline in the number of servant-servant relationships in the years after 1750. What lay behind this? The most likely explanation seems to involve not a change in sexual practices or attitudes, but a change in the nature of the servant class. The last half of the eighteenth century probably saw the beginnings of the feminization of domestic service, with a substantial decline in the numbers of men employed as servants.[58] This would naturally cause a decline in the number of servant-servant sexual relationships.

We have seen that the rise in illegitimacy occurs in none of the places where we might have expected it if Shorter's hypotheses about the sexual revolution were correct. Where then does the rise occur? It appears among the cases in which the woman was born and remained in a rural area. The proportion of such cases shows a dramatic rise in the years after 1750. Such cases formed only 35.1 percent of all lower-class cases and 17.8 percent of all

57 Sheppard, *Lourmarin*, 36.
58 We know literally nothing about domestic service in Aix in this period, although Sarah Maza of Princeton University is at work on a Ph.D. dissertation dealing with it. But the feminization of domestic service has been documented elsewhere in France. See Bernard Marcoul, "Les domestiques à Toulouse en XVIIIe siècle," unpub. D.E.S. thesis (University of Toulouse, 1960); Marc Botlan, "Domesticité et domestiques à Paris dans la crise, 1770–1790," unpub. paper. I wish to thank Theresa McBride for the last reference.

cases in our earlier period, but in the years from 1750 to 1789 comparable percentages are 50.0 and 33.0. The annual rate of cases in this category more than doubled, from 6.2 per year in the pre-1750 period to 14.6 cases per year from 1750 to 1789. Thus, although the gaps in our sample in the 1770s and 1789s (and the possibility of a change in reporting methods favoring rural areas) prevents us from drawing any firm conclusions, it would seem that the rise in illegitimacy in eighteenth-century Aix was fueled by a striking rise in rural illegitimacies.[59]

What caused this rise? Obviously urbanization was not at work. And apparently neither was a turn toward sexual adventurism on the part of rural lower-class women. These rural cases had always been the least permissive of our relationships of equality, and that did not change in the years after 1750. Women in these cases still showed a tendency to cluster in the upper-age brackets, as Table 6 of Appendix II shows. Table 7 reveals that these relationships continued to show the standard rural pattern of long courtships, promises of marriage, and ritual rape.

The most likely explanation seems to lie with the worsening economic condition of the Provençal peasantry in the last half of the eighteenth century. There seems little doubt that times were hard for the peasants of Provence in these years. After 1740, the population began to rise, leading to increased competition for land and work, while the notorious price rise of the last years of the Old Regime drastically raised the cost of living for the poor.[60] These trends made it much harder for a young couple to save enough to rent or own land of their own. Many couples may have started what they took to be legitimate courtships, only to discover in the end that they could not afford to marry. Also, the worsening economic conditions may have led to increased mobility among the rural lower classes, as farm laborers moved farther and farther afield in search of work. One slight indication of increased mobility for the peasants of Provence in this period comes from Lourmarin, where we find in these years an increasing

59 Depauw found a similar increase in rural cases in Nantes, although he ignored it and built his argument around illegitimacy as an urban phenomenon. Depauw, "Illicit Sexual Activity," 155.
60 For the economic condition of Aix and its environs in these years, see Fairchilds, *Poverty and Charity*, 132–133.

number of marriages in which one or both partners were strangers to the village.[61] Increased mobility would tend to drive up illegitimacies, for if young men were more likely to go farther looking for work, they were also more likely to forget about promises to return and marry the girl back home. Finally, the worsening economic conditions in the countryside may account for the other changes we can observe in Table 2, the rises in cases of rape and prostitution. Hard times may have forced more women into the occupations of harvest-hand and inn servant, where the risk of illegitimate pregnancy was high.

Aix would therefore seem to be a case in which the Scott, Tilly, and Cohen hypothesis of the persistence of old attitudes in changing economic circumstances explains the rise in illegitimacy, although it should be noted that these changes are not economic "modernization" but instead a simple worsening of conditions. It was not economic modernization but the lack of it that may have driven up the numbers of illegitimacies in eighteenth-century Provence. But before we accept this economic explanation wholeheartedly, we should consider one other possibility. The rise in illegitimacies may simply have been a by-product of changing courtship and marriage patterns. Obviously there were changes in marriage customs in rural Provence in this period. The drop in average age at marriage has been mentioned. Apparently women were not only marrying at younger ages than ever before, but also more of them were pregnant when they took their marriage vows. In Lourmarin, for example, over 18 percent of the first children of all marriages between 1681 and 1830 were premarital conceptions; in the last decade of the eighteenth century this figure was 34 percent.[62] Both the drop in the age of marriage and the increase in prebridal pregnancies would have had the effect of increasing the number of courtships that had the potential of going wrong and ending in an illegitimacy instead of marriage. Thus both might have contributed indirectly to the rise in illegitimacies.

What lay behind these changes in courtship is not clear. The lower age of brides may indicate the spread of a less prudential view of marriage, which may in turn be tied to the worsening

61 Sheppard, *Lourmarin*, 34.
62 *Ibid.*, 40–42.

economic conditions. Since the possibility of land of one's own probably seemed increasingly remote, more and more couples may have given up on the usual period of waiting and saving before marriage. And the increase in prebridal pregnancies may be a reflection of changing norms of family discipline, specifically the spread of a more "bourgeois," child-oriented notion of the family (this at any rate is the factor cited for the rise in prebridal pregnancies in colonial America in the same period).[63] Or it may reflect the declining efficacy of religious prohibitions of premarital sex, as dechristianization spread through the countryside.[64] Obviously much more research into the mentality, patterns of property-holding, and family discipline of the Provençal peasant is necessary before we can draw any firm conclusions. But it suggests that Shorter may be partially right about his "sexual revolution": attitudes toward courtship and marriage may have changed in very basic ways in the late eighteenth century. The rise in illegitimacy may have been the by-product of these changes. But it seems clear that Shorter is wrong in postulating as a major factor a change in the attitudes of women that encouraged them to undertake illicit sexual adventures. For what the *déclarations* show above all else is that lower-class women viewed illicit relationships in the context of marriage, and that a search for sexual fulfillment or notions of romantic love had little to do with their entering into such relationships.

FEMALE SEXUAL ATTITUDES AS REFLECTED IN THE DECLARATIONS
It is difficult to deduce how these women felt about sex from their *déclarations*. It is hard to disentangle how they actually felt at the moment they made love from how they said they felt when they looked back on it seven or eight months later, trapped in an unwanted pregnancy and forced to discuss embarassingly intimate matters with male, upper-class officials who probably radiated disapproval. Nonetheless it is possible to offer some hypotheses about sexual attitudes based on the *déclarations*. They show in both the years before *and after* 1750 little evidence of a search for sexual fulfillment. In both periods, for most women,

63   Smith and Hindus, "Premarital Pregnancy in America," 539.
64   For dechristianization in Provence see Michel Vovelle, *Piété baroque et déchristianisation en Provence au XVIIIe siècle: les attitudes devant la mort d'après les clauses des testaments* (Paris, 1973).

sex seems to have been instrumental rather than affective, a means to an end—marriage, economic advantage, or mere survival—rather than an end in itself.

This is not to say they never enjoyed it. Even in the *déclarations*, where the intimidating presence of the officials taking the statements would have inhibited frank avowal of sexual pleasure, that nevertheless comes through. Tulle Lemaye speaks of the "transports of love" she experienced, and we can read similar enjoyment between the lines of the countless stories like that of Marianne Verat, whose boyfriend forced himself upon her as she gathered fruit in an orchard. Marianne stated that she returned to the orchard the next day "eager to gather apricots," as she put it, when "again it happened."[65] These rather naive confessions that the woman, although she resisted at first, just happened to be around when her lover found another opportunity for sex—and another and another, recur repeatedly in the *déclarations*.

But there are in the *déclarations* suggestions that the sexual experiences of these women were not, on the whole, very enjoyable. Although the *déclarations* speak of the actual sexual acts only in very veiled terms, they give the impression that these acts were usually short and frequently brutal. Men apparently made few attempts to increase the enjoyment of their sexual partners; what might have been foreplay is mentioned in only four cases. Rape was of course frequent, even in cases of legitimate courtship. The litany of "he threw me on the ground, he stuck a handkerchief in my mouth, he lifted my skirts," recurs again and again even in cases of legitimate courtship. And even when outright force was not used, the threat of it was always there. Anne Pascal spoke for many when she said that she gave in to her lover's demands because she was afraid he would harm her if she did not.[66]

There was apparently in these relationships little of the paraphernalia of romantic courtship that might have cast a veil over the unattractive realities. Although there are some cases that show the traditional stuff of romance—gifts of flowers and jewelry and quiet walks in the countryside—and there are others in which the couple shows obvious signs of mutual affection and esteem, in

65 A.D. (Aix), XXH, E35, Déclarations de grossesse, 1752–57; XXH, E50, Déclarations de grossesse, 1785–86.
66 A.D. (Aix), XXH, E35, Déclarations de grossesse, 1752–57.

most of the cases we find brutality and an all-pervading masculine contempt for women. Instead of words of romance, there was verbal abuse. The best a woman could hope for in the way of tender words was the apparently standard line, "I have no other women but you." The worst was curses and obscenities. Ann Pascal, a peasant's daughter, had been courted for three years by a neighbor's son. When they finally made love he said: "You let strangers do it to you," and added "some indecent words."[67] Signs of the men's contempt for their women were frequent. Magdeleine Lus was raped in the woods by a soldier who joked when she screamed: "*Tais-toi*," he said. "Let me do my will. The king needs men."[68] And Marguerite Roche, one of the few upper-class women to make a *déclaration*, was thoroughly humiliated by her long-time suitor, a neighbor, Nicolas Rolland, who she thought "respected her like a sister." Rolland not only raped her, but did it in front of her maid.[69] We cannot tell how these women felt about the abuse and contempt that they received. Such treatment may have been all any lower-class women might ever expect from men, inside or outside marriage. Cases of wife-beating were certainly common on eighteenth-century police blotters.[70] But it seems probable that this atmosphere of brutality and abuse detracted from the pleasure that these women gained from their illicit sexual affairs.

It is also important to note that the pleasure these women found in sex was always ambivalent and riddled with guilt. Eighteenth-century France was a society in which the double standard flourished, and women seem to have internalized its values. At least evidence from the *déclarations* suggests this. These women, as well as their society, apparently valued virginity highly. Tulle Lemaye mentions that she "cried and made a thousand reproaches" to her lover the first time they had intercourse, and says that after he left her she lay awake beset by "mortal fears."[71] Another reflection of the reverence for virginity that these women seem to have shared with their society was the notion that once her virginity was lost outside marriage, a woman was little better

67 *Ibid*.
68 A.D. (Aix), XXH, IE45, Déclarations de grossesse, 1774–75.
69 A.D (Aix), XXH, E50, Déclarations de grossesse, 1785–86.
70 See above, note 23; Fairchilds, *Poverty and Charity*, 121.
71 A.D. (Aix), XXH, E35, Déclarations de grossesse, 1752–57.

than a prostitute. At least many of the women who made *déclarations* seem to have felt that, if society considered them abandoned, they might as well relax and enjoy the role. As one put it, "the first step having been taken, I no longer dreamed of resisting."[72]

In addition to a reverence for virginity, women seem to have shared with their society the notion that in sexual matters the initiative should always rest with the man. At least that is the pattern that emerges from the *déclarations*. However much the woman may admit to maneuvering so that the couple could be alone together ("I had to return to the orchard"; "I was alone in the house when he came") they *always* state that it was the man who made the first overt gesture that led to their intercourse (often this gesture took the form of force). The women may of course have lied, wishing to excuse themselves in the eyes of their judges, or in their own eyes. After seven or eight months of brooding over—of replaying in their mind the circumstances that led to their predicament—the temptation to shift the blame onto their false lovers must have been overwhelming. Yet the very fact that they felt compelled to make this kind of lie indicates, I think, how widespread were the notions of female modesty and masculine initiative in sexual matters and how guilty women would have felt if they had in fact violated them.

Thus women probably entered into illicit relationships burdened with guilt, and probably also oppressed by a fear of becoming pregnant, although this is more difficult to document from the *déclarations*. Whether these women feared pregnancy depends of course on whether birth control was widely practiced. This is a matter of much controversy at the moment. It is generally accepted that within marriage birth control through *coitus interruptus* was used only rarely, if at all, by the lower classes, especially in the south of France, in the eighteenth century, although its use increased in the century's last decades. But recently Flandrin has suggested that the religious prohibitions against birth control that discouraged its use applied only to its practice within marriage, and that its use in illicit affairs may have been widespread.[73] If this were true, it would greatly change our notions

72 A.D. (Aix), XXH, E50, Déclarations de grossesse, 1785–86.
73 Jean-Louis Flandrin, "Contraception, marriage, et relations amoureuses dans l'Occident chrétien," *Annales: E.S.C.*, XXIV (1969), 1370–1390; "Mariage tardif et vie

about female sexuality in this period, for it would mean that the women who made *déclarations* were only a hapless few too unsophisticated to insist that their partners practice birth control, and that most women in eighteenth-century France could indulge in illicit sex with impunity. But it is unlikely that Flandrin is correct. As his critics have pointed out, if the lower classes practiced birth control outside marriage, why on earth did they not carry over their expertise into the marriage bed?[74] Further, this form of birth control depends on masculine cooperation, and thus would entail a man's concern for his sexual partner that seems to be missing in most illicit relationships of the period. Finally, there is the evidence of the *déclarations* themselves. Admittedly, using the statements of women who so obviously did not practice birth control to argue that it probably was not practiced among the lower classes as a whole has some logical pitfalls. But it seems significant that the *déclarations* show nothing that would suggest that the pregnancies they record occurred when birth control was tried but failed. There is only one case in which the woman states that she thought she would not become pregnant; that concerned a hospital nurse who had an affair with an invalid patient.[75] And despite all the false promises that these men made, only one promised his partner that she would not become pregnant.

Therefore there is no solid evidence that birth control was widely used in illicit relationships. A woman probably entered such a relationship knowing that she stood a good chance of becoming pregnant. How good a chance we do not know. Flandrin suggests that on the average 8 out of every 100 acts of intercourse result in pregnancy, but this figure is for modern women.[76] Doubtless the malnutrition and generally poor health of working-class women in Old Regime France lowered the figure for them. A woman could obviously carry on an affair and escape pregnancy. But the possibility of pregnancy was always there.

Most women must have realized that the consequences of an illegitimate pregnancy were invariably disastrous. An illegiti-

sexuelle: Discussions et hypothèses de recherche," *ibid.*, XXVII (1972), 1351–1378. Flandrin repeats this assertion, although with more caution, in *Familles*, 214–215.

74 André Burguière, "De Malthus à Max Weber: le mariage tardif et l'esprit d'entreprise," *Annales: E.S.C.*, XXVII (1972), 1131.

75 A.D. (Aix), XXH, E34, Déclarations de grossesse, 1747–51.

76 Flandrin, "Mariage tardif et vie sexuelle," 1375.

mate pregnancy brought shame to the woman involved and to her family. In the *déclarations* women repeatedly state that they left home and came to the city to have their children to prevent their parents from knowing about their pregnancy or to keep disgrace from their families. And as we have said, illicit pregnancy brought in its train not only disgrace but unemployment, and it often set women on a downward path toward prostitution. Thus, for the lower-class women of Old Regime France, illicit sex seems to have meant frequent brutality, possible pregnancy, and consequent unemployment, disgrace, and damnation. Therefore it is hard to imagine that they would cherish romantic illusions about illicit sex, or use it as a means of self-expression. Whatever may have caused the rise in illegitimacy in the late eighteenth century, it was apparently not a change in women's attitudes toward sex.

APPENDIX I

Table 1   Social Status of the Fathers of the Women Who Made *Déclarations*

	1727–49		1750–89	
	TOTAL	%	TOTAL	%
Noble	0	0	2	.1
Bourgeois	61	8.4	68	4.7
Shopkeeper, master artisan	70	9.6	65	4.5
Artisan	190	26.1	359	24.7
Wage laborer	11	1.5	41	2.8
Substantial peasant	81	11.1	151	10.4
Agricultural laborer	278	38.2	643	44.3
Servant	10	1.4	20	1.4
Government employee	1	.1	26	1.8
Soldier	5	.6	28	1.9
Prisoner	4	.5	2	.1
Other	17	2.3	46	3.2
	728		1,451	

SOURCE: A.D. (Aix), XXH, G28–33, XXH, E33–34, 40, 43–52.

Table 2 Social Status of Putative Fathers of Illegitimate Children

	1727–49		1750–89	
	TOTAL	%	TOTAL	%
Churchmen	3	.3	2	.2
Nobles	26	3.0	44	3.3
Bourgeois	164	18.9	176	13.3
Shopkeepers	59	7.0	90	6.8
Artisans	141	16.2	346	26.1
Wage laborers	33	3.8	64	4.8
Substantial peasants	47	5.4	98	7.4
Agricultural laborers	77	8.8	214	16.1
Servants	233	26.8	198	14.9
Government employees	38	4.4	27	2.0
Soldiers	45	5.2	66	5.0
Prisoners	2	.2	2	.2
	868		1,327	

SOURCE: A.D. (Aix), XXH, G28–33, XXH, E33–34, 40, 43–52.

Table 3 Occupations of Unwed Mothers

	1727–49		1750–89	
	TOTAL	%	TOTAL	%
Servant	327	60.9	306	55.4
Widow	100	18.6	86	15.6
Wife	27	5.0	11	2.0
Laundress	5	.9	2	.4
Textile worker	6	1.1	12	2.2
Shop girl	8	1.5	19	3.4
Day laborer	4	.7	8	1.4
Farm servant	11	2.0	19	3.4
Harvest hand	11	2.0	40	7.2
Inn servant	25	4.7	38	6.9
Prisoner	7	1.3	1	.2
Beggar, handicapped	1	.2	6	1.1
Other	5	.9	4	.7
	537		552	

SOURCE: A.D. (Aix), XXH, G28–33, E33–34, 40, 43–52.

Table 4 Age Distribution of Unwed
Mothers

	1727–49	1750–89
Under 15	1	2
15–19	80	185
20–24	326	672
25–29	195	383
30–34	121	178
35–39	45	87
40+	3	11
Average	24.8	23.9
Median	24	24
Total	771	1,518

SOURCE: A.D. (Aix), XXH, G28–33, E33–34, 40,
43–52.

APPENDIX II

Table 1 Geographical Distribution of Women in Various Types of
Relationships, 1727–49

	RURAL	RURAL–URBAN	URBAN	TOTAL
Master–servant	10	23	3	36
Other relationships of inequality	66	88	39	193
Servant–servant	19	87	18	124
Other lower class relationships	142	164	99	405
Rape highly probable	9	1	3	13
Promiscuity highly probable	4	17	4	25
Total	250	380	166	796
Total Sample	1,142			
Chi square 10 df = 59.4, p < .001				

N.B. "Rural" means those women who were born and continued to live in a small town
(under approximately 5,000 in population) until they made their *déclaration*; "rural to
urban" refers to those women born in a rural area who conceived their babies in a large
town; and "urban" means those women who were born and continued to live in urban
areas.
SOURCE: A.D. (Aix), XXH, G28–31; XXH, E33–34

Table 2 Age Distribution of Women in Various Types of Relationships, 1727–49

	−15	15–19	20–24	25–29	30–34	35+	TOTAL
Master–servant	0	4	19	7	3	1	34
Other inequality	0	32	74	24	24	6	160
Servant–servant	0	7	38	48	15	6	114
Other lower class	1	20	124	95	59	53	352
Rape probable	0	3	3	4	2	0	12
Promiscuity probable	0	5	10	5	2	0	22
Total	1	71	268	183	105	66	694

Total sample   1,142

Chi square, 25 df = 82.9, p < .001

SUBCATEGORIES OF RELATIONSHIPS OF EQUALITY

	−15	15–19	20–24	25–29	30–34	35+
Rural women	1	6	40	27	22	11
Rural–urban	0	8	54	43	24	35
Urban	0	6	30	25	13	7

SOURCE: A.D. (Aix), XXH, G28–31; XXH, E33–34.

Table 3 Patterns of Courtship, 1727–49

	FORCE USED MAN UNKNOWN	FORCE USED MAN KNOWN	LONG COURTSHIP	PROMISE OF MARRIAGE	FORCE & PROMISE OF MARRIAGE	LIVING TOGETHER	TOTAL
Master–servant	0	1	1	5	0	3	10
Other inequality	0	0	0	1	0	0	1
Servant–servant	0	1	0	11	0	0	12
Other lower class	0	1	4	41	3	7	56
Rape probable	0	0	0	0	0	0	0
Promiscuity probable	1	0	0	0	0	0	1
Total	1	3	5	58	3	10	80
Total Sample	1,142						

This sample is too small to be statistically significant. I have drawn on it because it is the only information we have about methods of courtship in this period. A larger sample from the years after 1750 (Table 7) shows that courtship patterns do vary significantly with the type of relationship.

Table 4   Lengths of Relationships, 1727–49

	ONCE	UNDER 6 MONTHS	6 MONTHS +	TOTAL
Master–servant	0	6	6	12
Other inequality	1	13	5	19
Servant–servant	0	9	6	15
Other lower class	2	40	10	52
Rape probable	2	3	0	5
Promiscuity probable	0	1	1	2
Total	5	72	28	105
Total Sample	1,142			

Chi square 10 df = 25.5, p < .01

SUBCATEGORIES OF RELATIONSHIPS OF EQUALITY

	ONCE	UNDER 6 MONTHS	6 MONTHS +
Rural women	2	11	3
Rural–urban	0	14	3
Urban	0	15	4

SOURCE: A.D. (Aix), XXH, G28–G31; XXH, E33–34

Table 5   Geographical Distribution of Relationships, 1750–89

	RURAL	RURAL–URBAN	URBAN	TOTAL
Master–servant	43	14	6	63
Other inequality	131	70	79	280
Servant–servant	50	46	11	107
Other lower class	584	313	259	1,156
Rape probable	69	7	8	84
Promiscuity probable	46	27	9	82
Total	923	477	372	1,772
Total Sample	1,859			

Chi square, 10 df = 70.6, p < .001

SOURCE: A.D. (Aix), XXH, G32–G33; XXH, E40, E43–52.

Table 6   Age Distributions of Relationships, 1750–89

	−15	15–19	20–24	25–29	30–34	35+	TOTAL
Master–servant	0	9	36	11	2	1	59
Other inequality	0	46	103	66	29	18	262
Servant–servant	0	7	45	37	12	3	104
Other lower class	2	120	465	251	129	69	1,036
Rape probable	1	12	24	13	9	11	70
Promiscuity probable	0	8	29	21	10	3	71
Total	3	202	702	399	191	105	1,602

Total Sample   1,859

Chi square, 25 df = 52.4, p < .01

SUBCATEGORIES OF RELATIONSHIPS OF EQUALITY

	−15	15–19	20–24	25–29	30–34	35+
Rural women	1	46	224	110	68	41
Rural–urban	0	22	131	89	36	20
Urban	1	52	110	52	25	8

SOURCE: A.D. (Aix), XXH, G32–G33; XXH, E40, E43–52.

Table 7 Courtship Patterns in Relationships, 1750–89

	FORCE USED MAN UNKNOWN	FORCE USED MAN KNOWN	LONG COURTSHIP	PROMISE OF MARRIAGE	FORCE & PROMISE OF MARRIAGE	LIVING TOGETHER	TOTAL
Master-servant	0	3	3	2	0	1	9
Other inequality	0	6	8	15	2	2	33
Servant-servant	0	1	7	14	5	0	27
Other lower class	0	6	51	99	32	10	198
Rape probable	26	2	0	0	1	0	29
Promiscuity probable	1	0	0	2	0	1	4
Total	27	18	69	132	40	14	300

Total Sample 1,859

Chi-square, 25 df = 295.2, p < .001

SUBCATEGORIES OF RELATIONSHIPS OF EQUALITY

	FORCE USED MAN UNKNOWN	FORCE USED MAN KNOWN	LONG COURTSHIP	PROMISE OF MARRIAGE	FORCE & PROMISE OF MARRIAGE	LIVING TOGETHER
Rural women	0	4	48	61	28	5
Rural–urban	0	0	2	20	2	4
Urban	0	1	1	18	2	1

SOURCE: A.D. (Aix), XXH, G32–G33; XHH, E40, E43–52.

Table 8 Lengths of Relationships, 1750–89

	ONCE	UNDER 6 MONTHS	6 MONTHS +	TOTAL
Master–servant	0	9	4	13
Other inequality	3	24	4	31
Servant–servant	1	19	4	24
Other lower class	6	88	29	123
Rape probable	46	4	0	50
Promiscuity probable	4	15	0	19
Total	60	159	41	260

Total Sample

Chi square, 10 df = 176.8, p < .001

SUBCATEGORIES OF RELATIONSHIPS OF EQUALITY

	ONCE	UNDER 6 MONTHS	6 MONTHS +
Rural women	5	54	16
Rural–urban	1	17	7
Urban	0	17	6

SOURCE: A.D. (Aix), XXH, G32–G33; XXH, E40. E43–52.

Journal of Interdisciplinary History, ix:2 (Autumn 1978), 309–321.

Comment and Controversy

A Case of Naiveté in the Use of Statistics

The Editors:

For the past ten years I have held views about the sexual history of the West which conflict with those of Edward Shorter, and since I am not sure that my consideration of the growth of illegitimacy as evidence for the growing repression of female sexuality is entirely correct, I was especially interested to read Fairchilds' article, "Female Sexual Attitudes and the Rise in Illegitimacy."[1] I did find some original remarks in it, which ought to be compared with the results of other studies on the *déclarations de grossesse,* either in cities such as Grenoble, Lille, Lyon, Nantes, (and Carcassonne,) or in small towns in the French Department of the Ardèche, the Aude, the Seine-et-Marne, and the Côtes-du-Nord.[2] But I have not been convinced by her arguments against Shorter. On the contrary, if the figures given by Fairchilds supply a true image of sexual activities outside marriage in Aix-en-Provence and its country-side, it seems to me that this image supports Shorter.[3]

I wonder, indeed, whether Fairchilds is not confusing Shorter's first sexual revolution with his second. It was in the second revolution that girls were no longer marriage-oriented. In the first, "there was a good chance that engaged couples would begin having intercourse fairly early in their courtship" (Shorter, *Modern Family,* 119). If 80.9 percent of the girls having intercourse with men of their own social class intended to marry their sexual partner (Fairchilds, 641), this statistic would support Shorter's view, especially if the proportion of such girls were growing

1 Cissie Fairchilds, "Female Sexual Attitudes and the Rise of Illegitimacy: A Case Study," *Journal of Interdisciplinary History,* VIII (1978), 627–667. For my views, see Jean-Louis Flandrin, *Les Amours paysannes, XVI°–XIX° siècles* (Paris, 1975), 229–231, 243, 246.
2 Solange Sapin and Monique Sylvoz, "Les Rapports sexuels illégitimes au XVIII° siècle à Grenoble d'après les déclarations de grossesse," unpub. M.A. thesis (University of Grenoble, 1969); Alain Lottin, "Naissances illégitimes et Filles-Mères à Lille au XVIII° siècle," *Revue d'Histoire Moderne et Contemporaine,* XVII (1970), 278–322; Annick Thivollier and Pierre Laroque, "Filles-mères et naissances illégitimes à Lyon au XVIII° siècle," unpub. M.A. thesis (University of Lyon II, 1971); Jacques Depauw, "Amour illégitime et société à Nantes au XVIII° siècle," *Annales,* XXVII (1972), 1155–1182, trans. in R. Forster and O. Ranum (eds.), *Family and Society* (Baltimore, 1976), 145–191; see also Depauw, "Immigration féminine, professions féminines et structures urbaines à Nantes au XVIII° siècle," *Enquêtes et Documents publiés par le Centre de Recherches sur l'histoire de la France Atlantique,* II (1973); Alain Molinier, "Enfants trouvés, enfants abandonnés et enfants illégitimes en Languedoc aux XVII° et XVIII° siècles," in Société de Démographie Historique, *Hommage à Marcel Reinhard* (Paris, 1973), 445–473. The series for the Aude, the Seine-et-Marne, and the Côtes-du-Nord have been studied by Marie-Claude Phan; I presented some of the *déclarations* in *Les Amours paysannes,* 215–223.
3 Edward Shorter, *The Making of the Modern Family* (New York, 1975).

and if they began having sexual intercourse and marrying sooner in the late eighteenth century than they had prior to 1750.[4]

As evidence that girls involved in relationships of inequality were hardly consenting to intercourse, Fairchilds emphasizes that they were young, whereas in relationships of equality, which could lead to marriage, one finds mainly mature girls. But after 1750 this difference in age at pregnancy had dropped considerably, which suggests that the difference between the two types of sexual affairs had become obliterated. This fact, either because marriage was possible between lovers of different social classes, or because girls became voluntarily involved in affairs which could not result in marriages, still corroborates Shorter's theories.[5]

I do not think that it is useful to point out the other data supporting Shorter's view in spite of Fairchilds' conclusion, for any reader of the *Modern Family* can find them. What has led me to respond to Fairchilds' article is her surprising representation of some work of mine and of Marie-Claude Phan, my former student. Since this work is little known in America, I would like to show that Fairchilds has misunderstood it, and to point out how debatable are the figures supplied by the *déclaration de grossesse* in Aix-en-Provence.

When Fairchilds refers to my view of contraception (657), she makes five mistakes in a few lines. First, she represents as my recent view what I had said in 1969, whereas I have written several articles and books on the subject from 1969 to 1977. Second, she assumes that "the religious prohibitions against birth control . . . discouraged its use," whereas in my 1969 article I emphasized that "many Christians acquainted with the

---

4 The proportion of such girls grew from 66.5% in 1727–1749 to 71.2% in 1750–1789 (Fairchilds, 635, Table 1; 649, Table 2). Previous to 1750, only 40.8% of these girls were under 25 years of age whereas after this date 56.1% were (from Fairchilds, Tables 2 and 6 in Appendix II). As for the change in age at marriage, it seems to be even more dramatic, according to the figures for Lourmarin presented by Fairchilds on 651. In fact one must consider also the median age, which dropped only from 23.5 in 1726–1755 to 23 in 1756–1785, and the mean age at marriage which rose from 24.3 to 24.4: Thomas F. Sheppard, *Lourmarin in the Eighteenth Century: A Study of a French Village* (Baltimore, 1971), 36–38.

Fairchilds adds that "apparently women were not only marrying at younger ages than ever before, but also more of them were pregnant when they took their marriage vows. In Lourmarin, for example, over 18 percent of the first children of all marriages between 1681 and 1830 were premarital conceptions; in the last decade of the eighteenth century this figure was 34 percent" (653). One must know that prebridal pregnancy in Lourmarin began dropping from 23.3% in 1681–1710 to 10.3% in 1711–1770, then grew to 24.4% in 1771–1800 and 23.9% in 1801–1830: Sheppard, *Lourmarin,* 41, Table II-6. But, given the importance of the Protestants in Lourmarin, these figures may not be really significant from 1685 to 1747.

5 Before 1750, one finds 66.5% of women under 25 years among girls involved in relationships of inequality and only 40.8% in relationships of equality. After 1750 the figures became 60.4% and 56.1% (from Fairchilds, Tables 2 and 6, Appendix II).

doctrine not only did not follow it but did not accept it." Third, she claims that I had said that these religious prohibitions against birth control "applied only to its practice within marriage," whereas I specified that "all authors dealing with the subject unequivocally condemned contraceptive intercourse and that this condemnation made no exception for intercourse occurring extramaritally."[6]

Fourth, she declares that, according to me, contraceptive practices "in illicit affairs may have been widespread" even in centuries when they were not used within marriage. I must confess that at the end of my 1969 article, I suggested this without sufficient explanation. But, replying to Burguière's criticism in 1972, I pointed out that I had not claimed that young people, in the lower classes, practiced coitus interruptus outside marriage and then forgot this practice in their marital life. The evidence of the acceptance of a double standard concerned only the upper classes, and the evidence of the use of withdrawal in these classes concerned married women in adultery. As for young people of the lower classes, thanks to masturbation, petting, and prostitution, they could have sexual pleasure without giving birth to bastards.[7]

Fifth, these theories must be examined in the context of a debate that I had with Le Roy Ladurie and Burguière about the meaning of the French illegitimacy rates. They assumed that the very low rates of illegitimacy in French villages of the seventeenth century were indisputable evidence of continence and sexual repression—an interpretation which Shorter is claiming again, now—and that the growth of illegitimacy in the late eighteenth and the nineteenth centuries revealed the beginning of a sexual liberation.[8] The question was not at all about contraception in the late eighteenth century, since most of the French demographers have admitted that, in this period, even peasants began to practice birth control within marriage. Therefore, since Fairchilds is

6 I quote from the English version of my article, "Contraception, Marriage and Sexual Relations in the Christian West," in Forster and Ranum (eds.), *Biology of Man in Society* (Baltimore, 1975), 25, 41.

7 André Burguière, "De Malthus à Max Weber: le mariage tardif et l'esprit d'entreprise," *Annales*, XXVII (1972), 1128–1139, trans. in Forster and Ranum, *Family and Society;* Flandrin, "Mariage tardif et vie sexuelle: Discussion et hypothèses de recherche," *Annales,* XXVII (1972), 1351–1378. See also Flandrin, "Contraception . . . ," in Forster and Ranum, *Biology of Man,* 46–47, n. 68, n. 69. On contraception and masturbation, see Flandrin "Mariage tardif et vie sexuelle," 1351–1355, 1358–1366. On prostitution, *ibid.,* 1377–1378; Jacques Rossiaud, "Prostitution, jeunesse et société dans les villes du Sud-Est au XV° siècle," *Annales,* XXXI (1976), 289–326. On petting, see Flandrin, *Les Amours paysannes,* 122–127, 191–200, 241–242; *idem,* "Repression and Change in the Sexual Life of Young People in Medieval and Early Modern Times," *Journal of Family History,* II (1977), 196–210.

8 The debate will be found in the sum of the following books and articles: Emmanuel Le Roy Ladurie, *Les Paysans de Languedoc* (Paris, 1966), I, 644, n. 4; Flandrin, "Contraception"; Burguière, "De Malthus à Max Weber"; Flandrin, "Mariage tardif et vie sexuelle"; Shorter, *Modern Family,* esp. 98–108; Flandrin, "Repression and Change."

dealing with contraception in the late eighteenth century, her reference to my argument and to the criticism of Burguière is irrelevant.

This reference is especially surprising since, in *Familles*—a recent book to which she refers—I reacted against the belief of many French demographers and historians about the practice of coitus interruptus in late eighteenth-century France. I stressed, for instance, that this practice implies a sort of domestication of the man by the woman, which domestication, no doubt, did not occur at the same moment in every class, in every kind of sexual affair, and in every region.[9]

On Provence, only one demographic study is published: Sheppard's *Lourmarin*. I do not understand why Fairchilds does not refer to it when dealing with marital fertility, since she did when writing about age at marriage and prebridal pregnancy. Sheppard shows a continuous decline of family size in the late eighteenth century: from 4.9 children in 1726–1755, to 4.2 in 1756–1785, to 3.9 in 1786–1815. This is strong evidence of birth control, especially since the duration of marital life was growing in this period. Thus, the argument of Fairchilds against the likelihood of birth control in illicit affairs seems nonsense to me.[10]

When they declared their pregnancy to the judge, the girls made scarcely any allusion to birth control practices. This is true in Aix-en-Provence as well as elsewhere in France. But sometimes *déclarations de grossesse* can supply other clues such as the frequency of sexual intercourse and the length of the sexual relationship. The interval between first intercourse and the beginning of pregnancy among lovers who have had frequent intercourse should be compared with the interval between marriage and first pregnancy among married couples of the same age. Is such a comparison impossible to carry out in Aix-en-Provence? I do not know. But I am surprised that Fairchilds, when she deals with the possibility of birth control, does not make any allusion to the "many cases" of "long-standing liaison" of which she spoke (638). For example, Catherine Folie had been the mistress of Joseph Richaud for eleven years when she declared her first pregnancy. So long a period of sterility in a girl who was not definitively sterile is very strange: among the 1,239 married women of Meulan whose birth intervals we do know, I find none who had had her first child more than 7.5 years after marriage. Yet, it is certain that birth control was practiced among many of these married women in Meulan after 1750.[11]

Other facts reported in Fairchilds' article could indicate that contraception or abortion were practiced in Aix-en-Provence more frequently in the late eighteenth century than previously. For instance, if we assume that birth control was more frequent in the towns than in the countryside—which is likely—that could explain the growing proportion of

9 Flandrin, *Familles: parenté, maison sexualité dans l'ancienne société* (Paris, 1976), 214–217.
10 Sheppard, *Lourmarin*, 37–38.
11 Marcel Lachiver, *La population de Meulan du XVII° au XIX° siècle* (Paris, 1969), Table VIII, 275–312.

girls impregnated in the countryside and the declining proportion of girls impregnated in the city. If we assume that withdrawal was practiced first among the upper classes—which is likely too—that could explain the declining proportion of girls impregnated by men of the upper classes, more especially as we know that many of the known relationships of inequality "were long-standing liaisons" such as that of Catherine Folie and Joseph Richaud.[12] Finally, if we admit the assertion, made frequently in the late eighteenth century, that domestic service was the school of vice, we should not be surprised by the declining proportion of girls impregnated by male servants. I do not know if these facts resulted from the rise in contraceptive practices, and I do know that there are other likely explanations of them; but Fairchilds should have examined these hypotheses when dealing with the problem of contraception, rather than using rhetorical arguments to prove that contraception was not practiced.

I am surprised, too, by another reference to me, where Fairchilds considers "how good a chance" a woman had of becoming pregnant when entering into an illicit affair. "Flandrin suggests," she writes, "that on the average 8 out of every 100 acts of intercourse result in pregnancy, but this figure is for modern women. Doubtless the malnutrition and generally poor health of working-class women in Old Regime France lowered the figure for them" (658).

Here, again, her reference to me is irrelevant and she distorts what I have said. Many demographers have studied the risk of pregnancy according to sexual frequency and, since I am not an authority in this field, Fairchilds should have referred to their studies. From these studies of a very difficult problem, she would have found that, among modern women who do not practice birth control, the risk of pregnancy, *on average,* is much lower than 8 / 100. She would also have learned how doubtful is the effect of malnutrition on fertility.

In my 1972 article, I only tried to show that the *déclarations de grossesse* supply a statistically wrong image of the actual sexual activities outside marriage—a difficulty that Fairchilds prefers not to examine. Taking as an example the *déclarations de grossesse* from Grenoble, I wrote: "Let's admit, *since we are only trying to make clear a procedure,* that the girls told what really happened; let's admit, too, *provisionally,* the table on risks of pregnancy according to sexual frequency which J. Bourgeois-Pichat set up. One simple act of intercourse would stand 8 chances out of 100 of resulting in pregnancy. This means that the 137 affairs of this type having resulted in pregnancy may be considered as the known part of a much larger number of affairs of the same type. This number would be 137 × 100 / 8 = 1,713 rapes or other affairs with a single act of

12   Girls impregnated in the countryside grew from 17.8% to 33.0%; girls impregnated by men of the upper classes declined from 28.7% to 19.4% (Fairchilds, 635, Table 1; 649, Table 2).

intercourse." I then emphasized that Bourgeois-Pichat was "quite conscious of the theoretical character of his table," and that "actually the risks of pregnancy are much lower, even without any contraceptive practices." If pregnant girls had spoken the truth, there must have been a good many more than the 1,713 affairs of this type in early eighteenth-century Grenoble.[13]

I do not understand why, referring to my article, having such data as those from Grenoble available, trusting them more than I did, and daring to speculate about risks of pregnancy, Fairchilds did not go as far as I did five years ago. Whatever the actual risk of pregnancy in the eighteenth century, it was obviously lower in short-term encounters than in long-standing liaisons, if birth-control were not practiced, as she assumes. Therefore, the proportion of short-term encounters in the whole mass of sexual affairs is certainly much underestimated by figures set up from the *déclarations de grossesse,* in her Tables 1 and 2 (635, 649). Here was the main argument against Shorter's theories, especially since, in Aix-en-Provence, the proportion of rapes and other short-term encounters had been growing in the late eighteenth century. It appears that Fairchilds did not understand this point.

More important for her article is her misunderstanding of the study by Phan of the legal aspect of the *déclarations de grossesse* to which she refers in note 8.[14] First, it is clear, from the edict of Henri II itself, that it "did not oblige [girls] to make a formal *déclaration de grossesse*" (Phan, 76), which is the opposite of what Fairchilds claims in note 8.

Second, after 1556 there was no royal edict ordering girls to declare their pregnancies to a specified judge, so that "officers of justice had no right to constrain girls declaring their pregnancy" (Phan, 78, 77). They had no right, "except to exhort girls to make a *déclaration* or to order the vicars to exhort them" (note 122). Therefore, *déclarations de grossesse* were not "required by the French law," whereas Fairchilds asserts that they were (Fairchilds, 630).

Third, the pregnant girls were allowed to declare their pregnancies to any judge, even far from their residence, which means that the purpose of the law was not "that the humiliation involved in making a *déclaration* would discourage repetition of the sin," in contradiction to what Fairchilds writes in note 8. They were even allowed to make their declaration to a notary, and we know that they often did so, for instance in Grenoble. Declaration to the vicar was also common practice, although it was contested on legal grounds; and we know that more and more girls, in the late eighteenth century, made no declaration at all, either because of the growing indulgence of the judges toward the *recel de grossesse,* or because of "the development of the practice of being

---

13 Flandrin, "Mariage tardif et vie sexuelle," 1375–1377, n. 56.
14 Phan, "Les Déclarations de grossesse en France (XVIᵉ–XVIIIᵉ siècles): Essai institutionnel," *Revue d'Histoire Moderne et Contemporaine,* XXII-1 (1975), 61–88.

delivered in the house of a midwife." Midwives, indeed, were considered sworn witnesses. Besides, they took care of everything, offered children to be baptized, and then brought them either to a wet nurse or to the foundling hospital, according to the wealth of the mother or the attitude of her lover.[15]

Thus, the girls who declared their pregnancies in a city such as Aix-en-Provence were not all of those who either were delivered in the city or had been impregnated in it—to say nothing of the whole mass of those who had had sexual intercourse outside marriage. In the city of Lyon, for instance, only 27.7 percent of the women who were delivered at the Hotel Dieu, in 1727, had declared their pregnancies to the baillif of Lyon; and, in the years 1770, 1771, and 1772, there were only 10 percent of them.[16] I might hope that the proportion is better for Aix-en-Provence which is not so big a city; but Fairchilds has made no effort to prove this, and she seems to ignore the problem.

The problem is evident in Aix-en-Provence, at least for the declarations of the late eighteenth century: their number was declining while the number of illegitimate births was probably growing, as Fairchilds herself asserts.[17] This situation makes the results of her study dubious, because, whether on the basis of their social characteristics, or on the basis of their types of love affairs, it is unlikely that women who did not declare their pregnancies would be similar to those who did declare them.

Finally, it is difficult to admit that these *déclarations de grossesse* are "ideally suited for the task of exploring the sexual attitudes of the women who contributed to the rise in illegitimacy"; and I do not think it was a good idea to chose this sample "to test the hypothesis that urbanization and economic modernization lay behind the rise in illegitimacy" (623, 631).

Jean-Louis Flandrin
University of Paris

15 *Ibid.,* 78, 79, 86.
16 Thivollier and Laroque, "Filles-mèreset naissances illègitimes à Lyon," I, 83.
17 As a matter of fact Fairchilds presents no evidence of such a growth. The illegitimacy ratio in Lourmarin began to drop from 2.6 in 1726–1755 to 1.3 in 1756–1785, then grew in 1786–1815, but to 2.5 only. If Lourmarin supplies a good image of trends in Provence, as Fairchilds suggested when dealing with age at marriage and pre-bridal pregnancy, Provence would not be a good place for testing Shorter's views on the rise of illegitimacy in France and in Europe.

A Reply

The Editors:

I welcome this opportunity to reply to Flandrin's criticisms of my article, "Female Sexual Attitudes and the Rise in Illegitimacy," although I must say that I am rather surprised that Flandrin, rather than Edward Shorter, was the one to mount the first attack against it.[1] I am surprised because it seems to me that Flandrin and I share virtually the same views on the nature of female sexual attitudes during the late eighteenth century, views which are directly opposite to those of Shorter. In his latest article Flandrin says:

> I must emphasize that, in the eighteenth and nineteenth, as in earlier centuries, no woman became an unwed mother by choice: every unwed mother would have preferred to have intercourse and children within marriage. Thus, the rise of illegitimacy in this age is not in any sense evidence of women's sexual liberation: on the contrary it seems to be evidence of greater difficulty in effecting marriage with the men they had intercourse with.[2]

As readers of my article will note, this is precisely the point that I tried to make, in opposition to Shorter's suggestion that it was a newly emancipated attitude toward sex among women which fueled the rise in illegitimacy.

But despite our identity of views, Flandrin has chosen to criticize my work. The points that he has raised seem to me to fall into these categories: (1) that I misread or deliberately distorted his work and that of his student, Marie-Claude Phan; (2) that I ignored evidence in my sample which suggests that birth control was widely practiced in illicit relationships in the seventeenth and eighteenth centuries; and (3) that my sample was inadequate to test Shorter's notions about illegitimacy, and that even if it were adequate, what it showed supported rather than refuted Shorter's hypotheses. Let us take each of these points in turn.

1. On the question of distortion, let me say that I have nothing but respect for Flandrin's scholarship, especially for *Familles*, a sensitive and thought-provoking study which anyone interested in family history or the history of sexual attitudes will find rewarding.[3] If I have not done full justice to his ideas, it was due to lack of space, not malice. Flandrin's notions about sexuality among the lower classes are far-ranging and subtle and they have evolved considerably over the years, much as Shorter's have. To do full justice to them would take an article devoted

---

1 Cissie Fairchilds, "Female Sexual Attitudes and the Rise of Illegitimacy: A Case Study," *Journal of Interdisciplinary History*, VIII (1978), 627–667.

2 Jean-Louis Flandrin, "Repression and Change in the Sexual Life of Young People in Medieval and Early Modern Times," *Journal of Family History*, II (1977), 196–210, quotation from 203.

3 *idem, Familles: parenté, maison, sexualité dans l'ancienne société* (Paris, 1976).

only to that. I seized upon and discussed only the point—the possibility that birth control was practiced in illicit affairs—which was most relevant to my study.

The alleged misreading of Phan's work on the legal aspects of the *déclarations* will be discussed below.

2. The suggestion that my sample shows evidence that birth control was widely practiced in illicit relationships seems to me to be the most important issue raised by Flandrin's critique. In this regard Flandrin makes three points. He suggests first, that I should have made some attempt to analyze the interval between first coitus and pregnancy among the women of my sample, to see if contraception may have been employed. Second, he suggests that the long-standing liaisons found in my sample among relationships of inequality show that birth control was used by members of the upper classes in their extramarital liaisons. Third, Flandrin suggests that the gradual spread of birth control may have caused the changes which I found after 1750 in the types of relationships in my sample: that *this* was the cause of the decline of cases of relationships of inequality, of servant-servant relationships, and of relationships among the urban lower classes after 1750.

As to the first of Flandrin's points, the interval between first coitus and pregnancy, it would be useful if we could determine it. Unfortunately it is impossible to do so from my sample. In my *déclarations* the woman often stated how long her courtship had lasted, but it is not clear whether this referred to the interval since she first had become acquainted with her lover or the interval since they first had had intercourse. In some *déclarations* it seems to mean the first, in others the second. It is for this reason that I analyzed the length of "courtship," but did not try to be more specific.

As to the second of Flandrin's points, it is certainly possible that the number of long-standing liaisons which I found among my relationships of inequality indicate that birth control was practiced by upper-class men in their illicit relationships. But that is not necessarily the case. That a woman did not make a *déclaration* until years after her relationship had begun does not prove that contraception was employed. The woman may have borne other children before the one for whom the *déclaration* was made; I cite the case of Jeanne Telene (note 32) as an example. She may have made her earlier *déclarations* in a different town, or under a different name. She may have failed to declare her earlier children. And she may have aborted or miscarried in her earlier pregnancies. All of these seem to me to be more likely than the use of birth control.

In Flandrin's third point, he suggests that the decline in servant-servant relationships after 1750 was also due to the spread of birth control: that domestic service was a "school for vice," the conduit through which birth control lore was spread from the upper to lower classes. This is a most interesting suggestion, which may well be correct. But there are alternative explanations for the decline of servant-servant relationships which seem to me more persuasive. In my article I suggested that it was due to declining numbers of men in service after 1750. But at present I am less inclined to favor this explanation.

I am currently studying domestic servants in Old Regime France. Research on servants in Toulouse has shown a great increase after 1750 in the number of servant couples marrying and leaving service, an increase spurred by the dramatic rise in servants' wages in this period, and by a growth of servants' ambitions to better themselves. Therefore I would now suggest that the numbers of illicit relationships among servants declined because such relationships increasingly resulted in marriage.

As to Flandrin's suggestion that birth control was more likely to be practiced in towns than in the countryside, and that this explained the decline in the number of urban and rise in the number of rural cases in my sample, again this may well be true. But the earlier use of contraception in towns has not yet been proven, largely because no one has as yet undertaken the arduous task of reconstructing families in an urban population. As Flandrin himself points out, the only demographic study done for Provence is Sheppard's study of Lourmarin, a country village.[4] Flandrin chides me for not mentioning Sheppard's evidence that birth control was practiced by some married couples in Lourmarin after the middle of the eighteenth century. But if contraception had spread to the countryside in this period, as Sheppard's evidence suggests, then that destroys Flandrin's argument about the number of urban cases declining because towns and not the countryside practiced birth control after 1750. Flandrin cannot have it both ways.

In sum, Flandrin's hypotheses about the use of birth control in illicit relationships seem to be possible but not probable. The use of birth control in relationships outside marriage is difficult to prove since it leaves no traces on the historical record. But the most telling argument against it is the very rise in illegitimacies in this period. The amount of illicit sex must have been truly staggering if illegitimacies rose at the same time that the use of birth control in illicit relationships was spreading! Also, I would like to repeat a point that I made in my article: what we know about the attitudes of men toward women in illicit relationships makes it unlikely that contraception was used. As Flandrin has stated in his comment, the rise of coitus interruptus implies a "domestication of the man by the woman"; as I have stated, it "entails a man's concern for his sexual partner."[5] But, as I said in my article, there is little in illicit relationships to suggest that such concern was present. The keynote of most was the exploitation of the woman by the man. There was little reason why he should limit his pleasure because of a concern for her health or feelings. The alternative explanations that I sketched

---

4 Thomas F. Sheppard, *Lourmarin in the Eighteenth Century: A Study of a French Village* (Baltimore, 1974).

5 Flandrin, "A Case of Naiveté in the Use of Statistics," *Journal of Interdisciplinary History,* IX (1978), 312; Fairchilds, "Female Sexual Attitudes," 658.

to explain the changes in my sample are more probable than the use of contraception.

3. The final group of Flandrin's criticisms centers around the assertions that my sample is, first of all, inadequate to test Shorter's theories, and second, even if it were, what it shows tends to support rather than refute Shorter's position. Flandrin suggests at the beginning of his critique that I have ignored evidence from my sample which supports the existence of Shorter's so-called "first" sexual revolution, as outlined in *Making of the Modern Family*. Here the sexual revolution of the late eighteenth and early nineteenth centuries is defined as an increase in *premarital* sexual activity. But it should be noted that Shorter has written about "the sexual revolution" many times and defined it in many different ways. The definition in his book is, for example, directly opposite to the one in his article, *"Female Emancipation,"* where it is defined as an increase in sexual activity *undertaken with no thought of marriage*. It is the latter position that I challenged, and I feel justified in having done so because this position still lingers on in his book.[6] In fact, I agree with Shorter's suggestion that the rise in illegitimacy was the result of changing courtship and marriage patterns (as the remarks on page 653 of my article show). The problem is that *Shorter* does not always agree with this position.

Flandrin also suggests that I have ignored the implications of the increase in short-term sexual encounters which my sample shows for the last half of the eighteenth century. Flandrin says that since the risk of pregnancy is obviously lower in short-term encounters than in long-term liaisons, many more short-term encounters must have occurred than show up in my statistics. And since the statistics themselves reveal an increase in this type of relationship, there must have been much more sexual activity among the lower classes than even the rise in illegitimacy figures would indicate. All of this, Flandrin implies, supports Shorter's thesis that more and more women indulged in non-marital sexual activity after 1750.

But I would point out that most of the increase in short-term encounters in my sample occurs in those relationships where rape was probable.[7] Unless we take the often-held masculine view that all women who are raped have somehow "asked for it," a rise in instances of rape cannot be seen as evidence for a new and freer sexual morality among women. Therefore, I do no think that I have ignored evidence favorable to Shorter.

Flandrin is on firmer ground when he suggests that my sample may not be complete enough to show anything of value. Flandrin makes

6 Edward Shorter, *The Making of the Modern Family* (New York, 1975), 119. See the discussion of illegitimacy, 79–98. *Idem,* "Female Emancipation, Birth Control, and Fertility in European History," *American Historical Review,* LXXVIII (1973), 605–640.
7 They increase from 1–6% to 4–7% of the total cases: Fairchilds, "Female Sexual Attitudes," 649, Table 2.

three points in this regard. First of all, he suggests that I have ignored the work of Phan on the legal aspects of the *déclarations*. Since Phan showed that they were not "required" by law, and were enforced less and less strictly in the last half of the eighteenth century, my sample may include only a small proportion of all unwed mothers. In a related criticism, Flandrin chides me for not attempting to discover how many of the unwed mothers who were delivered at the Hôtel-Dieu in Aix had actually made *déclarations,* the implication again being that there were large numbers of unwed mothers who escaped my sample. Finally, Flandrin points out that since the number of *déclarations* in my sample declines after 1764, when the number of illegitimacies was probably increasing, the results of my study are "very dubious."

Let me say at the outset that no one is more conscious of the deficiencies of my sample than I am. But I think only the last of Flandrin's points is valid. As to the legal background of the *déclarations,* I based my remarks about this not only on Phan's work but also on that of Sabatier (see note 11 of my article), who discussed how the edict about *déclarations* was enforced in Provence. Sabatier shows that every effort was made to see that every unwed mother declared her pregnancy.[8] While some women doubtless avoided making *déclarations* and therefore escaped my sample, there is no reason to think that there was wholesale evasion of the law. And this is true even for the period after 1750. Officials may have been even more strict in enforcing the edict in that period, for by then the local communities in Provence had financial responsibility for the care of unwed mothers, and accurate *déclarations* were necessary for the proper apportioning of the financial burden.

As for my failure to discover how many unwed mothers gave birth at the Hôtel-Dieu in Aix without making a *déclaration,* I confess that I do not see how this can be done. The hospital registers, as I remember them, show only the names of patients admitted, not the reason for their admittance, and there are no separate registers for babies born out of wedlock. It would be possible to calculate the number of *enfants-trouvés* (abandoned children) in Aix each year, but since many of them were legitimate children abandoned by parents who could not afford to care for them, that would not be useful.[9] Again, there is every reason to believe that my sample is as complete as possible, at least until the 1760s.

After that date, there were many *déclarations* which no longer survive, as Flandrin points out. This does make the validity of my sample doubtful. But I would point out (a) that I revealed its short-comings to my readers, so that they could make their own judgments about the value of my work, and (b) that my real concern was less to disprove Shorter quantitatively than to distinguish varieties of relationships which

8 Nicole Sabatier, *L'Hôpital St.-Jacques d'Aix-en-Provence, 1519–1789* (Aix, 1964), III.
9 Fairchilds, *Poverty and Charity in Aix-en-Provence* (Baltimore, 1976), 83–85, deals with *enfants trouvés* in Aix.

might have led to illegitimacies, and to find out something about sexual practices and attitudes among lower-class women. It seems to me that the most important historical question involved in this debate is not why illegitimacy rose but, instead, the broader one of lower-class sexual attitudes and practices in general.

At present there are two opposing views of the nature of lower-class sexuality in early modern Europe: Shorter's and Flandrin's. Shorter sees a strict repression of sexual impulses until the liberating influence of his "sexual revolution," while Flandrin sees a multifaceted sexuality among the lower classes becoming not less but more repressed in the seventeenth and eighteenth centuries. The problem with both of these positions is lack of evidence. The dubiousness of Shorter's "liberation" leads one to doubt the repression that had supposedly gone before, but Flandrin's examples of sexual experiences (petting, masturbation, etc.) are ones which leave few traces for the historian. Given this situation, I think that the *déclarations de grossesse* can make a unique contribution to the question of sexual practices and attitudes, since they are a source in which one segment of the lower class actually described its sexual experiences. I hope that my work, imperfect though it is, will stimulate other historians to use the *déclarations,* not as the French have done, merely to quantify characteristics, such as the age and geographical origin of unwed mothers, but instead as I have done, to trace varieties of sexual experiences and attitudes.[10] I would suggest a suspension of polemics until more research is completed. When more is known about how people actually *behaved,* questions like why illetigimacy began to rise in the late eighteenth century will be easily answered.

Cissie C. Fairchilds
Syracuse University

10　To be fair, I should note that Flandrin pioneered this sort of analysis in *Les Amours paysannes (XVI-XIXe siècles),* (Paris, 1975).

Journal of Interdisciplinary History VI:3 (Winter 1976), 447–476.

Louise A. Tilly, Joan W. Scott, and Miriam Cohen

Women's Work
and European Fertility Patterns

During the nineteenth century most commentators on the "condition of the working classes" attributed large families and frequent illegitimacy among the poor to social, economic, or moral pathology. For Engels overpopulated working-class families were the offspring of industrial capitalism. For Malthus they were evidence of imprudence, of an inability to make rational calculations. For both, as for many government investigators and social reformers, high rates of fertility among married and single workers were both indicators and causes of misery and deprivation. Since the nineteenth century, of course, there have been many debates about the effects of industrialization on the standard of living of workers and on their demographic behavior. There have been some studies of family size among occupational groups and there have been attempts to describe and explain changes in working-class fertility patterns. Most of these studies lack the explicit moralizing of the nineteenth-century commentators, although some implicitly retain those biases. Few, however, maintain that large families and numerous bastards were positive developments.[1]

Now Edward Shorter has advanced such an argument. In an intriguing and provocative piece, Shorter speculates that "female emancipation" led to increased rates of legitimate and illegitimate fertility in Western Europe at the end of the eighteenth century.[2] His subject is not economic deprivation; indeed, that is an irrelevant consideration for him. Instead, he maintains that industrialization early led to the sexual emancipation of working-class women by offering employment opportunities outside the home. Work led to

Louise A. Tilly is Assistant Professor of History and Director of Women's Studies Program at the University of Michigan. She is the author of numerous articles on social history. Joan W. Scott is Associate Professor of History at the University of North Carolina, Chapel Hill and the author of *The Glassworkers of Carmaux: French Craftsmen and Political Action in a 19th-Century City* (Cambridge, Mass., 1974). Miriam Cohen is a Ph.D. candidate at the University of Michigan.

The authors would like to thank for their help Charles Tilly, Michael Hanagan, Lawrence Stone, Peter Laslett, Peter Stearns, Robert Lerner, Daniel Scott Smith, Ellen Sewell, Michael Marrus, Anne Bobroff and Kathryn Kish Sklar.

1 Friedrich Engels, *The Condition of the Working Class in England in 1844* (London, 1892); Thomas Malthus, *First Essay on Population 1798* (reprinted, Ann Arbor, 1959).
2 " Female Emanicipation, Birth Control and Fertility in European History," *American Historical Review*, LXXVIII (1973), 605–640.

sexual liberation, according to Shorter, by revolutionizing women's attitudes about themselves: They became individualistic and self-seeking; they rebelled against traditional constraints and sought pleasure and fulfillment in uninhibited sexual activity. In the absence of birth control, heightened sexual activity inevitably meant more children. Indeed, toward the end of the nineteenth century, as information about contraception became available, fertility rates sharply declined.

Shorter's is a novel interpretation with some important contributions to women's history as well as to demographic history. Above all, he must be commended for bringing together hitherto scattered evidence about European fertility patterns. He has established that from about 1750–90 there were widespread increases in illegitimate fertility rates in both urban and rural areas. He has collected evidence to suggest that there were also increases in legitimate fertility, especially among young married women in some areas of Western Europe and the United States. The question of marital fertility, however, is still unresolved, in spite of Shorter's definitive statements about it.[3] In addition, Shorter insists that the social and economic experiences of women are central to fertility changes. In so doing, he implicitly challenges the conventional view of women's history, which sees political emancipation as the source of all other changes in women's lives in the modern world. This view, which echoes some of the more simplistic literature on political development, suggests that a change in political consciousness during the nineteenth century led to political enfranchisement for women in the twentieth century, and, only then, to their expanded social and economic activity. Shorter, on the contrary, points out the social, economic, and demographic changes in women's lives that pre-dated political emancipation by more than 100 years.

Despite these contributions, however, Shorter's article is misleading. It confuses the connections between fertility patterns and women's experience instead of clarifying them. If Shorter accurately describes changes in illegitimate fertility, he nonetheless explains them

3 On illegitimacy see Edward Shorter, "Illegitimacy, Sexual Revolution and Social Change in Modern Europe," *Journal of Interdisciplinary History*, II (1971), 261–269. Shorter's general statement about the rise in illegitimacy is borne out most strongly in large cities and in German rural and urban areas. There is, however, a great deal more variety in French rural areas. On marital fertility see Shorter, "Female Emancipation," 633–640. As noted in the text, the marital fertility figures are incomplete. Some are ambiguous; others contradict his claims.

incorrectly. Although he is justified in insisting that women's history must be considered by historical demographers, he fails seriously to examine that history. The clarity and simplicity of Shorter's logic may be persuasive, yet the historical evidence that he offers is scant. In fact, his only evidence that attitudes changed is the *consequence* of that presumed change. In other words, increased illegitimacy rates are the only real proof which he has that women's attitudes and sexual behavior did change.

There is, despite Shorter's neglect of it, a growing body of evidence about women's role in pre-industrial and industrial society. This evidence was available to Shorter. We do not claim new and dramatic findings, yet we seriously question both Shorter's premise about the position of pre-industrial women and his central assertion that a change in popular attitudes led to increased illegitimate and, possibly, legitimate fertility.

In this article we first examine Shorter's hypothesis. Then we present the historical evidence about women's work experiences before and during industrialization. Finally, we offer an alternative model to explain fertility changes, which is based on that evidence.

SHORTER'S HYPOTHESIS   When Shorter began writing about illegitimacy, he attributed its increase between 1790 and 1860 to a sexual revolution, but he carefully related sexual behavior to social situations. Social instability, he suggested, would tend to decrease the likelihood that marriage would follow a sexual encounter; in stable social situations, however, marriage more regularly legitimized sexual relationships. The model which he constructed was more complicated than we have described and we have serious disagreements with it; but it is unnecessary here to review it at length. The important point is that in his earlier work Shorter indicated that sexual relationships and marriage patterns (hence, fertility rates) were extremely sensitive to social and economic realities and to changes in them.[4]

In his article in the *American Historical Review*, Shorter has sharpened and simplified this argument. He builds his case by correlating a number of events: industrialization, migration, changes in women's

4 Other articles by Shorter which treat the same question are "Sexual Change and Illegitimacy: The European Experience," in Robert J. Bezucha (ed.), *Modern European Social History* (Lexington, Mass., 1972), 231–269; "Capitalism, Culture and Sexuality: Some Competing Models," *Social Science Quarterly*, LIII (1972), 338–356. See also Shorter, John Knodel, and Etienne van de Walle, "The Decline of Non-Marital Fertility in Europe, 1880–1940," *Population Studies*, XXV (1971), 375–393.

work, changes in fertility rates, etc. He then argues that since they all involve fertility, they can be reduced to a single causal sequence, constructed on a premise about a change in women's attitudes. Structural considerations are pushed aside, and so are alternative explanations. According to Shorter, a change in fertility rates can only mean a change in sexual practices, which has to mean a change in attitudes, particularly of women. The sequence must be linear and direct. As Shorter argues:

> It seems a plausible proposition that people assimilate in the market place an integrated, coherent set of values about social behavior and personal independence and that these values quickly inform the non-economic realm of individual mentalities. If this logic holds true, we may identify exposure to the market place as a prime source of female emancipation.[5]

This statement, as its langugage clearly reveals, is based on a chain of reasoning, not on evidence. Shorter offers nothing to prove that more women worked in the capitalist marketplace in this period. He merely assumes that they did. Similarly, he assumes that women at the end of the eighteenth century had different family roles and attitudes from their predecessors. And he assumes as well that changes in work opportunities immediately changed values.[6] Ideas, in his opinion, instantly reflect one's current economic experience. Shorter employs a mechanistic notion of "value transfer" to explain the influence of changes in occupational structure on changes in collective mentalities: "In the eighteenth and early nineteenth centuries the market economy encroached steadily at the cost of the moral economy, and the values of individual self-interest and competitiveness that people learned in the market were soon transferred to other areas of life."[7]

For Shorter, sexual behavior echoes market behavior at every point. "Emancipated" women gained a sense of autonomy at work that the subordinate and powerless women of pre-industrial society had lacked. That work, created by capitalist economic development,

5 "Female Emancipation," 622.
6 The weakness of Shorter's evidence on these points is striking. For example, the source of his description of peasant and working-class women's roles in traditional society is Helmut Möller's study of the eighteenth-century petty bourgeois family in Germany (*Die kleinburgerliche Familie im 18. Jahrhundert: Verhalten und Gruppenkultur* [Berlin, 1966], 69). For his proposition about the free and easy sexuality of the early nineteenth-century European working class, Shorter draws his evidence from post-World War II West Germany.
7 "Female Emancipation," 621.

necessarily fostered values of individualism in those who participated in it, and individualism was expressed in part by a new desire for sexual gratification. Young women working outside the home, Shorter insists, were by definition rebelling against parental authority. Indeed, they sought work in order to gain the independence and individual fulfillment that could not be attained at home. It follows, in Shorter's logic, that sexual behavior, too, must have been defiant of parental restraint. As the market economy spread there arose a new, libertine, proletarian subculture "indulgent of eroticism." Once married, the independent young working women engaged in frequent intercourse because they and their husbands took greater pleasure in sex. Female "emancipation" thus began among the young and poor. In the absence of birth control, the sexual gratification of single working girls increased the illegitimate birthrate; that of married women (who worked or had worked) inflated the legitimate birthrate. In this fashion Shorter answers a central question of European historical demography. The fertility increase in the late eighteenth century was simply the result of the "emancipation," occupational and sexual, of working-class women.

Shorter then attributes the fall in fertility at the end of the nineteenth century to the diffusion of birth control knowledge and techniques. Middle-class women were the first to use birth control. Later, it was adopted as well by lower-class women "mentally prepared for small families" by their experiences with motherhood and work. Presumably single, lower-class women were even more willing to curb fertility once they knew how. Meanwhile, middle-class women became personally emancipated. The chronological coincidence of the search for individual autonomy, which originated among the lower classes, and of techniques of birth control, known first to the middle classes, caused the late nineteenth-century fertility decline. Shorter concludes by suggesting that the movement for women's political rights was the final outcome of the growth of capitalism, industrialization, and changes in women's work which had started more than a century earlier.

It is now time to examine the historical evidence that Shorter neglected on women's role in pre-industrial society; on the effects of industrialization on women's work and on their attitudes; and on the motives which sent young girls out into the "marketplace" at the end of the eighteenth and beginning of the nineteenth century. None of the evidence that we have found supports Shorter's argument in any way.

Women were not powerless in "traditional" families; they played important economic roles which gave them a good deal of power within the family. Industrialization did not significantly modernize women's work in the period when fertility rates rose; in fact, the vast majority of working women did not work in factories, but at customary women's jobs. Women usually became wage earners during the early phases of industrialization not to rebel against their parents or declare independence from their husbands, but to augment family finances. Indeed, women in this period must be studied in their family settings, for the constraints of family membership greatly affected their opportunities for individual autonomy. No change in attitude, then, increased the numbers of children whom working women bore. Rather, old attitudes and customary behavior interacted with greatly changed circumstances—particularly in the composition of populations—and led to increased illegitimate fertility.

Women eventually shed many outdated priorities, and by the end of the nineteenth century some working women had clearly adopted "modern" life styles. But these changes involved a more gradual and complex adaptation than Shorter implies. The important point, however, is that the years around 1790 were not a watershed in the history of women's economic emancipation—despite the fact that the locus of women's work began to move outside the home. These *were* the crucial years for the increases in fertility in Europe. All of the evidence is not in, by any means; what we offer, however, indicates that in this period, women of the popular classes simply were not searching for freedom or experiencing emancipation. The explanation for changed fertility patterns lies elsewhere.

WOMEN'S PLACE IN "TRADITIONAL" FAMILIES   In the pre-industrial family, the household was organized as a family or domestic economy. Men, women, and children worked at tasks which were differentiated by age and sex, but the work of all was necessary for survival. Artisans' wives assisted their husbands in their work as weavers, bakers, shoemakers, or tailors. Certain work, like weaving, whether carried on in the city or the country, needed the cooperation of all family members. Children and women did the spinning and carding; men ran the looms. Wives also managed many aspects of the household, including family finances. In less prosperous urban families, women did paid work which was often an extension of their household chores: They sewed and made lace; they also took odd jobs as carters, laundresses, and

street cleaners. Unmarried women also became servants. Resourceful-
ness was characteristic of poor women: When they could not find work
which would enable them to contribute to the family income, they
begged, stole, or became prostitutes. Hufton's work on the Parisian
poor in the eighteenth century and Forrest's work on Bordeaux both
describe the crucial economic contribution of urban working-class
women and the consequent central role which these women played
in their families.[8]

In the country, the landowning peasant's family was also the
unit of productive activity. The members of the family worked together, again at sex-differentiated tasks. Children—boys and girls—
were sent to other farms as servants when their help was not needed
at home. Their activity, nonetheless, contributed to the well-being of
the family. They sent their earnings home, or, if they were not paid
wages, their absence at least relieved the family of the burden of
feeding and boarding them. Women's responsibilities included care
of the house, barnyard, and dairy. They managed to bring in small net
profits from marketing of poultry and dairy products and from work
in rural domestic industry. Management of the household and, particularly, of finances led to a central role for women in these families.
An observer in rural Brittany during the nineteenth century reported
that the wife and mother of the family made "the important decisions,
buying a field, selling a cow, a lawsuit against a neighbor, choice of a
future son-in-law." For rural families who did not own land, women's
work was even more vital: From agricultural work, spinning, or
petty trading, they contributed their share to the family wage—the
only economic resource of the landless family.[9]

8 Olwen Hufton, "Women in Revolution, 1789-1796," *Past & Present*, LIII (1971),
93; Alan Forrest, "The Condition of the Poor in Revolutionary Bordeaux," *ibid.*, LIX
(1973), 151-152. See also Natalie Z. Davis, "City Women and Religious Change in
Sixteenth-Century France," in Dorothy Gies McGuigan (ed.), *A Sampler of Women's
Studies* (Ann Arbor, 1973), 21-22; Michael Anderson, *Family Structure in Nineteenth
Century Lancashire* (Cambridge, 1971), 96.
9 Y. Brekelien, *La vie quotidienne des paysans en Bretagne au XIXe siècle* (Paris, 1966), 69.
On the family basis of the peasant economy see Daniel Thorner, Basile Kerblay, and
R. E. F. Smith (eds.), *A. V. Chayanov on the Theory of Peasant Economy* (Homewood,
Ill., 1966), 21, 60; Teodor Shanin, "The Peasantry as a Political Factor," in Shahin (ed.),
Peasants and Peasant Societies: Selected Readings (Harmondsworth, 1971), 241-244;
Basile Kerblay, "Chayanov and the Theory of Peasantry as a Specific Type of Economy,"
in *ibid.*, 151. For Western Europe see "Giunta per la Inchiesta Agraria e sulle condizioni
della classe agricola," *Atti* (Rome, 1882), *passim*; Henri Mendras, *The Vanishing Peasant:
Innovation and Change in French Agriculture* (Cambridge, Mass., 1970), 74-76; Jean-Marie
Gouesse, "Parenté, famille et marriage en Normandie aux XVIIe et XVIIIe siècles,"

In city and country, among propertied and propertyless, women of the popular classes had a vital economic role which gave them a recognized and powerful position within the household. It is impossible to guess what sort of sexual relations were practiced under these circumstances. We *can* say, however, that women in these families were neither dependent nor powerless. Hence, it is impossible to accept Shorter's attempt to derive women's supposed sexual subordination from their place in the pre-industrial household.

WHY WOMEN WORKED   Shorter attributes the work of women outside the home after 1750, particularly that of young, single women, to a change in outlook: a new desire for independence from parental restraints. He argues that since seeking work was an individualistic rebellion against traditionalism, sexual behavior, too, reflected a defiance of parental authority. The facts are that daughters of the popular classes were most often sent into service or to work in the city by their families. Their work represented a continuation of practices customary in the family economy. When resources were scarce or mouths at home too numerous, children customarily sought work outside, generally with family approval.

Industrialization and urbanization created new problems for rural families but generated new opportunities as well. In most cases, families strategically adapted their established practices to the new context. Thus, daughters sent out to work went farther away from home than had been customary. Most still defined their work in the family interest. Sometimes arrangements for direct payment in money or foodstuffs were made between a girl's parents and her employer. In other cases, the girls themselves regularly sent money home. Commentators observed that the girls considered this a normal arrangement—part of their obligation to the family.[10]

Annales E.S.C., XXVII (1972), 1146–1147 and Annexe V, 1153–1154; Martin Nadaud, *Mémoires de Léonard, ancien garçon maçon* (Paris, 1895; reissued, 1948), 130; Michael Drake, *Population and Society in Norway, 1735–1865* (Cambridge, 1969), 137–144.

10   Rudolf Braun, "The Impact of Cottage Industry on an Agricultural Population," in David Landes (ed.), *The Rise of Capitalism* (New York, 1966), 61–63; R.-H. Hubscher, "Une contribution à la connaissance des milieux populaires ruraux au XIXᵉ siècle: Le livre de compte de la famille Flauhaut, 1881–1887," *Revue d'histoire économique et sociale*, XLVII (1969), 395–396; Evelyne Sullerot, *Histoire et sociologie du travail féminin* (Paris, 1968), 91–94; Anderson, *Lancashire* 22; Peter Stearns, "Working Class Women in Britain, 1890–1914," in Martha Vicinus (ed.), *Suffer and Be Still* (Bloomington, Ind., 1972), 110; Marie Hall Ets, *Rosa, The Life of an Italian Immigrant* (Minneapolis, 1970), 138–140; Frédéric Le Play, *Les Ouvriers européens* (Paris, 1855–78), V, 122.

In some cases the conditions of migration for young working girls emphasized their ties to family and in many ways limited their independence. In Italy and France, factory dormitories housed female workers, and nuns regulated their behavior and social lives. In the needle trades in British cities, enterprising women with a little capital turned their homes into lodging houses for piece-workers in their employ.[11] Of course, these institutions permitted employers to control their employees by limiting their mobility and regulating their behavior. The point is not that they were beneficient practices, but that young girls lived in households which permitted them limited autonomy. Domestic service, the largest single occupation for women, was also the most traditional and most protective of young girls. They would be sent from one household to another and thus be given security. Châtelain argues that domestic service was a safe form of migration in France for young girls from the country. They had places to live, families, food, and lodgings and had no need to fend for themselves in the unknown big city as soon as they arrived.[12] It is true that servants often longed to leave their places, and that they resented the exploitation of their mistresses (and the advances of their masters). But that does not change the fact that, initially, their migration was sponsored by a set of traditional institutions which limited their individual freedom.

In fact, individual freedom did not seem to be at issue for the daughters of either the landed or the landless, although clearly their experiences differed. It seems likely that peasant families maintained closer ties with their daughters, even when the girls worked in distant cities. The family interest in the farm (the property that was the birthright of the lineage and not of any individual) was a powerful influence on individual behavior. Thus, farm girls working as domestics continued to send money home. Married daughters working as domestics in Norwegian cities sent their children home to be raised on the farm by grandparents. But even when ties of this sort were not maintained, it was seldom from rebellious motives. Braun describes the late eighteenth-century situation of peasants in the hinterland of Zurich. These peasants were willing to divide their holdings for their children

11 Ets, *Rosa*, 87–115; Italy, Ufficio del Lavoro, *Rapporti sulla ispezione del Lavoro (1 dicembre 1906–30 giugno 1908)* (Milan, 1909), 93–94; Sullerot, *Histoire*, 91–94, 100; Jules Simon, *L'Ouvrière* (Paris, 1871), 53–54. Eileen Yeo and E. P. Thompson, *The Unknown Mayhew* (New York, 1972), 116–180.

12 Abel Châtelain, "Migrations et domesticité feminine urbaine en France, XVIIIe siècle-XXe siècle," *Revue d'histoire économique et sociale*, XLVII (1969), 508.

228 | TILLY, SCOTT, AND COHEN

because of new work opportunities in cottage industry. These young people married earlier than they would have if the farm had been held undivided, and they quickly established their own families. Braun suggests that the young workers soon lost touch with their parents. The process, as he describes it, however, was not rebellion; rather, the young people went into cottage industry to lessen the burden that they represented for the family. These motives were welcomed and encouraged by the parents. Family bonds were stretched and broken, but that was a consequence, not a cause, of the new opportunities for work.[13]

Similarly, among urban artisans, older values informed the adaptation to a new organization of work and to technological change. Initially, artisans as well as their political spokesmen insisted that the old values of association and cooperation could continue to characterize their work relationships in the new industrial society. Artisan subculture in cities during the early stages of industrialization was not characterized by an individualistic, self-seeking ideology, as Thompson, Hufton, Forrest, Soboul, Gossez, and others have clearly shown.[14] With no evidence that urban artisans adopted the values of the marketplace at work, Shorter's deduction about a "libertine proletarian subculture" has neither factual nor logical validity. It seems more likely that artisan families, like peasant families, sent their wives and daughters to work to help bolster their shaky economic situation. These women undoubtedly joined the ranks of the unskilled who had always constituted the urban female work force. Wives and daughters of the unskilled and propertyless had worked for centuries at service and manufacturing jobs in cities. In the nineteenth century there were more of them because the proportions of unskilled propertyless workers increased.

Eighteenth- and early nineteenth-century cities grew primarily by migration. The urban working class was thus constantly renewed and enlarged by a stream of rural migrants. Agricultural change drove rural laborers and peasants cityward at the end of the eighteenth century, and technological change drove many artisans and their families into the ranks of the unskilled. Women worked outside the

13 Drake, *Population*, 138; Braun, "Impact of Cottage Industry," 63–64.
14 Hufton, "Women in Revolution"; Forrest, "Condition of the Poor"; Albert Soboul, *Les Sans-Culottes parisiens en l'an II* (Paris, 1958); Rémi Gossez, *Les Ouvriers de Paris* (Paris, 1967), I; E. P. Thompson, *The Making of The English Working Class* (London, 1963).

home because they had to. Changed attitudes did not propel them into the labor force. Family interest and not self-interest was the underlying motive for their work.

WOMEN'S WORK   What happened in the mid-eighteenth century with the spread of capitalism, the growth of markets, and industrialization? Did these economic changes bring new work experiences for women, with the consequences which Shorter describes? Did women, earning money in the capitalist marketplace, find a new sense of self that expressed itself in increased sexual activity? In examining the historical evidence for the effects on women's work of industrialization and urbanization, we find that the location of women's work did change—more young women worked outside the home and in large cities than ever before. But they were recruited from the same groups which had always sent women to work.

The female labor force of nineteenth-century Europe, like that of seventeenth- and eighteenth-century Europe, consisted primarily of the daughters of the popular classes and, secondarily of their wives. The present state of our knowledge makes it difficult to specify precisely the groups within the working classes from which nineteenth-century women wage earners came. It is clear, however, that changes in the organization of work must have driven the daughters and wives of craftsmen out of the family shop. Similarly, population growth (a result of declining mortality and younger age at marriage due to opportunities for work in cottage industry) created a surplus of hands within the urban household and on the family farm. Women in these families always had been expected to work. Increasingly, they were sent away from home to earn their portion of the family wage.[15]

Shorter's notion that the development of modern capitalism brought new kinds of opportunities to working-class women as early as the middle of the eighteenth century is wrong. There was a very important change in the location of work from rural homes to cities, but this did not revolutionize the nature of the work that most women did. Throughout the nineteenth century, most women worked at traditional occupations. By the end of the century, factory employment was still minimal.

Domestic service, garment-making, and textiles had long been

15   For an elaboration of this see Joan W. Scott and Louise A. Tilly, "Women's Work and the Family in Nineteenth Century Europe," *Comparative Studies in Society and History*, XVII (1975), 36–64.

the chief non-agricultural employers of women. This continued to be the case during the nineteenth century. In France, in 1866, 69 percent of women working outside agriculture were employed in these three fields; in 1896, the figure was 59 percent. In England, the occupational opportunities for women were similarly stable. In the 1840s, Pinchbeck notes, women served in traditional female occupations—the largest percentage were in domestic service, the next largest in textiles, the next in clothing manufacture. In her study of women in the labor force in 1915, Hutchins noted that as late as 1911, two-thirds of working women were in the same three fields: domestic service (including laundry) 35 percent; textiles 19.5 percent; and garment making 15.6 percent.[16]

It is worthwhile to examine the case of England more closely. England was the first country to industrialize and its fertility rates probably rose with industrialization.[17] Yet, contrary to Shorter's assumption that new work experiences for women led to increased illegitimacy, nothing indicates that women's work there changed significantly. During the early phases of British industrialization the proportion of women entering the workforce did not increase; nor did women work in factories in significant numbers in the crucial late eighteenth-century period when fertility rates began to rise. (And it is this factory experience, particularly, that Shorter emphasizes as "liberating.")

Aggregate statistics on the number of women workers before 1841 do not exist, but several studies have shown that opportunities for women to participate in the economy actually shrank with early industrialization. The reorganization of agriculture displaced women who had worked on the family plot. (A portion of these women became wage laborers toward the end of the eighteenth century, but only temporarily. Their numbers declined toward the middle of the nineteenth century as did all employment in agriculture.) In the manu-

16 T. Deldycke, H. Gelders, and J.-M. Limbor, *La Population active et sa structure* (Brussels, 1969), 169. Ivy Pinchbeck, *Women Workers and the Industrial Revolution, 1750–1850* (New York, 1930), 84. Similar distributions can be found in Germany and Italy; see Adna Ferrin Weber, *The Growth of Cities in the Nineteenth Century* (New York, 1967), 375; Louise A. Tilly, "Women at Work in Milan, Italy, 1880–World War I," unpub. paper, read to the American Historical Association (1972). B. L. Hutchins, *Women in Modern Industry* (London, 1915), 84.

17 Shorter, "Female Emanicpation," 633. See also Peter Laslett and Karla Oosterveen, "Long-term Trends in Bastardy in England: A Study of the Illegitimacy Figures in the Parish Registers and in the Reports of the Registrar General, 1461–1960," *Population Studies*, XXVII (1973), 255–286.

facturing sector, the mechanization of cotton spinning at the end of the eighteenth century first deprived women of that age-old occupation. Until the second decade of the next century, women had to compete with children for jobs assisting men who operated the large new machines. It was not until after the power loom was introduced into the factory (after 1820) that opportunities were created for large numbers of women to participate in the factory workforce. The experience of wool workers was similar. As the industry was concentrated into workshops, long before power-driven machinery was introduced, women were excluded from the preparation process. Although some women competed with men as handloom weavers in the early nineteenth century, it was not until the 1860s that the power loom brought many women into the wool factories. Because the mill-based woolen industry was concentrated in Yorkshire and Nottinghamshire, many female domestic wool workers elsewhere were left permanently unemployed.[18] Finally, as a consequence of changes in the organization of craft work, many artisans' wives who had heretofore taken an active part in their husbands' work were deprived of their occupations.

Not all women employed in manufacturing were engaged in textile spinning and weaving. Women's occupations also included millinery, corset, boot- and shoe-making, dress and artificial flower-making, bookbinding, food production and canning, and match-making. Such were the industries which employed women, primarily in London and other cities. In Birmingham, an unusual number of women engaged in small metal trades. In the course of the nineteenth century, many of these activities were moved into small workshops and larger factories, but this happened long after the factory organization of textile production.[19] Thus, it was primarily in the textile industry, and then only after the 1820s, that the number of women factory workers increased.

In England women moved very slowly into "modern occupations." Let us compare the number of women in the British population from 1841 to 1911, the number of women in the labor force outside agriculture as a whole, and the number of women who were occupied in work other than domestic service. Our category for

---

18 Pinchbeck, *Women Workers*, 117–121, 152–153, 155–156; Neil Smelser, *Social Change in the Industrial Revolution: An Application of Theory to the British Cotton Industry* (Chicago, 1959), 184, ff.

19 Edward Cadbury, M. Cecile Matheson, and George Shann, *Women's Work and Wages: A Phase of Life in An Industrial City* (Chicago, 1907), 44–46; Gareth Stedman Jones, *Outcast London* (Oxford, 1971), 83–87. Pinchbeck, *Women Workers*, 315.

modern occupations, it should be noted, is a rough one, including all non-servant, non-agricultural occupations. This includes not only factory jobs, but all manufacturing jobs, in whatever kind of setting, and non-manufacturing jobs, such as those in commerce and the professions. The following facts are evident. First, the number of women in the labor force outside agriculture at the middle of the nineteenth century was relatively small (24.4 percent); the non-agricultural female workforce did not increase apace with the female population after mid-century. In 1841 as in 1891, the largest proportion of women was engaged in domestic and other personal service occupations such as laundering. There was an increase in non-servant occupations between 1841 and 1851 but between 1861 and 1891 servants increased at approximately the same rate as all other occupations. Until 1891, the growth in modern occupations absorbed neither the natural increase in the female population nor the increase of unemployed females which, as noted above, resulted from structural changes in industry and agriculture. In mid-nineteenth-century England, a century after Shorter's supposed revolution in women's work experience, a large proportion of working women were still in domestic service, and most others were still engaged in traditionally organized industries. Throughout the greater part of the nineteenth century, women's factory work was almost exclusively in textiles, and the number of women employed in factories was a small proportion of the entire female work force. The major early effect of industrialization and urbanization on the fields of work open to women was to increase the numbers of women in domestic service, and in the artisan industries which were being transformed by the new division of labor.

In cities, matters were no different. Urban women remained in traditional occupations. Domestic service persisted as the most important, claiming in 1891, one-third of all working women. In 1910, the London County Council reported a similar proportion. The next largest occupation was dressmaking, then laundering and tailoring. Of the manufacturing enterprises, many were still domestic endeavors. A report on women's employment in Birmingham based on the 1901 census showed a relatively high proportion of women in the labor force: 37 percent. Of these, almost half were engaged in domestic service, charring, the professions, or commerce. This meant that even in this manufacturing city, about 20 percent of women were employed in industry, with about half that number still in domestic outwork.[20]

20 Cadbury, Matheson, and Shann, *Women's Work*, 44–45.

Fig. 1 Percentage Participation of Women in the British Labor Force

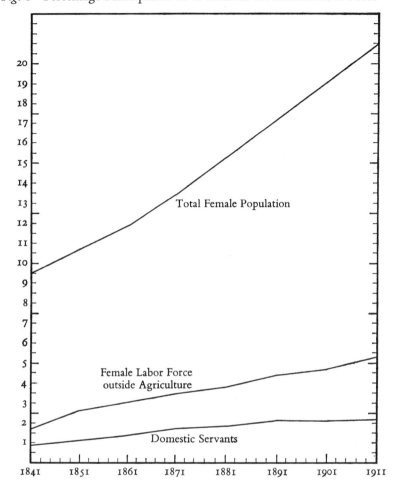

SOURCE: Deldyke et al., *La Population active*, 181–193.

Shorter is also incorrect in his assumption that the working woman was able to live independently of her family because she had the economic means to do so. Evidence for British working women indicates that this was not the case. Throughout the nineteenth century, British working women's wages were considered supplementary incomes—supplementary, that is, to the wages of other family members. It was assumed by employers that women, unlike men, were not responsible for earning their own living. Female wages were always far lower than male. In the Lancashire cotton mills in 1833, where female wages were the highest in the country, females aged 16–21 earned 7/3.5 weekly, while males earned 10/3. Even larger differentials obtained among older workers. In London in the 1880s, there was a similar differential between the average earnings of the sexes: 72 percent of the males in the bookbinding industry earned over 30/- weekly; 42.5 percent of women made less than 12/-. In precious metals, clocks, and watch manufacturing, 83.5 percent of the males earned 30/- or more weekly; females earned 9–12/-. Women in small clothing workshops earned 10–12/- weekly, while women engaged in outwork in the clothing trades made only 4/- a week. In Birmingham, in 1900, the average weekly wage for working women less than age 21 was 10/-, for men 18/-. Women's work throughout this period, as in the eighteenth century, was for the most part unskilled. Occupations were often seasonal or irregular, leaving women without work for many months during the year.[21] Is it possible that there were many single women who could enjoy a life of independence when the majority could not even afford to live adequately on their personal wages?

Finally, throughout the period, British women tended to give up work outside the home when they married, although many worked at home or moved in and out of the labor force when necessary. This demonstrates that women, married or single, were motivated to work by economic necessity and not by a drive for "liberation" in Shorter's sense. We can cite only a few examples here, based mostly on age evidence. In 1833, the bulk of women in the Lancashire cotton mills were between the ages of 16 and 21. In 1841, in six out of seven districts in Lancashire 75 percent of the female workforce in the cotton mills was unmarried. In the woolen mills of the north and in Gloucestershire, 50 percent of working women left the mills after age 21; of those remaining, few were married. Retirement of married women from the labor force was most noticeable in the textile industry. In mill towns, children could be employed at young ages and the family could count on their wages to take the place of the mother's. In London in the 1880s, the greatest number of women in the female workforce were between ages 15 and 25. In 1911, in all of Great Britain only 9.6 percent of the entire married female population was employed.[22]

21 Pinchbeck, *Women Workers*, 193; Charles Booth, *Life and Labour of the People of London* (London, 1895), IV, *passim*; Cadbury, Matheson, and Shann, *Women's Work*, 121; Stedman Jones, *Outcast London*, 83–87.
22 Pinchbeck, *Women Workers*, 219; Booth, *Life and Labour*, IX, 52; Deldycke, et al., *La Population*, 185.

Among the married women who did work, domestic industry provided occupations for the largest number. In East London in the 1880s, Booth's survey found that most employed married women worked at home. In Birmingham, twenty years later, married women were the largest part of the domestic labor force, as indeed married women had been for decades in most countries of Western Europe.[23] In contrast to middle-class women, who could afford servants, the work experience for lower-class wives was neither psychologically nor economically rewarding, except in the sense that it supplemented an inadequate family wage. If these women worked, they were torn between the cares of a mother and those of a worker. It is no wonder that they much preferred to stay home and supervise their own families—a preference amply documented by the labor force statistics.

Women's work from 1750 to 1850 (and much later) did not provide an experience of emancipation. Work was hard and poorly paid and, for the most part, it did not represent a change from traditional female occupations. Those women who traveled to cities did find themselves free of some traditional village and family restraints. But, as we shall see, the absence of these restraints was more often burdensome than liberating. Young women with inadequate wages and unstable jobs found themselves caught in a cycle of poverty which increased their vulnerability. Having lost one family, many sought to create another.

THE ORIGINS OF INCREASED ILLEGITIMACY   The compositional change which increased the numbers of unskilled, propertyless workers in both rural and urban areas and raised their proportion in urban populations also contributed to an increase in rates of illegitimacy. Women in this group of the population always had contributed the most illegitimate births. An increase in the number of women in this group, therefore, meant a greater incidence of illegitimacy.

A recent article by Laslett and Oosterveen speaks directly to Shorter's speculations: "The assumption that illegitimacy figures directly reflect the prevalence of sexual intercourse outside marriage, which seems to be made whenever such figures are used to show that beliefs, attitudes and interests have changed in some particular way, can be shown to be very shaky in its foundations." Using data from Colyton, collected and analyzed by E. A. Wrigley, they argue that

23 Booth, *Life and Labour*, I, *passim*; Cadbury, Matheson, and Shann, *Women's Work*, 14.

one important component in the incidence of illegitimacy is the existence of illegitimacy-prone families, which bring forth bastards generation after generation. Nevertheless, they warn, "this projected sub-society never produced all the bastards, all the bastard-bearers."[24]

The women who bore illegitimate children were not pursuing sexual pleasure, as Shorter would have us believe. Most expected to get married, but the circumstances of their lives—propertylessness, poverty, large-scale geographic mobility, occupational instability, and the absence of traditional social protection—prevented the fulfillment of this expectation. A number of pressures impelled young working girls to find mates. One was the loneliness and isolation of work in the city. Another was economic need: Wages were low and employment for women, unstable. The logical move for a single girl far from her family would be to find a husband with whom she might re-establish a family economy. Yet another pressure was the desire to escape the confines of domestic service, an occupation which more and more young women were entering.

Could not this desire to establish a family be what the domestic servants, described by the Munich police chief in 1815, sought? No quest for pleasure is inherent in the fact that "so many young girls leave service . . . . But they do little real work and let themselves be supported by boyfriends; they become pregnant and then are abandoned."[25] It seems a sad and distorted version of an older family form, but an attempt at it, nevertheless. Recent work has shown, in fact, that for many French servants in the nineteenth century, this kind of transfer to urban life and an urban husband was often successful.[26]

Was it a search for sexual fulfillment that prompted young women to become "engaged" to young men and then sleep with them in the expectation that marriage would follow? Not at all. In rural and urban areas premarital sexual relationships were common.[27] What Shorter interprets as sexual libertinism, as evidence of an in-

24 Laslett and Oosterveen, "Long-term Trends," 257–258, 284.
25 Quoted in Shorter, "Female Emancipation," 618. Sex ratios discussed in Weber, *Growth of Cities*, 285–300, 320, 325–327.
26 Theresa McBride, "Rural Tradition and the Process of Modernization: Domestic Servants in Nineteenth Century France," unpub. Ph.D. diss. (Rutgers University, 1973).
27 Shorter, Knodel, and van de Walle, "Decline of Non-Marital Fertility," 384; Le Play, *Les Ouvriers*, V, 150–154. Pierre Caspard attacks Shorter's notion of a sexual revolution as the cause of increased prenuptial conceptions in "Conceptions prénuptiales et développement du capitalisme dans la Principauté de Neuchâtel (1678–1820)," *Annales E.S.C.*, XXIX (1974), 989–1008.

dividualistic desire for sexual pleasure, is more likely an expression of the traditional wish to marry. The attempt to reconstitute the family economy in the context of economic deprivation and geographic mobility produced unstable and stable "free unions."

Free or consensual unions had two different kinds of consequences for those who entered into them, but both resulted in illegitimate children. One consequence, the more stable, was common-law marriage, a more or less permanent relationship. The other was less stable and involved desertion of the woman, or a series of short-lived encounters, or prostitution. Middle-class observers were most disturbed by the unstable side of consensual union, and especially by the increase in the numbers of abandoned pregnant women and prostitutes.

When asked how she let herself get into difficult and immoral situations, the woman most frequently answered that the man had promised to marry her. In Nantes, in the eighteenth century, information drawn from declarations to midwives at childbirth shows that mothers of illegitimate children were, for the most part, servants and working women. These women testified that promises of work and of marriage usually preceded intercourse with the fathers of their bastards. In Aix in 1787–88, according to Fairchilds, the *declarations de grossesse* show that the vast majority of all illegitimate pregnancies were preceded by promises of marriage. A needleworker explained her plight to Henry Mayhew in 1851: "He told me if I came to live with him he'd care I should not want, and both mother and me had been very bad off before. He said he'd make me his lawful wife . . . ."[28]

The absence of traditional constraints—family, local community, and church—led to the disappointment of many marital expectations. What Shorter deems "freedom" here, in all of its normative implications, is in fact the opposite, for the absence of traditional constraints increased women's vulnerability. Lack of money or a lost job, the opportunity for work in a distant city, all kept men from fulfilling their promises, and the women's families were nowhere at hand to enforce them. Eighteenth-century evidence from Lille, also based on women's declarations during childbirth, shows that most unmarried mothers had

28 Shorter, "Sexual Revolution and Social Change," 258; Jacques DePauw, "Amour illégitime et société a Nantes au XVIIIᵉ siècle," *Annales E.S.C.*, XXVII (1972), 1163–1166; M. Cl. Murtin, "Les abandons d'enfants à Bourg et dans le département de l'Ain à la fin du XVIIIᵉ siècle et dans la première moitée du XIXᵉ," *Cahiers d'histoire*, II (1965), 135–166. Cissie Catherine Fairchilds, "Poverty and Charity in Aix-en-Provence 1640–1789," unpub. Ph.D. diss. (Johns Hopkins University, 1972). Yeo and Thompson, *Mayhew*, 148.

come to the city as textile workers or as servants, all poorly paid occupations. Fully 70 percent of these women came from families broken by the death of at least one parent. The men involved were in professions marked by unstable tenure, such as servants, traveling workers, or soldiers. Lottin concludes that work outside the family weakened traditional family authority and "facilitated the emancipation of the girls." But like Shorter, his evidence for this statement is illegitimate birth statistics only. Lottin's other point seems more likely in light of the evidence about the occupations and backgrounds of the women whom he studied: "All the same, seducers could pursue their ends more easily, because they did not fear an avenging father, often violent, ready to make them pay for the dishonor."[29]

Cobb's sympathetic evocation of lower-class life during Year III of the French Revolution notes that "women and girls born in the provinces were easier to recruit to prostitution and were less protected. (They were also much more exposed to seduction and to unemployment...)... prostitution witnesses for the feminine population as a whole, emphasizes its fluidity, its insecurity, the enormous risks encountered by the provincial girl...." In 1836, in Paris, Parent-Duchâtelet reported that the majority of the prostitutes whom he studied were recent migrants. Almost one third were household servants and many had been initially seduced by promises of marriage and then abandoned, pregnant or with an infant. He also remarked on the instability of women's employment which drove them to prostitution when they could not find work. Some years later, and across the Channel, abandoned women told Mayhew some of the reasons that their hoped-for marriages never took place: Sometimes there was no money for a proper wedding; sometimes the men moved on to search for work; sometimes poverty created unbearable emotional stress.[30] Overall, the traditional contexts which identified and demanded "proper" behavior were absent. There is obviously much still to be learned about young working girls and about the behavior and motives of their suitors. The central point here is that no major change in values or mentality was necessary to create these cases of illegitimacy.

29 Alain Lottin, "Naissances Illégitimies et filles-mères à Lille au XVIIIᵉ siècle," *Revue d'histoire moderne et contemporaine*, XVII (1970), 309 (authors' translation).
30 Richard Cobb, *The Police and the People: French Popular Protest 1789–1820* (Oxford, 1970), 235, 238; Alexandre Parent-Duchâtelet, *De la Prostitution dans la Ville De Paris* (Paris, 1836), 73–75, 93–94. Yeo and Thompson, *Mayhew*, 116–180. See also Massimo Livi Bacci, *A Century of Portuguese Fertility* (Princeton, 1971), 71–73.

Rather, older expectations operating in a changed context yielded unanticipated (and often unhappy) results.

If they were left far from their families with illegitimate children, young women were forced to become independent. But theirs was an independence or self-reliance based on desperation and disillusionment, and not on the carefree, self-seeking individualism of Shorter's description. Evidence for this can be found in the reasons for their prostitution given by women in the Year III: "to get bread"; "to be able to live"; "to feed my child"; "to pay for a wet nurse." "What are we?" exclaimed a Paris prostitute; "Most of us are unfortunate women, without origins, without education, servants, maids for the most part . . . ." These bitter tones are echoed by the London working girls who told Mayhew that they "went wrong" in order to support their children.[31]

Prostitution, in turn, produced more illegitimate children. Many prostitutes were domestic servants or girls from the garment industry out of work—women whose need sent them into the streets. In an ironic way, even this kind of activity had its historical roots. Hufton's catalog of the resources developed by lower-class women in pre-Revolutionary France in their roles as providers of food includes begging, the renting out of their children to other beggars, flirtation, and sexual favors. Many of the girls testifying to Mayhew of their "shame" explained it as the only way to provide food for their children and keep them out of the workhouse. This attitude would have been recognizable to peasant women, although they would have found the life-style associated with it unfamiliar and abhorrent: A woman's body was her last resource in a desperate effort to support her family.

The sheer increase in the numbers of prostitutes and deserted pregnant women was not alone responsible for the increase in illegitimacy rates. Charitable institutions, developed at this time for the care of illegitimate children, lengthened their lives or, at least, registered their births. From the mid-seventeenth century on, reformers who established new foundling hospitals or improved old ones explicitly defined their goal as the elimination of infanticide. St. Vincent de Paul's work in Paris, for example, culminated in the dedication of the Bicêtre for this purpose in 1690. A Foundling Hospital was opened in Dublin in 1704. And, in 1739, the London Hospital was incorporated, "to prevent the frequent murders of poor miserable children at their

31 Cobb, *Police and the People*, 234, 237, 238. See also Henry Mayhew, *London Labour and the London Poor* (London, 1851; reprinted, 1967), IV, 220, 255, 256.

birth, and to suppress the inhuman custom of exposing new-born infants to perish in the streets." Similarly such hospitals were opened in Strasbourg (in 1748) and in Moscow and St. Petersburg during the reign of Catherine. Malthus, in fact, criticized the Russian institutions for discouraging marriage by making it too easy for illegitimate children to be cared for by others.[32] The incidence of infanticide in the sixteenth and seventeenth centuries has never been quantified, as far as we know, but qualitative evidence suggests that death was the common fate of children of illicit unions, whether the mother was deserted or the parents simply too poor to support another child. The hospitals, of course, often simply institutionalized infanticide, but they guaranteed registration of the birth in their baptismal records. The eighteenth-century foundling hospital "civilized" the care of illegitimate children by baptizing them, but it failed in the majority of cases to nurture these children to adulthood.

Domestic servants, prostitutes, and deserted women were not the only mothers of illegitimate children in the eighteenth and nineteenth centuries. Often bastards were the products of stable consensual unions which sometimes even ended in legal marriage. Although we do not yet have hard evidence, it seems likely that the number of these unions increased as the population of unskilled, propertyless workers grew in cities. These unions were not a new phenomenon; instead, they represented the continuation of a practice long common with the urban working-class. From mid-seventeenth-century Aix comes this comment on the urban poor: "They almost never know the sanctity of marriage and live together in shameful fashion."[33] Ford characterizes mid-eighteenth-century Strasbourg as "a society where cohabitations frequently began with the formal announcement of intended marriage. This practice did not enjoy full social or religious approval to be sure, but neither did it create any particular scandal." Children born out of wedlock were frequently legitimated by marriage, Ford says, but

32 *Encyclopedia Britannica* (New York, 1911), X, 746–747, "Foundling hospitals"; Franklin Ford, *Strasbourg in Transition* (New York, 1966), 177–179. The graph of illegitimacy in Paris supplied by Shorter, "Sexual Revolution and Social Change," 265, is based on figures in E. Charlot and J. Dupaquier, "Mouvement annuel de la population de la Ville de Paris de 1670 à 1821," *Annales du Demographie historique*, I (1967), 512–513. See also William Langer, "Checks on Population Growth: 1750–1850," *Scientific American*, CCXXVI (1972), 92–99; J. F. Terme et J.-B. Monfalcon, *Histoire des enfants trouvés* (Paris, 1840).

33 Fairchilds, "Poverty and Charity," citing *La mendicité abolie dans la ville d'Aix par l'Hôpital général ou Maison de charité*, an undated pamphlet which she dates from the late seventeenth century.

even when this did not happen, the mother's family recognized its responsibility for her child. Similar practices were noted by Frederic Le Play in his biographies of urban workers in the middle of the nineteenth century and by novelists of working-class life such as Emile Zola. Agulhon also describes the existence of free unions among the working class of Toulon before 1849.[34]

Free unions seem to have increased as more and more young men and women left their native towns and villages and moved to larger towns or cities. For some, there was no point in legalizing a union because there was no property to protect. For others, consensual union was the prelude to marriage—the period during which women worked and accumulated the dowry required for a "proper" marriage. Children born in this period were legitimated at the wedding ceremony. Often young people did not marry because they did not know priests or ministers to perform the ceremony. Many, too, scorned the rituals of the church. Others simply were too busy working, and, if they were migrants, they may well have been ignorant of the place where one went to secure a civil act. In some German states, marriage was forbidden to those without sufficient economic resources. Couples simply lived together without the blessing of the state.[35]

Illegitimacy was the product of free unions, and free unions seem to have increased during the late eighteenth and early nineteenth centuries, most probably because industrialization and urbanization moved many people out of their traditional occupational, social, and geographic contexts. Mobility, in fact, was the recurring experience for those people responsible for increased illegitimacy from about

---

34 Ford, *Strasbourg*, 178; Maurice Agulhon, *Une Ville ouvrière au temps du socialisme utopique. Toulon de 1815 à 1851* (Paris, 1970), 99. See also Pierre Pierrard, *La Vie ouvrière à Lille sous le Second Empire* (Paris, 1965), 118–120; Edith Thomas, *Les Petroleuses* (Paris, 1963), 20–23; Richard Cobb, "The Women of the Commune," in his *Second Identity: Essays on France and French History* (London, 1969), 231.

35 The whole question of the place and meaning of legal sanctification of marriage needs further exploration. There may have existed among the poor a moral concept of the family, similar to the "moral economy" described by E. P. Thompson. Indeed, common-law marriage in England and consensual union in France were both recognized in law. It may well be, despite the laws imposed by centralizing states and churches, that a popular tradition of non-legal, non-sanctified marriage continued. See John Knodel, "Law, Marriage and Illegitimacy in Nineteenth-Century Germany," *Population Studies*, XX (1966–67), 279–294; U. R. Q. Henriques, "Bastardy and the New Poor Law," *Past & Present*, XXXVII (1967), 103–129; Régine Pernoud, "La vie de famille du Moyen Age à l'ancien Régime," in Robert Prigent (ed.), *Renouveau des idées sur la famille* (Paris, 1954), 29: E. P. Thompson, "The Moral Economy of the English Crowd in the Eighteenth Century," *Past & Present*, L (1971), 76–136.

1750 to 1850. Geographic mobility meant that men and women left familiar and family settings and therefore lost the protection and constraint they provided. Shorter himself describes this kind of situation, in discussing the factors which led to illegitimacy in rural areas. Itinerant workers seduced young girls and then moved on. "The hapless young girls were still giving the traditional response to what they thought was the customary signal." Shorter here acknowledges the traditionalism of the rural women's responses, but he insists that the *men* had changed their attitudes. Again the evidence for this alleged mentality change is the consequence of it—abandoned pregnant women. But it is equally plausible, and more congruent with the evidence, that the economic pressures on young men prevented them from fulfilling their obligations.[36]

Rising rates of illegitimacy, then, did not signify a "sexual revolution." They followed, instead, from structural and compositional changes associated with urbanization and industrialization. There is no evidence, moreover, that these changes immediately gave rise to changes in attitude. On the contrary, men and women engaged in intercourse with established expectations, but in changed or changing contexts. As a result, illegitimacy increased.

A MODEL FOR THE RISE AND FALL OF EUROPEAN FERTILITY RATES
We have dealt so far with the rise in illegitimate fertility which occurred in most of Europe toward the end of the eighteenth century. Shorter also sees this as the central issue to be explained, but he places it in a much larger context: the rise of all illegitimate fertility, and possibly legitimate fertility in the eighteenth century, and the decline of both kinds of fertility at the end of the nineteenth century. His model is wrong. We offer an alternative to it.

We start with declining mortality. Early in the eighteenth century, in much of Western Europe, mortality began to drop, presumably as a result of increased food supply. Subsistence crises ended, and the rate of population growth increased. The growth in population was almost surely distributed differentially by class. In the wealthy and upper levels of the popular classes (propertied peasants and prosperous

---

36 Shorter, "Capitalism, Culture and Sexuality," 342; Shorter accepts the initial importance of population growth in "Sexual Change and Illegitimacy," 249, as well as the connection of migration and increased illegitimacy and the end of the linkage of marriage and property settlement.

artisans), adult and child mortality decreased earlier in time than it did in poor and unpropertied classes. As more of these children survived to adulthood, the problems of "placing" them and of avoiding fragmentation of property became acute. Thus, the ranks of the propertyless were swelled with the surplus children of more prosperous families, who were forced to seek a living with no expectation of inheritance.

Fortunately, new occupational opportunities were another byproduct of population growth. Increasing population meant increased demand. This, together with a complex of technological and agricultural changes, launched in England the process which became industrialization. But even in England, and *a fortiori* throughout the rest of Western Europe, the early effect of increased demand was the expansion of cottage industry, of market agriculture, and of consumer and service industries in administrative and commercial cities. Despite their abundance, however, these jobs often turned out to be quite unstable, as British stocking frame knitters and handloom weavers or French cotton textile workers learned after 1780. In consumer services and domestic service, as in cottage industry, employment fluctuated enormously according to seasons and business cycles.

Far from home, cut off from possible property ownership, no longer required by craft organizations to postpone marriage until the completion of long apprenticeships, and in difficult economic straits, the men and women in cottage, consumer, and service industries acted in what contemporaries called "improvident" ways: They married younger and did not control their fertility as compulsively as peasant and artisan families had tended to.[37] Why? A number of related factors were involved. The abandonment of late marriage itself represented the relinquishing of the chief means that families had used to control fertility. Associated with this was a decline in the numbers of those who never married. Stearns has reminded us that in pre-industrial society fertility was controlled through the celibacy of a large minority of men and women. The likelihood that such celibacy could be enforced decreased with propertylessness and with migration; hence, the rates of partnerships of all sorts, including marriage, were likely to increase, and with them, the number of children born. The economic necessity which required both partners to work for the survival

---

37 On improvident marriages, see Henriques, "Bastardy," 111–112; Braun, "Impact of Cottage Industry," 59; Matti Sarmela, *Reciprocity Systems of the Rural Society in the Finnish-Karelian Culture Area with Special Reference to Social Intercourse of the Youth* (Helsinki, 1969), 57.

of the family led young mothers to relinquish the practice of nursing their own young. This, and high levels of infant mortality which also reduced the nursing period shortened the interval between successive births.[38] The possibility of employment for young children encouraged families to continue high fertility strategies even as child mortality fell. Above all, however, high rates of infant mortality determined family strategies of high fertility. In order to guarantee the the survival of one or two children, families experiencing high rates of infant mortality had traditionally produced many children. This continued to be the case.

Le Play's example of the Parisian carpenter's family well illustrates the pressures which led to high fertility. The carpenter's wife worked in the early years of her marriage. She sold fruits and vegetables at Les Halles and polished metal at home. In a period of eight years she bore six children. Four of them were bottle-fed, and all died before the age of 18 months. Bottle feeding (a necessity for a mother working away from home who could not afford or did not want to send her baby to a wet nurse) was undoubtedly a factor in the short interval between the births as well as in the deaths. This high rate of infant mortality made a strategy of high fertility appropriate, especially if a son were to live to inherit his father's membership in the carpentering trade, but also if two or three children were to survive to an age when they could earn wages and thus free their mother of the need to work.[39]

Illegitimate fertility increased, too, because of a growth in the population of propertyless working men and women. In rural areas, geographically mobile men established relationships with women, became betrothed, engaged in intercourse, and then moved on. In cities, engagement often led to abandonment, or to a free union. In all cases, illegitimacy was a by-product. The migration of these "surplus" children, then, resulted in an even larger population of mobile men and of sexually vulnerable women, far from the protection of their families. The consequences of the increase in this population were increased incidence of abandoned pregnant women; increased prostitution of abandoned or unemployed women; increased incidence and duration

38 Peter Stearns, private communication, 30 Nov. 1973. *Annales de l'Assemblée Nationale*, T. XXXII, 5 juin-7 juillet 1874, Annexe No. 2446 (Paris, 1874), annexe, 48-133; see esp. 54, 59, 74, 84-85. See also, Margaret Hewitt, *Wives and Mothers in Victorian Industry* (London, 1958). John Knodel, "Two and a Half Centuries of Demographic History in a Bavarian Village," *Population Studies*, XXIV (1970), 353-376.
39 Le Play, *Les Ouvriers*, V, 427.

of consensual or free union. All three of these alternatives produced illegitimate children.

Illegitimate and legitimate fertility rose simultaneously, then, because of a complex of changes stemming from declining mortality during the eighteenth century. These changes increased the numbers of young people physically and materially removed from their families and from work within the traditional household. They were also removed from the constraints on personal and marital behavior of property; for many of them, the link between legal marriage and property had been broken. There is little evidence to indicate, however, that changes in sexual attitudes, particularly those of women, preceded these developments. Instead, the various attempts at union whether successful or not, represented the pursuit of older goals, an endorsement of established male–female relationships. In every kind of situation, the woman's goal, at least, seems to have been to reestablish the family economy, the partnership of economic enterprise and of social and, perhaps, emotional sustenance. These women sought not sexual fulfillment, but economic cooperation and all of the other things which traditional marriage implied. That they often failed to find them, and that their attempts to establish a family took a variety of forms does not prove anything about their motivation. The form of male–female relationships was created not by the revolutionized sexual attitudes of the partners, but by a complex interaction of values and expectations and changing social and economic circumstances. And it is those circumstances that must be examined if rising rates of fertility are to be explained.

Why did fertility decline toward the end of the nineteenth century? Above all, because infant mortality declined among the working classes as economic prosperity increased. The explanation offered by Banks for the decline of middle-class fertility applies at a later date to working-class marital fertility. He argues that middle-class family size shrank because of the parents' expectations about their own standard of living and because of their rising ambitions for their children.[40] Among the working classes, child mortality declined in the nineteenth century. For the first time, the children of working-class

40 James A. Banks, *Prosperity and Parenthood: A Study of Family Planning among the Victorian Middle Classes* (London, 1954). See also Charles Tilly, "Population and Pedagogy in France," *History of Education Quarterly*, XIII (1973), 113–128. See also H. J. Habakkuk, *Population Growth and Economic Development since 1750* (New York, 1971), 63; Michael Young and Peter Wilmott, *The Symmetrical Family: A study of Work and Leisure in the London Region* (London, 1973), 39.

families, once they survived infancy, were not subject to continuing high mortality risk. As long as children could work, though, fertility does not appear to have fallen. As factory legislation reduced possibilities of child labor and educational opportunity became available to the working classes after 1870, family outlooks changed. Finally, the standard of living of workers improved during this period with two important results: Many mothers of young children could withdraw from outside work because the family could live on the husband's wages; children were no longer needed as additional wage earners. With fewer children, a man's wages went farther and there would be more money for the education of children. (An investment in education was a contribution to a child's future and might function as apprenticeship and property had earlier.) At this point, the working-class family acted on what was clearly its own interest by adopting family limitation, and its marital fertility fell.[41]

What about illegitimate fertility? In an article written with Knodel and van de Walle, Shorter peremptorily discounts any kind of prosperity model.

> It is unlikely that higher incomes moved unwed mothers to curb their illegitimate fertility so as to plan better the educational future of their bastards on hand. Possibly improvements in the standard of living during the last quarter of the nineteenth century restricted illegitimate fertility through some other mechanism. But *ad hoc* rummaging about for alternate linkages in an "economic prosperity" model is unlikely to result in any generalizable kind of explanation.[42]

Shorter and his associates assume here that individual decisions—of unwed mothers—lay behind falling illegitimacy rates. Yet, it can be shown that *fin-de-siècle* prosperity did bring about some compositional changes in European populations that tended to reduce the size of the population which produced illegitimate births. First, the number of

41 It appears that decisions about family strategy were more important than the technology of birth control. Most evidence indicates that workers used age-old methods, particularly *coitus interruptus*. The technological revolution appears to have reached the lower class at a much later date than Shorter implies. See, for example, R. P. Newman, "Industrialization and Sexual Behavior: Some Aspects of Working Class Life in Imperial Germany," in Bezucha (ed.), *Modern European Social History*, 270–298. Infant mortality did not fall decisively in the nineteenth century until fertility began to decline. Public health measures and increased parental awareness improved the life chances of infants. See E. A. Wrigley, *Industrial Growth and Population Change: A Regional Study of the Coalfield Areas of North-West Europe in the Later Nineteenth Century* (Cambridge, 1961), 102–103; Great Britain, National Health Insurance Medical Research Committee, *The Mortalities of Birth, Infancy and Childhood* (London, 1917), xiii–xiv.

42 Shorter, Knodel, and van de Walle, "Decline of Non-Marital Fertility," 393.

women in sexually vulnerable situations, particularly servants and other female migrants to cities, began to wane. From about the last decade of the nineteenth century the rate of increase of women in domestic service began to drop; eventually the number of domestic servants absolutely declined.[43] Both the increase in factory jobs for women and the increase in working-class prosperity reduced the number of women working on their own, far from their families. Second, increased prosperity led to a decrease in the number of extremely mobile, propertyless men restlessly moving about in search of work. Third, increased prosperity led to a new emphasis on marriage, as the urban working classes began to acquire goods and even landed property in working-class suburbs. Formal and legalized marriage which spelled out the disposition and use of this property led to a decline in consensual unions. In addition, children's work was limited by law, and there was greater educational opportunity for them. Unwed mothers whose illegitimate children were the results of seduction and abandonment or of prostitution might not be able to decide to marry, but it behooved couples whose children were equally illegitimate to reach the altar when conventional marriage meant improved opportunity for themselves and their children. Regular employment and better wages clearly opened up new vistas for workers and the custom of free union became less widespread.

The movement to the cities, of course, did not end with the nineteenth century. Why did later urbanization and geographic mobility not result in compositional changes like those of the late eighteenth and early nineteenth centuries? They probably did, but migrants were a smaller proportion of the population. Furthermore, cities were no longer the same types of administrative and commercial centers with greatest employment opportunity in unstable areas. Industrial growth broadened and changed occupational opportunities in twentieth-century cities. Also, most rural migrants to these cities were not as economically vulnerable as their nineteenth-century predecessors. They now came from rural areas where fertility was also controlled. Their families thus had greater resources with which to sponsor their migration and maintain contacts with them.

Women's work in the late eighteenth and early nineteenth centuries was not "liberating" in any sense. Most women stayed in established

---

43　See the historical tables on labor force composition for France, England, Germany, and Italy in Deldycke, et al, *La Population active*, 165–177, 181–193, 129–139, 106–107, for the proportionate decline in domestic service as a woman's occupation.

occupations. They were so poorly paid that economic independence was precluded. Furthermore, whether married or single, most women often entered the labor force in the service of the family interest. The evidence available points to several causes for illegitimacy, none related to the "emancipation" of women: economic need, causing women to seek work far from the protection of their families; occupational instability of men which led to *mariages manqués* (sexual intercourse following a promise of marriage which was never fulfilled). Finally, analysis of the effects of population growth on propertied peasants and artisans seems to show that the bifurcation of marriage and property arrangements began to change the nature of marriage arrangements for propertyless people.

Our alternative model has the advantage of being built on evidence. Much more of this evidence is needed before the model can be confirmed. Nevertheless, the negative evidence which we have offered for Shorter's model and his own lack of evidence lead us to believe that less sensational but no less dramatic, more complex but less speculative explanations are in order for the fertility changes in Europe from 1750 to 1900. This examination of the history of working-class women and their families in the eighteenth and nineteenth centuries has shown that *continuities* in mentality mark the fertility rise. The fertility fall, a consequence of economic prosperity and family limitation, opened the way for a changed consciousness among women.

Journal of Interdisciplinary History, VII:4 (Spring 1977), 637–653.

George D. Sussman

Parisian Infants and Norman Wet Nurses in the Early Nineteenth Century:
A Statistical Study
Statistical studies of the wet-nursing business, a peculiarly French institution which flourished in the eighteenth and nineteenth centuries, have usually depended upon either of two types of sources, both of which have their weaknesses. First, there are the studies based upon a systematic exploitation of the parish register for a rural commune where urban babies were placed with wet nurses. The limitation with such studies is that they only inform us about those *nourrissons* who died while out to nurse, so there is no direct evidence concerning, for instance, the length of stay for the survivors nor the mortality rate for all *nourrissons*. Secondly, there are studies based upon the records of urban agencies which placed infants with wet nurses in the country. These records, although more informative about the survivors, generally encompass only a special section of the wet-nursing business, namely infants receiving public assistance and, particularly, the foundlings. The bulk of the wet-nursing business was not charitable, but served the needs of urban mothers who were prevented from feeding their own infants by their employment and who therefore paid rural women monthly wages to replace them in this function. And most of the infants placed in the country did not die there, but returned to their natural mothers in the city after the period of their nursing.

An examination of a register from the Direction or Bureau of Wet Nurses of the City of Paris provides new information. The municipal bureau was founded in 1769 and abolished in 1876. Until about 1828 it had an exclusive legal right to operate a lodging and hiring center for rural wet nurses who came to the capital looking for infants. Parents, mostly of a modest artisanal or shopkeeping background, came to the bureau to select a wet nurse and to negotiate the wages they would pay her. The nurse then took

George D. Sussman is Assistant Professor of History at Vanderbilt University.

I am grateful to the National Endowment for the Humanities and the Vanderbilt University Research Council for support, respectively, for the research and writing of this article. I would also like to thank my colleague, Donald L. Winters, who patiently guided my first steps in the use of the computer for historical studies.

the infant to her village for the duration of the nursing period. In the first two decades of the nineteenth century, approximately 5,000 Parisian infants were placed this way each year. They constituted about one quarter of the infants born in the capital each year and one-half of those who were nursed commercially.[1]

The bureau's register is far from satisfactory as a source of information about the social, demographic, and economic aspects of the wet-nursing business, but it is the only source on individual placements by the municipal wet-nursing bureau of Paris in the nineteenth-century to have survived the fires of 1871 or routine bureaucratic disposal of old papers.[2] It was evidently prepared around 1822 as a part of the general reorganization of the Direction and straightening out of its books, and it was kept up until 1825. The register contains information on individual placements from 1814 through 1825 in four of the rural arrondissements where the Direction recruited its nurses: Evreux and Louviers in the Department of the Eure, Epernay in the Department of the Marne, and Fontainebleau in the Department of Seine-et-Marne. For each infant placed the register contains spaces for the following information: an identification number, the child's name, the nurse's name, her commune and canton, the date when the child was put out to nurse, what happened to the child—whether he died, was returned, was purged from the books (probably because the nurse and parents came to a private arrangement), or was still with the nurse in 1825— the date of the child's return or death, and the amount of the monthly wage the parents agreed to pay the nurse. There are also spaces to record the payments made and these are only filled in from 1822. There is no information on the occupations of the child's parents or the nurse's husband, or the birthdate or age of the nurse, the child, or the nurse's own child (the *frère de lait*), or on the parents' address in Paris.

The register contains information on 1,648 placements during

1 The Foundling Hospital placed others, while wealthier families found wet nurses through private arrangements. A reorganization of the municipal bureau in 1821 had the effect of driving away wet nurses and parents to unauthorized and poorly policed private placement bureaus. On all of this introductory material, see Sussman, "The Wet-Nursing Business in Nineteenth-Century France," *French Historical Studies,* IX (1975), 304–328.
2 The manuscript register is entitled: "Administration générale des hôpitaux, hospices et secours de la Ville de Paris. Direction des Nourrices. Service extérieur. Payement des mois de nourrices et dépenses accessoires. Contrôle du Bureau." It may be found in the Archives de l'Assistance publique à Paris (hereafter, Arch. Asst. pub.), 224.

the years 1814–1825, about 3 percent of the total number of placements by the Direction of Wet Nurses during these twelve years. Out of 1,653 infants placed in the four arrondissements (including five stray placements before 1814), 438 or 26.5 percent of the total died while they were out to nurse in the country (see Table 1). I recorded on computer punch cards for further analysis the data concerning 826 children placed in the Arrondissement of Evreux, almost all between 1814 and 1824, and this analysis is the subject of the remainder of this article.

Table 1   Placements and Deaths in Four Arrondissements

ARRONDISSEMENT (YEARS)	PLACEMENTS	DEATHS	MORTALITY
Epernay (1814–25)	451	133	29.5%
Evreux (1806, 1812–24)	826	204	24.7%
Fontainebleau (1813–25)	269	78	29.0%
Louviers (1814–23)	107	23	21.5%
Totals	1653	438	26.5%

The area around Evreux in Normandy was a major wet-nursing region for the city of Paris for two centuries. In addition to the children placed in the Arrondissement by the Direction of Wet Nurses and private placement bureaus, the service of the Enfants-Trouvés of the capital placed foundlings in the region from 1690 until the 1850s. In 1820 there were 687 Parisian foundlings in the Arrondissement. Before the railroad a national highway connected Paris with Evreux and the coach covered this distance in seventeen hours. Wet nurses, however, would have traveled in slower vehicles and would probably have had to walk from Evreux to their villages.[3]

The Arrondissement of Evreux, like the entire Department of the Eure, was a populous region in the early nineteenth century, but with no large cities.[4] The 826 infants placed in the Arrondissement in the years 1814–1824 by the Direction of Wet Nurses were dispersed among at least 172 distinct communes. Only twenty-five communes received ten or more children from the

3   Albert Dupoux, *Sur les pas de Monsieur Vincent, Trois cents ans d'histoire parisienne de l'enfance abandonnée* (Paris, 1958), 270–273. Jean Vidalenc, *Le département de l'Eure sous la monarchie constitutionnelle, 1814–1848* (Paris, 1952), 522–523.
4   *Ibid.*, ix–x.

municipal bureau over this eleven-year period, and only two communes received twenty or more (Vernon, twenty, and Evreux, twenty-nine).

Within the Arrondissement of Evreux there were roughly two economic zones. In the east and south (the cantons of Vernon, Pacy, Saint André, Nonancourt, Damville, and Verneuil) the principal activity was agriculture, especially wheat and barley production associated with sheep-raising. Two-thirds of the wet nurses in the Arrondissement came from these cantons. It seems likely that they belonged to the population of agricultural laborers who worked six or seven months a year for task wages or daily wages of 1–1.5 francs.[5] The western parts of the Arrondissement (the cantons of Evreux, Conches, Breteuil, and Rugles) had another resource in the state forests of the region and the small metallurgical and hardware industry which flourished around them. Most of the wet nurses from these western cantons probably came from the poorer families who lived a quasi-legal existence around the forests as woodcutters, charcoal-burners, and scavengers of one sort or another. "What cultivable soil there is in the area is worked by poor farmers," wrote an observer of the forest population in 1838:

> the other inhabitants are woodcutters or workers somehow involved with wood, and also a number of indigent people who live almost entirely off the forest or who keep foundlings for the hospitals of Rouen or of Paris.[6]

The register of the Direction of Wet Nurses gives almost no direct information about the women who nursed Parisian infants for a wage. Only their names and communes appear, and for thirty-one placements, 3.8 percent of the total, the clerk noted that the wet nurse was a "fille," unmarried. Each wet nurse received the basic monthly wage of 10 francs, which was guaranteed by the Direction, and usually 1–2 francs more depending on the contract that she had made with the parents and the parents' readiness to meet their obligations. The mean contracted wage for the wet nurses of Evreux in the years 1814–1824 was 11.6 francs. If the mean wage is compared for various smaller groups, it turns out that there are no important differences in the wages contracted by

5 *Ibid.*, 404; 437–439.
6 Quoted in *ibid.*, 486. I am responsible for the translation of this and other French passages quoted in this article.

women from different cantons nor between unmarried women and the sample as a whole. Nor does there appear to be any relationship between the wage contracted and the treatment the child received, measured by whether he died or survived. The treatment might have varied in relationship to the wage actually paid, but I do not have the information to assess that relationship. The mean contracted wage does appear to have fluctuated with the month in which the contract was made: the lowest mean was 11.3 francs for children put out in May and the highest was 12.0 francs for children put out in August. The availability of seasonal employment harvesting grain in August certainly accounts for the relatively high prices the rural wet nurses received that month. Year-by-year fluctuations in the mean contracted wage show one unusually low year, 1816, with a mean wage of 11.2 francs, and a series of notably high years at the end of the period, 1821–1824, when the mean wage ranged from 11.9 to 12.3 francs. The low figure for 1816 might be related to an abundance of nurses in a year of high food prices and military occupation. The rise in the *mois de nourrice* (the nurse's monthly wage) after 1821 is probably related to the reorganization of the Direction that year. When salaried employees replaced the commissioned *meneurs* as intermediaries for the bureau between Parisian parents and rural wet nurses, the *meneurs* began to operate on their own, offering the nurses higher wages and thus raising the general price level.[7]

Wet-nursing was an important source of supplementary income for many women, and many tried to make it a regular and enduring source of income as well, despite the unusual physiological demands it imposed. Assuming that where the nurse's surname and commune are identical, the nurse is the same, 274 of the 826 placements, one-third of the total, were with women who nursed more than one child for the bureau between 1814 and 1824. Eighty-six women nursed two Parisian children each, twenty-five nursed three, four nursed four each, one woman nursed five different children, and one woman nursed six children not her own in a period of eleven years (four of the last babies survived).

7 Arch. Asst. pub., 709[1], *Instruction sur le service des préposés à la surveillance des enfans placés dans les départemens par l'intermédiaire de la Direction des Nourrices* (Paris, 1823), 15.
    In parts of the Parisian Basin in the eighteenth century the price of a wet nurse doubled in August. Marcel Lachiver, "Tarif des mois de nourrice dans le Bassin parisien en 1771," *Annales de démographie historique, 1968* (Paris, 1968), 383–384. See also Sussman, "The Wet-Nursing Business," 315–317.

There were three distinct patterns of placements with these multiple nurses. In some instances there was a long enough lapse of time between two placements with the same woman for her to have given birth in between to a child of her own, who may have died, been put out with another nurse, or been weaned before the mother took another commercial *nourrisson*. Then there were many cases of what I call serial nursing with two Parisian infants: that is, when the lapse of time between the first child's death or return and the next child's placement with the same nurse is greater than zero and less than six months. A woman by the name of Bourgeois from the village of Mouettes took an infant on September 10, 1819, and returned him to Paris on June 7, 1820; took another child on July 16 and returned him on May 5, 1821; and took a third child on June 23 and returned him on March 3, 1823. In this example of serial nursing, three children were apparently on the same milk over a period of at least two years of nearly continuous nursing. A third possibility, which appears to violate the municipal bureau's rule against nursing more than one child at a time, occurred where the dates of two placements with one nurse overlapped. But the bureau seems to have permitted this situation rather often, either where the two babies were twins (César and Colas Lardi, both placed with a woman named Ste. Beuve on April 23, 1820, and both returned May 13, 1822) or where the first child had probably been weaned but still remained with the nurse (a woman named Malard from Pacy took one child March 31, 1818, then another nine months later on January 11, 1819, returning the first child in May 1819 and the second in December, 1820). With the eighty-six women who nursed two children commercially, there were twenty-two instances where the two placements overlapped in time, thirty-three where the two placements were in series, and thirty-one where the two placements were separated by more than six months. Among all the women who nursed more than one child, I counted fifty-nine instances of serial intervals between two placements and thirty-seven instances of overlapping placements. Both patterns, then, were not unusual.[8]

Of the 826 Parisian babies placed by the municipal bureau in

8 Both patterns were also found to be common in a small sample of women who nursed foundlings from Reims in the late eighteenth century. See Antoinette Chamoux, "L'enfance abandonnée à Reims à la fin du XVIIIᵉ siècle," *Annales de démographie historique, 1973* (Paris, 1973), 274–276.

the Arrondissement of Evreux during the first decade of the Restoration, 204 died, 598 were returned, sixteen were purged from the books, five were still with their nurses in 1825, and there is no information on three others. The mortality rate, then, on those for whom we have information, was 24.8 percent, a quarter of the babies, a relatively low rate for the Direction of Wet Nurses in the nineteenth century.[9]

For those babies who died while out to nurse, the mean length of time elapsing between their placement and their death was 144 days, nearly five months, but the median, the term by which half of the deaths had already occurred, was sixty-nine days, about ten weeks. Of all the babies placed 21.4 percent died within one year of their placement. There are several problems about comparing this first-year mortality with a true infant mortality. In the first place, the register does not specify the age of the infants but only allows us to calculate the time they spent with their wet nurses. In practice there was probably no more than a day or two difference between an infant's age at the time of his death or return and the length of his placement, since parents placed the infants immediately after birth.

Assuming, then, that the duration of the placement was nearly equivalent to age, there are still two problems in comparing first-year mortality of any group of *nourrissons* with the infant mortality of an ordinary population. The first-year mortality of the *nourrissons* does not take account, on the one hand, of the considerable mortality of the first several days of life before the infants were placed with the nurses, and, on the other, it does not take account of deaths that occurred among infants returned to their parents before they reached the first anniversary of their placement, a group that totaled about 30 percent of our sample. The first omission is more serious than the second because infant deaths are so heavily concentrated in the earliest part of the first year. In a group of nearly 2,000 infant deaths which occurred in nineteen parishes in the southern *banlieue* of Paris in the late eighteenth century among children who were born and died in the same parish, 13.2

9   The annual mortality among all the infants placed by the Direction of Wet Nurses, that is, the number who died each year as a percentage of the number placed the same year, ranged between 25.2 percent and 34.8 percent in the years 1813–1822. Over the whole ten-year period mortality was 29.8 percent. For the sources for these figures on deaths and placements, see Sussman, "The Wet-Nursing Business," n. 36.

percent of the infant deaths occurred in the first day of life and 28.7 percent in the first week; fewer deaths occurred in the last seven months of the first year (27.8 percent) than in the first seven days. Thus the first-year mortality of the *nourrissons* of the Eure (21.4 percent), which is already three or four percentage points higher than the general French figure for infant mortality in this period, would have to be significantly inflated before it could be legitimately compared with true figures of infant mortality.[10]

Assuming the age of the *nourrissons* in the Eure to be identical with the length of their placement, there is a sharp contrast between the age-distribution of their deaths and that of the deaths of other groups of *nourrissons*, mostly from the eighteenth century, discovered in the parish registers of the villages where they were nursed. In the sample from the Arrondissement of Evreux, 5.8 percent of all fatalities for which the length of placement is known occurred in the first week, 33.8 percent occurred in the first four weeks, 71.4 percent in the first six months, and 89.3 percent in the first year (see Table 2). The age at death here is younger than that found for other groups of *nourrissons* (see Table 3). In three villages of the Beauvaisis where Ganiage found 259 *nourrissons* who died in the years 1740–1799, only 20 percent of the deaths occurred in the first month and 70 percent in the first year. In Meulan, where 529 *nourrissons* died between 1670 and 1869, 16.8 percent of the deaths occurred in the first month, 42.8 percent in the first six months, and only 61.8 percent in the first year. Among 795 infants who died while with wet nurses in nineteen parishes of the southern *banlieue* of Paris in the years 1774–1794, 17.4 percent died in the first month of life, 38.7 percent in the first six months, and 58.0 percent in the first year. The figures most nearly like my own for the age of death of *nourrissons* were obtained by Bideau in a study of the small provincial town of Thoissey-en-Dombes. Considering the 249 children of the

10 Paul Galliano, "La mortalité infantile (indigènes et nourrissons) dans la banlieue sud de Paris à la fin du XVIIIe siècle (1774–1794)," *Annales de démographie historique, 1966* (Paris, 1967), calculated from table on 149. Dominique Dinet calculated infant mortality to be 18.5 percent in the First Empire: Dinet, "Statistiques de mortalité infantile sous le Consulat et l'Empire," in *Hommage à Marcel Reinhard, Sur la population française au XVIIIe et XIXe siècles* (Paris, 1973), 215–218. Galliano found infant mortality to be 17.7 percent among over 11,000 babies born in the southern *banlieue* of Paris in the late eighteenth century and raised at home: "La mortalité infantile," 149–150.

Table 2 Age of Infants at Time of Death or Return

		1ST WK.	2ND WK.	3RD WK.	4TH WK.	2ND MO.	3RD MO.	4TH MO.	5TH MO.	6TH MO.	7TH MO.
Deaths	number	11	22	26	5	27	13	10	10	11	4
	% of row	5.8	11.6	13.8	2.6	14.3	6.9	5.3	5.3	5.8	2.1
	% of table	1.4	2.8	3.3	.6	3.4	1.6	1.3	1.3	1.4	.5
Returns	number	3	0	0	1	4	4	4	16	21	24
	% of row	.5	.0	.0	.2	.7	.7	.7	2.7	3.6	4.1
	% of table	.4	.0	.0	.2	.5	.5	.5	2.0	2.7	3.0

		8TH MO.	9TH MO.	10TH MO.	11TH MO.	12TH MO.	2ND YR. 1ST QTR.	2ND YR. 2ND QTR.	2ND YR. 3RD QTR.
Deaths	number	4	6	5	7	8	8	6	2
	% of row	2.1	3.2	2.6	3.7	4.2	4.2	3.2	1.1
	% of table	.5	.8	.6	.9	1.0	1.0	.8	.3
Returns	number	25	35	40	20	45	95	58	52
	% of row	4.3	6.0	6.8	3.4	7.7	16.3	9.9	8.9
	% of table	3.2	4.4	5.1	2.5	5.7	12.0	7.3	6.6

		2ND YR. 4TH QTR.	3RD YR.	4TH YR.	OVER 4 YRS.	TOTALS
Deaths	number	2	2	0	0	189
	% of row	1.1	1.1	.0	.0	23.9[a]
	% of table	.3	.3	.0	.0	
Returns	number	45	64	17	12	585
	% of row	7.7	10.9	2.9	2.1	74.1[a]
	% of table	5.8	8.1	2.2	1.5	

a The discrepancies between figures in the individual column and the total column resulted from the rounding off of figures. This applies also in Tables 4 and 5.

Table 3 Comparative Age Distributions of *Nourrissons* at Death

SAMPLE GROUP	NO. OF DEATHS	% OF DEATHS OCCURRING		
		UNDER 1 MO.	UNDER 6 MOS.	UNDER 1 YR.
Arrondissement of Evreux, 1814–24	189	33.8	71.4	89.3
3 Villages of Beauvaisis, 1740–99	259	20.0		70.0
Meulan, 1670–1869	529	16.8	42.8	61.8
Parishes around Thoissey-en-Dombes, 1740–1814	249	33.7	67.1	88.0
Southern *banlieue* of Paris, *nourrissons* only, 1774–94	795	17.4	38.7	58.0

SOURCES: See note 11.

bourgeois and artisans of Thoissey who died in the years 1740–1814 while out to nurse in nearby parishes within seven kilometers of their homes, he found that 33.7 percent of the deaths occurred in the first month, 67.1 percent in the first six months, and 88.0 percent in the first year of life.[11]

There are three reasons which might explain the general discrepancy between the age at death of Parisian *nourrissons* placed in the Eure in the nineteenth century and that of Parisian *nourrissons* placed at Meulan, in the Beauvaisis, and in the southern *banlieue* of the capital, mostly in the eighteenth century. In the first place, all of the age distributions derived from parish registers would only include deaths that occurred after the babies arrived in the nurses' villages where those registers were kept, whereas the register from the municipal wet-nursing bureau probably also includes deaths which occurred on the journey from Paris to the nurses' villages. If this is so, it would certainly add to the number of deaths in the

11 Jean Ganiage, *Trois villages d'Ile-de-France, étude démographique* (Paris, 1963), 75; Marcel Lachiver, *La population de Meulan du XVIIᵉ au XIXᵉ siècle (vers 1600–1870), étude de démographie historique* (Paris, 1969), 126–128. (I calculated the percentages from the table on 126); Galliano, "La mortalité infantile" (I calculated the percentages from the table on 159); Alain Bideau, "L'envoi des jeunes enfants en nourrice. L'exemple d'une petite ville: Thoissey-en-Dombes, 1740–1840," in *Hommage à Marcel Reinhard*, 49–58. (I calculated the percentages from the table on 53).

first month. But this explanation is surely insufficient in itself, for (among other reasons) not many infant deaths could have been missed on the short trip from Paris to the parishes of the southern *banlieue*, where Galliano also found a very low first-month mortality for *nourrissons*. The other two possible explanations are that Parisian *nourrissons* in the nineteenth century (and those of Thoissey in the eighteenth century) were, in comparison with Parisian *nourrissons* of the eighteenth century, either put out to nurse at a younger age, or brought back to their parents' homes at a younger age, or both. With more babies aged under one month with their nurses and fewer aged over one year, there would have been more chances of death occurring among the *nourrissons* in the youngest age groups and fewer in the oldest. We shall return to this hypothesis later when we examine the direct evidence on the length of time which the survivors spent with their wet nurses.

In arranging the fatalities of the *nourrissons* of the Eure by the month in which they occurred, a startling pattern appears (see Table 4). In every one of the first six months of the year but January there were fewer fatalities than the mean, and January had exactly the mean. The lowest mortality occurred in February followed by May. Altogether 19.0 percent of the year's fatalities occurred in the first quarter, winter, 18.0 percent in the second quarter, spring, or 37.0 percent in the first half. Sixty-three percent of the deaths, then, occurred in the second half of the year, and these fatalities were about evenly divided between the third quarter, summer, with 31.7 percent of the annual mortality, and the fourth quarter, autumn, with 31.2 percent. The highest monthly mortality was in December, followed by July and September. Every month of the second half contributed more than the monthly mean to the total mortality.

The seasonal pattern of mortality for the infants being nursed in the Eure only partially resembles the pattern which Galliano found for native infants and *nourrissons* in the southern *banlieue* of Paris. There the three summer months were even more deadly, accounting for 33.7 percent of the year's fatalities, but the three autumn months were about on a level with the winter and spring months (autumn 21.8 percent, winter 22.8 percent, spring 21.7 percent). Galliano found the highest infant mortality in August, followed by September, and the lowest in May, followed by February. For Galliano the explanation for the high summer mortality

Table 4 Month and Season of Deaths (%)

	JAN.	FEB.	MAR.	APR.	MAY	JUN.	JUL.	AUG.	SEP.	OCT.	NOV.	DEC.
Arrondissement of Evreux, 1814–1824 (189 deaths)	8.5	2.6	7.9	6.9	4.2	6.9	11.1	9.5	11.1	9.5	9.5	12.2
	1st quarter 19.0			2nd quarter 18.0			3rd quarter 31.7			4th quarter 31.2		
Banlieue sud of Paris, natives & *nourrissons*, 1774–1794 (2,224 deaths)	7.8	6.9	8.0	7.8	6.7	7.2	8.8	12.9	12.0	7.6	7.1	7.1
	1st quarter 22.8			2nd quarter 21.7			3rd quarter 33.7			4th quarter 21.8		

SOURCE: Galliano, "La mortalité infantile," 161–164. I calculated some of the percentages from the table on page 162.

Table 5 Month and Season of Placements in the Eure

	JAN.	FEB.	MAR.	APR.	MAY	JUN.	JUL.	AUG.	SEP.	OCT.	NOV.	DEC.
Number (total 813)	81	87	76	60	68	66	57	54	76	54	59	75
Percentage	10.0	10.7	9.3	7.4	8.4	8.1	7.0	6.6	9.3	6.6	7.3	9.2
Percentage by quarters	1st quarter 30.0			2nd quarter 23.9			3rd quarter 23.0			4th quarter 23.1		

among infants was the preoccupation of the women—nursing mothers and commercial wet nurses—with outdoor work in the harvest months, resulting in neglect and premature weaning. This explanation would be more valid for the country around Evreux than for the suburban area which Galliano studied. Did women's outdoor labor in the Eure carry further into the autumn than outdoor labor in the Seine—perhaps gathering fuel or shearing sheep—or is there another explanation for the high mortality of the *nourrissons* in the Eure in the last quarter of the year?

The seasonal distribution of mortality does not appear to have any relationship to the seasonal distribution of placements, unless it is inverse. The month-by-month fluctuations in the percentage of placements are smaller than those for mortality, partly because there is a larger number of placements (813 placements for which the month is known) than of deaths which number 189 (see Table 5). Whereas mortality was concentrated in the third and fourth quarters of the year, placements are concentrated in the first quarter, the winter months, when 30.0 percent of all placements occurred. Among the other seasons the distribution is more or less equal. The winter peak of placements began in December and extended through March. In addition to those four months only September had above-average placements. The lowest number of placements occurred in July, August, and October. The conclusion seems to be that wet-nursing was a seasonal occupation. Rural women journeyed to Paris to collect babies in greater numbers in the winter months, when there was little work to be done in the fields, than in the summer months, when work was abundant.[12] They also appear to have taken better care of their charges in the winter months when they were not occupied with outdoor work.

---

12 The seasonal distribution of placements is not related to the seasonal distribution of births in Paris. The latter, as reported by Villermé for the Department of the Seine over the years 1807–1816, shows very little month-by-month fluctuation, at least in comparison to the fluctuation of placements in the Eure. The monthly percentage of births ranged from a low of 7.7 percent in June to a high of 9.2 percent in March. By seasons the distribution of Parisian births was 26.0 percent in the three winter months, 25.0 percent in the spring months, 24.6 percent in the summer, and 24.4 percent in the autumn: L.-R. Villermé, "De la distribution par mois des conceptions et des naissances de l'homme," *Annales d'hygiène publique et de médecine légale*, V, pt. I (1831), 55–155. I calculated the percentages from the table on 128–129.

Three out of four infants placed through the municipal bureau of wet nurses in the Arrondissement of Evreux in the years 1814–1824 returned to their parents' home in Paris. The normal pattern appears to have been for the child to be restored to his parents soon after his first birthday (see Table 2). The median length of stay in the country, for those who survived, was 406 days or about 13.5 months. The number of babies returned before the end of the fourth month was insignificant, only 2.8 percent of the eventual returnees. From the fifth through the twelfth month there was a slow, mounting movement of returns, from 2.7 percent of all returns occurring in the fifth month to a peak of 7.7 percent in the twelfth. By the end of the first year 41.4 percent of all returns had occurred. Another 16.3 percent of returns occurred in the first quarter of the second year (compared to 17.9 percent in the fourth quarter of the first year), then the rate began to taper off: 9.9 percent in the second quarter of the second year, 8.9 percent in the third quarter, 7.7 percent in the fourth quarter. By the second birthday 84.2 percent of all returns had taken place. Most of the remainder (10.9 percent) returned in the third year. Considering the total population put out to nurse in the country, those who died and those who survived, at the end of one year 21.4 percent of the *nourrissons* had died and 30.6 percent had been returned to their parents; at the end of two years 23.7 percent had died and 62.2 percent had been returned. Most of the deaths occurred early in the first year; the returns were about evenly divided between the latter part of the first year and the second year.

With the Parisian babies placed by the Direction of Wet Nurses, an important influence on the length of time that they spent in the country was the duration of the bureau's guarantee of wages to the wet nurses. Both to give the nurses security and to protect the infants' lives, the bureau paid the nurses 10 francs a month, whether or not the parents paid the bureau the amount they had agreed upon with the nurse. If the parents failed to pay, the baby was only returned at a certain age, after the guarantee had run out. It is difficult to determine what the duration of the guarantee was before 1821. One administrator who was involved in straightening out the bureau's books from this period stated that the bureau would advance up to three months' wages when the parents did not pay, but rarely more. After the reorganization of the municipal bureau in 1821 the duration of the guarantee was ten months, which would mean that children whose parents did not pay would be returned after eleven months, since all parents paid the first month directly to the nurse in advance. Does this mean that the Bureau regarded eleven months as a suitable age for a baby to be weaned? Probably it was expected that the child would have been weaned a month or two before his return. The nurse's own child was expected to be suckled at least seven months, for if her most recent child were alive, no woman was accepted as a nurse until that child was seven months old (nor after he was eighteen months old).[13]

Earlier, in noting the later age at death of eighteenth-century *nourrissons* in comparison with the nineteenth-century sample from the Eure, I hypothesized that, before the Revolution, infants were placed with wet nurses at a later age, or returned to their parents' home at a later age, or both. In the sample from the Eure the mean length of placements for those who returned was 493 days, about 16.5 months. The eighteenth-century hospital administrator Tenon found the mean length of placement for all infants placed by the municipal bureau in the years 1770–1776 and returned to their parents' home to range between nineteen and twenty-one months.[14] The difference of about four months, although significant, is hardly enough to account for the substantially later age at death for the *nourrissons* discovered in the eighteenth-century parish registers. Eighteenth-century infants must also have been placed somewhat later (a few days would probably suffice) than those of the nineteenth century.

Galliano, who made a comparative study of mortality among native children and *nourrissons* in the southern *banlieue* of Paris in the years 1774–1794, tried to calculate the normal length of stay for the *nourrissons*. Assuming that the mortality rates were the same for the two groups of children, an assumption partly justified by the observation that the seasonal distribution of mortality was nearly identical for the two groups, Galliano prepared an index for each interval of life (days to the first week, weeks to the

13   Arch. Asst. pub., 592[6], L. Faulcon, "Notice sur la direction des nourrices," n.d.; *ibid.*, 592[6], Vée, Report of January 7, 1863, 17; *ibid.*, 709[2], *Instruction sur le service des médecins et chirurgiens chargés de la surveillance des enfans placés dans les départemens par l'intermédiaire de la Direction des Nourrices* (Paris, 1823), 10.

14   Tenon (ed. A. Chamoux), "Mise en nourrice et mortalité des enfants légitimes," *Annales de démographie historique, 1973* (Paris, 1973), 419.

first month, months to the first year, years thereafter) consisting of a ratio of deaths of *nourrissons* in that age interval compared to deaths of native children in the same age interval. He found that this ratio rose to a plateau by the end of the second week of life, then stayed on this plateau until the end of the first year, when it began to fall off at a fairly steady rate until the end of the fourth year. From these observations Galliano concluded, with due expressions of caution, "that in our region, it was between fifteen days-one month, on the one hand, and nearly two years, on the other, that the largest number of children stayed with the nurse."[15] In the nineteenth century the children of the artisans and shop-keepers of Paris—a humbler group than Galliano's sample and nursed at a greater distance from home—were probably placed with their nurses a few days earlier and returned (three out of four of them) a few months earlier.

What emerges from this study of 826 placements of Parisian infants with wet nurses from the Arrondissement of Evreux in the years 1814–1824? For peasant women, wet-nursing was a seasonal occupation, a supplement to agricultural employment and to lean rural incomes. When agricultural employment lessened, especially in the months from December through March, those women who could became wet nurses. When agricultural employment again became available, in the summer and fall months, the wet nurses became scarce in the city and, perhaps also, less attentive to the infants whom they were keeping.

For working women in the cities, the resort to rural wet nurses was probably a necessity, but not a very attractive one. One in four infants sent away would never return. Although it is difficult to translate this figure into an infant mortality, it is clear that the *petits Paris* (as the *nourrissons* were called in the country) had substantially less chance of survival than the ordinary French child of the early nineteenth century.

Those *nourrissons* who did survive returned shortly after their first birthday.[16] There is some direct evidence and strong indirect evidence (resulting from comparisons with various studies of the

---

15 Galliano, "La mortalité infantile," 159–161.
16 Unfortunately our sources provide no information about the physical condition of the *nourrissons* upon their return or their subsequent mortality. Such information, if it were available, would provide an important supplementary measure of the quality of the care provided by wet nurses.

age at death of the *nourrissons* who died in the country) that fifty years earlier, before the Revolution, Parisian children of comparable social status were placed in the country a few days later and left there with their wet nurses for a significantly longer period of time. The later age at placement may be somewhat of an illusion resulting from a difference of sources—the rural parish registers in the eighteenth century and the municipal bureau's register, kept in Paris, for the nineteenth-century sample; it may also point to an improvement in the efficiency of placement services in the nineteenth century or a real difference in nursing customs.

I think that there is an economic explanation for the younger age of infants returning from rural wet-nursing in the nineteenth century. As the population of Paris increased, and with it the number of women working outside their homes who were unable to nurse their own babies, there was greater competition for the services of good wet nurses within reasonable proximity to the capital. This competition, I think, drove the cost of wet-nursing up so high as to put it out of the reach of the urban poor for any period longer than absolutely necessary to suckle the child or longer than the period when the municipal bureau guaranteed the wet nurse's wages. Rural wet-nursing was to become still more expensive and more dangerous before pasteurization and the possibility of safe bottle-feeding began to relieve the plight of working mothers in French cities in the last decade or two of the nineteenth century.[17]

17 This argument is presented more fully in Sussman, "The Wet-Nursing Business."

Journal of Interdisciplinary History, v:4 (Spring 1975), 669–686.

William L. Langer

The Origins of the
Birth Control Movement in England
in the Early Nineteenth Century
The early nineteenth century, in England as in Europe generally, was a period of almost chronic depression and social crisis. To the far-reaching dislocations of the Industrial Revolution were added the costs of the great wars, the widespread unemployment following the demobilization of the armies, and the phenomenal increase in the size of the population after 1760. Despite all efforts to combat the prevalent poverty, the numbers of the destitute continued to multiply and the costs of relief, which devolved upon the parishes, assumed frightening proportions. Where in 1750 they had totalled only some £600,000, by the 1780s they had reached £2 million and by 1812 surpassed £8 million. There was every reason to fear an impending upheaval and many members of the upper classes recalled the revolt of the French lower classes during the recent Revolution.[1]

The problem of poverty had long exercised the thoughts of social philosophers. Indeed, it is not unfair to say that by 1798, when the Rev. Thomas Malthus published his slim *Essay on the Principle of Population*, just about all of the principal points of his argument had already been made by one or another of his predecessors.[2] This fact in no way diminishes the significance and importance of Malthus' *Essay*, which appeared in 1803 in a second, vastly enlarged, and documented edition and, through the cogency of its argument and the beauty of its style, made the author almost overnight the chief exponent and recognized leader of a school of social thought. Of the so-called

William L. Langer is Archibald Cary Coolidge Professor, Emeritus, at Harvard University. His most recent book is *Political and Social Upheaval, 1832–1852* (New York, 1969).

The essence of the present essay derives from an address delivered by the author at the annual meeting of the Association of American Physicians, in Atlantic City, 1973. It is now printed with the permission of the Association.

1 The immense literature on this subject has produced of late the excellent studies of J. R. Poynter, *Society and Pauperism* (Toronto, 1969); Brian Inglis, *Poverty and the Industrial Revolution* (London, 1971).
2 The Rev. Joseph Townsend, parson, geologist, physician, and social scientist, published his *Dissertation on the Poor Laws* in London in 1786, the very year in which he undertook his fascinating *Journey through Spain* (London, 1791; 3v.). In these works he discussed the relationship of population and poverty, providing a neat digest of what became known as the Malthusian doctrine (II, 360ff.).

"political economists" who at this time established what amounted to a monopoly of social theory, there was hardly a one, from Jeremy Bentham and David Ricardo onward, who did not adhere to the Malthusian doctrine.

Bentham, born in 1748, was by 1800 already famous as an analyst and critic of political and social institutions. He had made his home the Mecca of a brilliant group of young men fully his juniors. Prominent among them were James Mill and his son John Stuart Mill, Ricardo, Nassau Senior, George Grote, Malthus, and Francis Place. Since Bentham was a close friend of the Rev. Joseph Townsend and had himself attempted to set up a scientific system of classifying parish paupers so as to make the distribution of relief more equitable and cheaper,[3] the pressing population problem must have been frequently discussed in the circle of the Philosophical Radicals, particularly in the critical years of crop failure and desperate want in 1816–17. It has been suggested that Bentham, in his 1797 essay, first broached the subject of birth control in his discussion of the limitation of population.[4] Himes rests his case on a passage, apparently addressed to his friend Townsend, in which Bentham speaks of the use of a "spunge," but like so much of Bentham's writing, the passage is obscure and unconvincing:

> When I speak of *limitation* [of the poor rates], do not suppose that limitation would content me. My *reverend* friend, hurried away by the torrent of his own eloquence, drove beyond *you*, and let drop something about a *spunge*. I too have my spunge: but that a slow one, and not quite so rough a one. Mine goes, I promise you, into the fire, the instant you can show me that a single particle of necessity is deprived by it of relief.[5]

These enigmatic remarks, buried in an article on improvement of the poor laws, in an agricultural publication, can hardly be termed a clarion call to adopt contraception. It is quite likely that Bentham sympathized with the later efforts of his friends in this direction, but so far as is known, he had no special interest in the problem of redundancy of the working classes and never referred to the subject in the remaining decades of his life. Himes, for all his critical scholarship, in

3 Bentham, "The Situation and Relief of the Poor," in Arthur Young (ed.), *Annals of Agriculture*, XXIX (1797).
4 Norman E. Himes, "Bentham and the Genesis of Neo-Malthusianism," *Economic History*, III (1937), 267–276.
5 Bentham, "Situation and Relief," 423.

this instance has stretched the tenuous evidence much too far. Only in the very last years of his life did Bentham, in a letter to Francis Place, express agreement with the latter's "overpopulation-stopping expedient."[6]

It must not be supposed, from this digression on Bentham's "spunge," that contraception was unknown and unpracticed in the late eighteenth century. *Coitus interruptus* was an obvious, simple, and effective method of forestalling impregnation. It was probably known even among the peasants and employed by them in times of stringency when it was important to avoid producing more mouths to be fed. The fact that the Church consistently denounced and condemned it, along with abortion and infanticide, suggests that even in reasonably normal times the limitation of population was not entirely unknown.[7] From Pepys' *Diary* and other literature we learn that the sheath or condom was also used, though chiefly as a safeguard against the contraction of disease in intercourse with prostitutes. It seems likely that by the end of the eighteenth century population pressures were resulting in more general use of contraceptives, especially among the upper classes in France, England, and other countries.[8]

One might think that Malthus, with his conviction that the root cause of pauperism was the excessive procreation of the lower classes, would have welcomed any reasonable plan for the limitation of population through measures of birth control. But this was not so. The only remedy that he suggested was education of the workers, leading them to recognize the cause of their plight and inducing them to exercise "moral restraint," which he defined as "restraint from marriage from prudential motives, which is not followed by irregular gratifications." He realized that "there is no period of human life at which nature more strongly prompts to a union of the sexes than from seventeen or eighteen to twenty." For that reason he did not

6 Himes, "Bentham," 267–276.
7 John T. Noonan, Jr., *Contraception* (Cambridge, Mass., 1965); Jean-Louis Flandin, "Contraception, mariage, et relations amoureuses dans l'Occident chrétien," *Annales*, XXIV (1969), 1370–1390.
8 Richard Carlile, *The Republican*, XI (May 6, 1825), 545–576, asserted that the vaginal sponge and the sheath were known to have been in common use by the British aristocracy for at least the previous century. Recent research by French scholars shows evidence that the French upper and middle classes practiced withdrawal; see Hélène Bergues (ed.), *La prévention des naissances dans la famille* (Paris, 1960); J. Duparquier and M. Lachiver, "Sur les débuts de la contraception en France," *Annales*, XXIV (1969), 1391–1397; Pierre Goubert, "Historical Demography and the Reinterpretation of Early Modern History," *Journal of Interdisciplinary History*, I (1970), 29–48. On other countries see Hans Ferdy, *Sittliche Selbstbeschränkung* (Hildesheim, 1904), 17ff.

delude himself as to the probable acceptance of his program. But he did believe that over the long term, recognition of the inexorable facts would make an impression. After all, he argued, the upper classes were already deferring marriage for financial reasons, and many indeed remained celibate for life. How they found sexual satisfaction he did not say.[9]

Few if any of Malthus' friends and admirers saw much hope in the admonition to "moral restraint," and he was roundly rebuked by William Cobbett and other popular writers for wanting to deprive the workers of marital happiness so as to ensure the enjoyment of luxuries to the wealthy drones of society. When, eventually, the issue of contraception was raised by others, Malthus declared himself positively opposed to all "artificial" means to prevent conception, declaring such methods immoral and tending to remove a necessary stimulus to industry on the part of the workers. The reasons for his unalterable attitude were probably due primarily to his position as a clergyman, for in the years following 1820 he not only lent effective support to the plans of Robert Wilmot Horton for state support of the emigration of paupers to Canada, but continued to agitate for the abolition or at least the fundamental amendment of the poor laws, and to advocate government restrictions on the marriage of the poor, such as existed in many German states.[10] With respect to birth control, so much at least must be said for Malthus: He never publicly criticized or opposed the doctrines advanced by some of his good friends.

The opening gun, so to speak, of the birth control movement was fired in 1818 by James Mill, the close friend and collaborator of Bentham, who at this time was actually living with Bentham on his estate at Ford Abbey. In an article on "Colony" written for the supplement of the *Encyclopedia Britannica*, Mill ventured the remark that

> the best means of checking the progress of population is the most important practical problem to which the wisdom of the politician and moralist can be applied. . . . If the superstitions of the nursery were

9 Malthus, *Essay* (London, 1806; 3rd ed.), 128, 322, 327.
10 J. D. H. Cole, *The Life of William Cobbett* (New York, 1924), 119, 285; Herman Ausubel, "William Cobbett and Malthusianism," *Journal of the History of Ideas*, XIII (1952), 250–256; G. N. Ghosh, "Malthus on Emigration and Colonization," *Economica*, XXX (1963), 45–62; Edward Bryan, "The Emigration Theories of Robert Wilmot Horton," *Canadian Journal of History*, IV (1969), 45–65; Hugh M. Johnston, *British Emigration Policy, 1815–1830* (Oxford, 1972). The question of restrictions on the marriage of the poor is discussed in William L. Langer, "Checks on Population Growth," *Scientific American*, CCII (Feb. 1972), 92–99.

disregarded and the principle of utility kept steadily in view a solution might not be very difficult to be found, and the means of drying up one of the most copious sources of human evil might be seen to be neither doubtful nor difficult to be applied.[11]

Mill could hardly have expected to reach a large workingmen's audience through the supplement of the staid *Britannica* and there is in fact no evidence that these general remarks elicited any significant response. He published nothing further on the subject, nor did any other member of the Benthamite circle. The subject of intimate sex relations was completely tabu, even in Georgian society, and Mill, a man with a large family and only slender resources, apparently felt unable to face the controversy and obloquy that were certain to follow extended discussion.

Only after several years, which included the tragic clash between the armed forces and the workingmen demonstrators at Peterloo, was a more forceful effort made, this time by Francis Place, the self-educated master tailor, the champion of the laborers, and the mentor of their leaders. Place, a man of humble birth, had at age 19 married a girl under age 17 and over the years had sired fifteen children. He knew from experience how agonizing poverty and unemployment could be. Even after he had built up a successful tailoring establishment and in 1818 was wealthy enough to turn over the business to his son, he remained a workingman at heart and his one great interest was in promoting the welfare of the lower classes. A long-time friend of both Mill and Bentham, he was probably the leading proponent of contraception as a remedy for pauperism.

Place was a confirmed Malthusian, except for the fact that he regarded "moral restraint" as utterly illusory. Far from advocating

11 See article on "Colony" in *Supplement to the Fourth, Fifth and Sixth Editions of the Encyclopedia Britannica* (Edinburgh, 1824; 6v.), III, 257–273 (quote on 261). The principal source for the early history of the birth control movement is the voluminous collection of Francis Place papers in the British Museum. These were first studied by James A. Field for his articles "The Early Propagandist Movement in English Population Theory" (1910) and "The Beginnings of the Birth Control Movement" (1916), both reprinted in his *Essays on Population* (Chicago, 1931), 91–129, 206–214. The papers were more systematically and critically exploited by Himes for a series of valuable monographic studies in the 1930s and for his authoritative account, *The Medical History of Contraception* (Baltimore, 1936; reprint, New York, 1963). Among more recent treatments, Maurice Chachuat, *Le mouvement du "Birth Control" dans les pays anglo-saxons* (Lyons, 1934), is scholarly but adds almost nothing to what was already known. Peter Fryer, *The Birth Controllers* (New York, 1966), is a competent, semi-popular account; Alfred Sauvy, *La prévention des naissances* (Turin, 1962) is a superb and all-too-brief historical and critical survey of the subject.

deferment of marriage among young workers, he wished young people could marry early, while their sexual passions were at the flood. He could not see why early marriages should not be possible since methods of birth control were known to exist. "It is time," he wrote in his *Illustrations and Proofs of Population* (London, 1822) "that those who really understood the cause of a redundant, unhappy, miserable and considerably vicious population, and the means of preventing this redundancy, should clearly, freely, openly and fearlessly point out the means." Despite the apprehensions, but with the consent of his friends, he published his little book as a primer on the population problem for young workers.

The larger part of the *Illustrations* was an exposition of Malthusian doctrine: The miseries of the poor were due primarily to the superfluity of their numbers: there were simply more workers than there were jobs available. Only in the concluding passage of the book did he come to grips with his message:

> If it were clearly understood, that it was not disreputable for married persons to avail themselves of such precautionary means as would, without being injurious to health, or destructive of female delicacy, prevent conception, a sufficient check might at once be given to the increase of population beyond the means of subsistence.

Great benefits would accrue to the workers from the practice of birth control: "If means were adopted to prevent the breeding of a larger number of children than a married couple might desire to have, and if the labouring part of the population could thus be kept below the demand for labour, wages would rise so as to afford the means of comfortable subsistence for all, and all might marry."[12]

To supplement his argument with more concrete information, Place in 1823 prepared three handbills, addressed chiefly to workers, which for the first time spelled out exactly what he had in mind. These handbills were distributed in large numbers, especially among the stricken handloom weavers of Spitalfields and in the industrial districts of the north. Young men of the Benthamite circle (including the seventeen-year-old John Stuart Mill) were so assiduous in their activity that they were apprehended by the police, locked up, and released only after they had been permitted to explain their conduct to the Lord Mayor.[13]

12 Place (ed. Norman E. Himes), *Illustrations* (Boston, 1930), 164ff., 311.
13 Michael S. Packe, *The Life of John Stuart Mill* (London, 1954), 56ff.

This episode raises the question of how much support Place had in his campaign. He was a man of some means, but hardly enough to finance the operation single-handed. He was later to refer to "some hundreds" of converts that he had made among the editors of popular journals, among politicians and people in high places, and presumably among financial well-wishers. His supporters were, understandably, eager to remain anonymous, and so nothing specific can be said on this important point. Richard Carlile, the radical free-thinker and champion of freedom of the press, was one of Place's converts. He was later to speak often in his paper, *The Republican*, of the eminent persons in many professions who subscribed to the birth control movement. He was even inclined to include in this category members of the Cabinet, in which case it would be easy to understand the tolerant treatment meted out to young Mill and other enthusiasts.

It stands to reason that Place, though his authorship of the "diabolical handbills" was not certainly known, was roundly abused for the foul and devilish attempt to corrupt the youth of both sexes; but presently his convert Carlile was to draw most of the fire. Carlile, a brash and fearless journalist, was serving a long term in Dorchester Gaol for defying the press laws. He was slow to support Place, for the simple reason that, by his own confession, he had not read Malthus and had no particular interest in the population problem.[14] Deprived in jail, however, of the company of his wife, he gave much thought to the questions of sex relations which had been raised in Place's handbills. In one of his lengthy anti-religious harangues, he went so far as to attack the commandment forbidding adultery. "What is love," he queried, "but that species of lust which is here denounced?":

> Where violence and undue control and injury are studiously avoided, and the health of individuals consulted, there cannot be too much of that lust or love which is here denounced as a Christian crime; nor even too much of the gratification of that lust. It is the very source of human happiness, and essential alike to health, beauty and sweetness of temper.

With greater freedom in sex relations, he argued, the woman would no more be injured than the man so long as conception did not follow and "anyone may now prevent it that wishes."[15]

---

14 Carlile, *The Republican*, XIII (April 26, 1826), 487ff.

15 *Ibid.*, XI (May 6, 1825), 545ff. In these views he was not far removed not only from Place in his advocacy of early marriage, but even from Malthus, who at times extolled the beauties of married (i.e., "virtuous") love (*Essay*, II, 304ff.).

274 | WILLIAM L. LANGER

Place was by no means gratified by Carlile's independent procedure. As an expert promoter, Place had remained in the background
and had quitely encouraged several editors of popular papers to take
an interest and actually to reprint the handbills. The same role had been
envisaged for Carlile, who was a daring publicist with a substantial
following. But Carlile, far from interesting himself in the Malthusian
theories of redundant worker population, had seized on the idea of
contraception as opening the way to sexual freedom without consideration of the possible consequences. No doubt with the best
intentions, he had shifted the objective of Place's propaganda campaign
and had laid both himself and Place open to the public attack which
Place and his friends had so scrupulously avoided.

The agitation initiated by Carlile's original article quickly assumed
larger and larger dimensions. In response to many letters asking him
to spell out the methods by which conception could be avoided, he
felt obliged to publish a much longer essay entitled, "What is Love?"
(*The Republican*, XI [May 6, 1825], 545-576), in which he elaborated
his argument for freedom in sex relations with emphasis on the fact
that these relations need not be clouded by fear of an unwanted child.
To make matters worse, he declared that some of the wisest of men,
such as James Mill and Place, had circulated specific information in
the form of handbills, which Carlile proceeded to reprint and urge
upon the attention of all working-class leaders.

So great was the demand for this longer treatment and for an
abridgment by Godfrey Higgins that in February 1826 Carlile announ-
ced the forthcoming publication of his essay in pamphlet form under
the title *Every Woman's Book, or What is Love?* As a special attraction,
the frontispiece was to depict Adam and Eve in the nude. The pamphlet
was immediately a best seller: 5,000 copies were sold in the first six
months. Carlile, well satisfied with his achievement, was unmoved by
the attacks made upon it and declared it "the most important political
pamphlet that had yet appeared, a pamphlet containing instruction
more socially moral and more morally effectual towards the amelioration of the condition of the human race, than any or all pamphlets
put together that have yet appeared." [16]

Place, seeing what was coming, had disapproved of Carlile's

[16] *The Republican*, XIII (May 19, 1826), 622, and, esp., Carlile's statement ending
publication of his paper (*ibid.*, XIV [Dec. 29, 1826], 771). The sales of the pamphlet were
discussed by Field, *Essays on Population*, 118ff., and more recently by Fryer, *Birth
Controllers*, 77, and his letter to the *Times Literary Supplement*, June 20, 1968.

article and tried to forestall the publication of the pamphlet. Presently Cobbett, Carlile's principal rival and a writer who detested Malthus (and, in fact, most of the Benthamite circle), lost no time in proclaiming that at last a monster in human shape had been found to recommend to the wives and daughters of the laboring classes the means of putting Malthusian ideas into practice, in fact "openly and avowedly [to teach] young women to be prostitutes before they are married." The instructions were being imparted in terms "so filthy, so disgusting, so beastly, as to shock the mind of even the lewdest of men and women."[17]

The dispute between these two doughty writers continued for years. Carlile complained, with some justification, that his opponent insisted on identifying him with "the monstrous" Malthus, though in fact he was as anti-Malthusian as Cobbett himself. Carlile was not fully convinced of the threat of a redundant population while Cobbett could see no surplus except the idlers who lived off peoples' taxes.[18]

Carlile derived some consolation from Cobbett's attacks in the thought that they increased the demand for *Every Woman's Book*, the sales of which doubled in less than two years. There would be no point in reviewing this vituperative exchange. The important thing is that Carlile had, for the time being, squelched the birth control movement and had diverted the argument from the issue of population to that of sexual freedom. Place himself appears to have dropped his effort for a time until a more suitable coadjutor appeared in the person of Robert Dale Owen, son of Robert Owen of New Lanark fame. The younger Owen in 1827 returned to England from the United States, where he had taken over from his father the management of the experimental community of New Harmony. While in London his attention was called to the fact that Carlile, in his pamphlet, had attributed the initiation of the entire birth control movement to the elder Owen. The latter, according to Carlile, had paid a visit to the Continent in 1817, and while there had obtained from French physicians the information about contraception which he then incorporated in the "diabolical handbills," of which he was believed to be the author. The elder Owen, who himself had only recently returned from abroad, learned of Carlile's imputation some two years after it was made. He at once

17 Cobbett, *Weekly Register*, April 15, 1826, reprinted by Carlile in *The Republican*, XIII (April 21, 1826), 487ff. See also John W. Osborne, *William Cobbett, His Thought and His Times* (New Brunswick, N.J., 1966), 114ff.
18 Carlile, *The Lion*, I, no. 1 (Jan. 4, 1828).

called on Carlile and extracted from him the admission that he had been misinformed and an apology.[19]

Robert Dale Owen, although finding Carlile's pamphlet offensive and in some respects inaccurate, nonetheless paid tribute to his courage and was deeply impressed with the argument advanced in his writings.[20] On his return to America, he wrote appreciatively of the English birth control movement and emphasized the fact that it enjoyed the support of many influential people. But his article at once provoked an anonymous attack (later shown to have been written by Thomas Skidmore, a New York labor leader) entitled *Robert Dale Owen Unmasked by his own Pen* (New York, 1830). The author denounced the passages cited by Owen from the Carlile pamphlet as "destructive to conjugal happiness, repulsive to the moral mind, equally of man and woman, and recommending the promiscuous intercourse of sensual prostitution"(1).

Coming from a labor leader this unreasoned and uncritical attack was a severe blow to a cause to which the younger Owen had become committed. He penned an immediate reply, which before the end of 1830 was published as a pamphlet of fewer than seventy pages with the rather strange title *Moral Physiology*. This little booklet, clearly and dispassionately written, beautifully organized, and persuasively presented may well be called a minor classic of social literature, and is certainly the most attractive of all of the early writings on birth control. Its success was immediate. Within the first five months it sold 1,500 copies and by June, 1831 appeared in a fifth edition. Republished at once in England, it enjoyed the same popularity there.[21]

Writing in the spirit of Francis Place, Owen addressed himself to the humble folk who were afflicted and impoverished by too large a family. Like Place, too, he fully subscribed to Malthus' concept of overpopulation as the root cause of pauperism. But he rejected outright the program of education in "moral restraint." Sex relations, he argued,

19 The story appears to have originated with Place, for reasons that are still obscure— possibly in order to cloak his own role. Owen was anything but a Malthusian and referred to the specter of overpopulation as "hobgoblin" talk. Yet, the story of his involvement continued to enjoy credence until finally laid to rest by Himes ("The Place of John Stuart Mill and of Robert Owen in the History of English Neo-Malthusianism," *Quarterly Journal of Economics*, XLII [1928], 627–640). The episode is well reviewed by Rowland H. Harvey, *Robert Owen, Social Idealist* (Berkeley, 1949), 64ff.

20 Robert Dale Owen, in the preface to *Moral Physiology* (Boston, 1875; 10th ed.).

21 Norman E. Himes, "Robert Dale Owen: The Pioneer of American Neo-Malthusians," *American Journal of Sociology*, XXXV (1930), 529–547; Richard W. Leopold, *Robert Dale Owen* (Cambridge, Mass., 1940), 60ff., 76ff.

should have more than a purely procreative purpose, for they constitute one of the most beautiful of human relations and should, if possible, be relieved of the fear of too many children. He noted, from his own experience, that in France large families were but rarely met with even among the working classes. From his discussions with French and English physicians he was convinced that control over sexual relations was possible, that

> men and women may, without injury to health, or the slightest violence done to moral feelings, and with but small diminution of the pleasure which accompanies the gratification of the instinct, refrain at will from becoming parents.

In conclusion he spoke briefly of various methods to accomplish this end.[22]

Owen's booklet could well have been written by Place himself, had he been anywhere near as competent a stylist. In any case, one can understand that he was delighted with it and frequently presented copies of it to his friends and to those whom he hoped to interest. Meanwhile, Owen's essay suggested the problem of contraception to Charles Knowlton, a New England physician in good standing and, like Place, Carlile, and Owen, a free-thinker and secularist. Like his predecessors, he put no stock in the idea of "moral restraint." He was a great admirer of Owen's booklet, but as a physician was dissatisfied with Owen's recommendations as to method, viz., withdrawal or drawback (*coitus interruptus*), as practiced by the French. In the introduction to the fourth edition of his own tract (1839) he tells us that he spent many nights and days in reflection on the technique of contraception before he hit upon a better method, which turned out to be the vaginal syringe, with or without some chemical additive in the water.

Knowlton's contribution, anonymously published in New York in 1832 under the title *The Fruits of Philosophy*, has none of the charm of Owen's essay, but had the distinction of being the first study of contraceptive techniques since the writings of Soranos in the second century A.D. He had the further, questionable distinction of being the first known person in the Western world to be tried and convicted for distributing birth control literature.[23] On the other hand, he had the

22 Owen, in the Preface to *Moral Physiology* (Boston, 1831; 3d ed.). I have also used his Preface to the 10th edition (New York, 1858).
23 After two mistrials he was finally sentenced to three months in jail by a Massachusetts court.

satisfaction of knowing that his tract was probably the most influential of all of the early writings on the subject. Republished and pirated in England in 1833 and 1834, it sold briskly, due no doubt to the prestige of the author as a professional medical man. In terms of information it went beyond Carlile or Owen in the description of the generative organs and the entire process of impregnation, subjects about which at the time and even much later there was a degree of popular curiosity exceeded only by professional ignorance.[24]

In reviewing the early birth control movement in England it cannot be too strongly emphasized that it grew out of the conviction of almost all economists that the increasing poverty was due to a superabundance of workers.[25] But even the most whole-hearted supporters of Malthus had no faith in the efficacy of "moral restraint" as a remedy for this overriding problem. Aware of various methods of contraception, they looked upon the practice as the long-range solution of the problem. But so intense was public feeling about the discussion of sex matters that even Place, himself a member of the working classes and a man enjoying the confidence of labor leaders, decided to operate anonymously. The experience of young John Stuart Mill evidently made a life-long impression. He never wavered in his belief in the rightness of birth control, but avoided all public involvement and, in a letter written as late as 1868, expressed doubt as to the wisdom of general publication. He thought that it was up to medical men to provide guidance to their patients.[26] It is truly remarkable, however, that in England there were no prosecutions until the Bradlaugh-Besant case (1877), which suggests that the movement enjoyed at least the tacit approval of many influential persons.

What success the Place propaganda may have had can never be known. Of the wide dissemination of both the handbills and the pamphlets by Carlile, Owen, and Knowlton there can be no reasonable

24 Copies of the earlier editions of Knowlton's tract are far more rare than those of Owen's booklet, partly because the former kept publication to 3,000 copies until 1839, when he was finally convinced of the soundness of his method. See the article by Norman E. Himes in the *Dictionary of American Biography* (New York, 1933), 471–472, and, esp., Himes' introduction to a modern edition of *The Fruits of Philosophy* (Mt. Vernon, N.Y., 1937), which for unknown reasons has become just about as rare as the early editions.

25 A. J. Taylor, "Progress and Poverty in Britain, 1750–1850," *History*, XLV (1960), 16–31, came to the conclusion that there was in fact a superabundant labor supply at that time.

26 Norman E. Himes, "John Stuart Mill's Attitude toward Neo-Malthusianism," *Economic History*, I (1929), 457–484.

doubt. They were sold by the tens of thousands, were passed from hand to hand, read aloud in the pubs and discussed in the workingmen's press.[27] The question is whether all of this discussion and literature made the desired impression. Carlile, who so confused the issue with his *Every Woman's Book*, admitted that many of his readers who supported the secularist position reacted negatively to his espousal of sexual freedom.[28] At least some of the popular leaders would have nothing to do with the notion that workingmen should limit their numbers. "Is it reasonable," wrote the influential *Trades Newspaper*, "to expect that the labouring man alone should propagate on general principle, and consult the population tables every time he goes to bed?" Even Thomas Carlyle could not conceive of twenty million workers simultaneously striking against further procreation: "passing in universal trade union a resolution not to beget any more children till the labour market becomes satisfactory." Even much later many workingmen continued to regard the sequence of babies as an act of God: "One would imagine," wrote John Stuart Mill, "that children were rained down upon married people, direct from heaven, without their being art or part in the matter."[29]

The reaction to the birth control literature was no doubt influenced by the lack of agreement among the proponents as to the best method for attaining the desired end. Place was convinced that French women were using the vaginal sponge, and this was the device so ardently urged in the "diabolical handbills." But it was at best a clumsy arrangement, hardly feasible among the lower classes who lived seven or eight in a room, without privacy, without running water, and without even the most primitive conveniences. Robert Dale Owen, on the other hand, had been educated in Switzerland and France and had many personal contacts on the Continent. He insisted that Place was misinformed and that the method used in France was *coitus interruptus*, which was the simplest, most obvious, and most reliable as well as the cheapest method known. Knowlton, who studied the question as none before him had done, finally proposed the vaginal syringe or douche

27 The radical paper *Black Dwarf* in 1819 reached a circulation of 12,000–13,000, which about equalled that of the *Edinburgh Review* and the *Quarterly Review* in their heyday. See Arthur Aspinall, *Politics and the Press, c.1789–1850* (London, 1949), 24ff.; Richard D. Altick, *The English Common Reader, 1800–1900* (Chicago, 1957), 322ff.
28 *The Republican*, XIV (Dec. 29, 1826), 771; *The Lion*, I, no. 1 (Jan. 4, 1928).
29 Patricia Hollis, *The Pauper Press* (Oxford, 1970), 230ff.; Carlyle, *Chartism* (London, 1839), quoted by Mark Blaug, *Ricardian Economics* (New Haven, 1958), ch. 6; Mill, *Principles of Political Economy* (London, 1848), I, 445ff.

with the use, if possible, of some germicide in the water—a scientific but hardly a simple procedure.[30]

Most important was the innate distrust of the workers for the upper classes. The early socialists, almost to a man, rejected the Malthusian notion of a superfluity of the labor market as the basic cause of pauperism. They insisted and for the better part of another century continued to insist that the workers' misery was due to the unequal and unjust distribution of the world's goods. Not the workers, but the institutions were at fault. The Malthusian doctrine of poverty reduced "the whole matter to a question between mechanics and their sweethearts and wives [rather than] to a question between employed and employees.[31] Robert Owen of New Lanark was convinced that the productive power of mankind was far greater than the population increase and the eminent socialist William Thompson completely rejected the notion of a surplus population.[31]

Malthus and his doctrine were anything but popular among the ordinary citizenry. "His name was already spitten upon by almost every decent and religiously-minded man and woman in the country. To doubt that 'God sent food for every mouth which he sent into the world' was blasphemous; to inquire further was obscene." As for Place, "his name, for twenty years, was hardly ever mentioned in print without some reference, deprecatory or abusive, to his notorious opinions. . . . Among the leaders of the workmen he met with but little success."[32]

Also important was the fact that latent class antagonisms had been fanned into flames of hatred by the Industrial Revolution and the trials of the revolutionary age. So great was the mutual distrust that while the propertied classes lived in constant dread of social upheaval

---

30 Recent studies have shown that even in the twentieth century, when contraception has become common, some 70% of French and British users employ withdrawal; see Jacques Bertillon, *La dépopulation de la France* (Paris, 1911); Philippe Ariès, "Interprétation pour une histoire des mentalités," in Bergues, *La prévention des naissances*, 311–328: For England see Griselda Rountree and Rachel M. Pierce, "Birth Control in Britain," *Population Studies*, XV (1961), 3–31, 99–101; John Peel, "The Manufacture and Retailing of Contraceptives in England," *ibid.*, XVII (1963–64), 113–125.

31 *Trades Newspaper* (1825), quoted by E. P. Thompson, *The Making of the English Working Class* (London, 1963), 776ff., and Hollis, *Pauper Press*, 231ff; John F. C. Harrison, *Quest for a New World: Robert Owen and the Owenites in Britain and America* (New York, 1969), 68; William Thompson, *An Inquiry into the Principles of the Distribution of Wealth* (London, 1824; reprint, New York, 1963); Richard K. P. Pankhurst, *William Thompson* (London, 1921), 66ff.

32 Graham Wallas, *The Life of Francis Place* (New York, 1919), 169–170.

by the redundant (i.e., unemployed) workers, the latter were convinced that their masters, under the guidance of Malthus, were aiming at making it all but impossible for the poor to marry and start families, and that they were preparing to "shovel out" the paupers into the colonial wilderness. The discussions preceding the amendment of the poor law (1834) gave rise to rumors that those on relief were to be deprived of their children, that families were to be broken up, that paupers were to be put on starvation rations. From Devon one of the new poor law commissioners reported in 1836 that the people were frightened and determined to resist:

> Among the ridiculous statements circulated, the peasantry fully believed that all the bread was poisoned, and that the only cause for giving it instead of money was the facility it afforded of destroying the paupers; that all young children and women under eighteen were to be spared; that if they touched the bread they would instantly drop dead.[33]

The suspicion and distrust of the workers was highlighted by other specific episodes. During the first great cholera epidemic (1831–1832) the lower classes all over Europe believed that physicians had been employed by the upper classes to poison the water supply so as to reduce the numbers of the indigent by increasing the mortality.[34] By 1838 the hysteria came to a climax with the publication of *An Essay on Populousness* (London, 1838) by "Marcus." This effusion blandly proposed infanticide as a simple and effective way of disposing of superfluous children. They were to be painlessly asphyxiated, leaving the mother with the satisfaction of having born a child without condemning it to a miserable existence. To make the plan more attractive "Marcus" suggested the erection of a "repository" for the "privileged remains of those infants unadmitted to life." There was to be nothing "funereal" about it, on the contrary it was to be made cheerful by being gently warmed in winter and kept fresh in summer, "verdant always, yet not expensive in exotics ... let this be the infants' paradise."

33 Richard E. Rose, *The English Poor Law, 1780–1930* (London, 1971), 104–105, quoting the *Second Annual Report of the Poor Law Commission*, Appendix B, no. 9; Nicholas C. Edsall, *The Anti-Poor Law Movement, 1834–1844* (Manchester, 1971), 32ff.
34 Melitta Schmideberg, "The Role of Psychotic Mechanisms in Cultural Development," *International Journal of Psychoanalysis*, XI (1930), 387–418; René Baehrel, "La haine de classe au temps d'épidémie," *Annales*, VII (1952), 351–360.

This ingenious proposal was at once snapped up by the Rev. Joseph R. Stephens, the Chartist leader, who attributed the authorship to the Commissioners of the Poor Law. Edwin Chadwick, the principal artisan of the amended poor law, at once repudiated the charge (*The Times*, Jan. 10, 1839), but Stephens stuck to his guns and identified Chadwick with the Benthamite circle, and especially with his "bosom friend Mr. Francis Place." The Marcus book soon disappeared, but rumors persisted that secret instructions had been issued by government officials or their henchmen to restrict the numbers of the poor by exterminating surplus infants. Presently pirated editions of the pamphlet appeared and, in 1841, the original was reissued under the title *The Book of Murders: a Vade Mecum for the Commissioners and Guardians of the New Poor Law*, with a preface roundly abusing both Malthus and Place. One might look upon the whole incident as something of a hoax. Yet the Commissioners reported that it was believed by many workers, and indeed prominent Chartist editors (like Feargus O'Connor of the *Northern Star*) took it up and made the most of it.

The lack of interest of almost all socialist writers in the population problem and their vehement denial of all redundancy of the working class persisted until almost the end of the century. G. A. Gaskell, who claimed an intimate acquaintance with the laborers, expressed the opinion in 1890 that the vast majority of the workers would not curb their procreative powers, either for the welfare of society or for their own domestic comfort. Society meant little to them: "The state offers no assistance and imposes no restraints, and the common man resents the interference with his liberty of having as many children as he pleases."[35]

There is no firm evidence, then, that the early birth control movement had much impact on working–class circles. It does seem, though, that during the mid-century contraception spread among the educated middle classes, with the professional people taking the lead.[36] By the mid-century contraceptive doctrine had been adopted by many free-thinking, secularist circles, as illustrated by the agitation of Charles

35 Gaskell, *Social Control of the Birth Rate and Endowment of Mothers* (London, 1890).
36 As early as May, 1835, an anonymous correspondent of Carlile's *Republican* wrote that apparently nine out of ten English medical men practiced birth control, judging from the size of their families. Somewhat later, Robert Dale Owen remarked that while the practice had been adopted by some working people, it had also been taken up "by persons who live genteel lives on narrow incomes" (quoted by Field, *Essays on Population*, 121ff.). It may be regarded as something of a mystery that Malthus himself fathered only three children in the course of thirty years of married life.

Bradlaugh and more particularly by the anonymous appearance in 1854 of one of the most comprehensive and competent treatments of the subject ever to see the light: *The Elements of Social Science, or Physical, Sexual and Natural Religion.*[37] The author was a young physician, a confirmed Malthusian, and an active member of the Secularist Society, George R. Drysdale by name.

The Elements proved to be extremely popular, despite its six-hundred pages and its rather dense style. By 1892 it had reached the twenty-ninth edition and had sold 77,000. Quickly translated into many European languages, it was perhaps the chief stimulus to revival of the birth control movement. The reasons for its popularity are fairly obvious, for it provided a competent review of the entire Malthusian doctrine, followed by an interesting review of Malthus' influence both in England and abroad, a detailed discussion of the physiology of sex, and, particularly, a review of all known or suspected venereal diseases. Only in the briefest fashion did the author analyze various methods of what he called "preventive intercourse." So well did Drysdale fill the bill that his book is still interesting reading a century later.[38]

The Drysdale book served as the prelude to the spectacular Bradlaugh-Besant trial of 1877, by which time the striking decline in the size of French families had already aroused much discussion in England.[39] Charles Bradlaugh and Annie Besant were Secularist leaders already known as champions of birth control. They provoked their arrest by publishing and selling copies of Knowlton's *Fruits of Philosophy* with illustrations definitely pornographic in character. The defendants were charged with the wicked intention "to incite and encourage the said subjects [of Her Majesty] to indecent, obscene, unnatural and immoral practices" by selling "a certain indecent, lewd, filthy, bawdy, and obscene book."[40] They were convicted, but the case was presently dismissed on a technicality. A year later the Secularist publisher Edward Truelove was tried for issuing a new edition of

---

37 The first two editions were entitled *Physical, Sexual and Natural Religion.*
38 Karl Kautsky, *Der Einfluss der Volksvermehrung auf den Fortschritt der Gesellschaft* (Vienna, 1880), 171ff.; Georges Hardy, *Malthus et ses disciples* (Paris, 1912), 26ff.
39 The average number of births per French family sank from 4.2 in 1800 to 4.0 in 1820, to 3.11 in 1851–1853, and to 3.03 in 1881–1885 (Emile Levasseur, *La population française* [Paris, 1889–92], III, 150ff.; David V. Glass, "World Population, 1800–1950," in the *Cambridge Economic History of Europe* [Cambridge, 1965], VI [1], 60–138).
40 *The High Court of Justice: The Queen v. Charles Bradlaugh and Annie Besant* (London, 1878).

Robert Dale Owen's *Moral Physiology*, but escaped conviction through the failure of the jury to agree. In the course of the trial the defense counsel made the following interesting and unchallenged statement, that

> There is a very large number of persons—more influential than you think, more wealthy than you would perhaps believe—a large number of individuals who believe that the doctrine of limitation of families is—if I may so express it—the one doctrine which renders morality practicable to a large part of the population.[41]

Even if some allowance is made for the lawyer's rhetoric, it remains true that by 1878 the British birthrate also had begun to decline and that contraception was already an established practice among the upper and middle classes. The Bradlaugh-Besant trial, although it did not inaugurate the birth control movement, certainly gave it wide publicity and created a demand for more information.[42] The renewed interest is attested by the fact that in the few years from 1876 to 1881 some 200,000 copies of the Knowlton tract were sold in England, while Annie Besant's own excellent little book, *The Law of Population* (London, 1877) sold 175,000 copies by 1891. The Malthusian League (founded in 1877) began publication of *The Malthusian* in 1879 and thus provided a clearing house for the entire European Neo-Malthusian movement.[43]

At the present time, when contraception is being practiced almost universally in the Western world and when governments are spending huge sums of money to promote birth control throughout the world, it is already clear that this revolution in social thinking and practice will stand as one of the major departures in the history of human society. Its beginnings lie in the early nineteenth century, when the main objective was to counteract growing poverty. Today, though no doubt there are other considerations in the spread of contraception, we can still argue that there are too many people and that the conquest of poverty and, indeed, starvation hinges on the limitation of population growth.

41 *The Queen v. Edward Truelove* (London, 1878).
42 Marie C. Stopes, *Early Days of Birth Control* (London, 1923; 3rd ed.), did her best to minimize the importance of the trial, but see J. A. Banks and Olive Banks, "The Bradlaugh-Besant Trial and the English Newspapers," *Population Studies*, VIII (1954), 22–34.
43 For an excellent review and analysis of the crucial period of the 1870s see J. A. Banks, *Prosperity and Parenthood* (London, 1954), which interestingly relates the development of birth control to the changing economic conditions.

Peter Laslett

Age at Menarche in Europe
since the Eighteenth Century
Age at sexual maturation is of obvious interest to historians of the family. It determines the point at which children reach the crisis of adolescence and begin the process of asserting their independence from their parents, and from the family of origin generally. It marks the stage at which they become capable of full sexual intercourse, and, for girls, of experiencing menstruation, both of which stages are often of crucial psychological significance. It introduces the possibility of procreation, which immediately implies stringent social control. For no community at any period, whatever its resources, can ever allow individuals to reproduce at will. In most societies known to me—certainly in all societies belonging to the Christian tradition, and perhaps in almost every other, too—sexual maturation is an essential preliminary to marriage for both sexes.

This is a subject which must affect the historian of social structure generally even more than most of those which concern the family group. If children mature late, then presumably parental supremacy endures longer. This has implications for societies organized on patriarchal lines which are easy to see. Furthermore there are the indications that age at sexual maturation may differ between social classes, and this implies a distinction in the fundamental process of personality development between bourgeoisie and workers, or, in the past, between lords and ladies, gentlemen and gentlewomen, as compared to common folk.[1] Yet almost nothing numerical is known about age at sexual maturity for any society before the twentieth century, and what fragments of information we have mostly concern only one of the conspicuous developments which occur at this time to one of the sexes. This is menarche, the onset of menstruation or of the "flowers," as our ancestors more elegantly phrased it. Some statistical information is available on the heights and weights of both sexes in nineteenth century Europe, and it may be that documents will be found which

Peter Laslett is co-founder of the Cambridge Group for the History of Population and Social Structure and is Reader in Politics and the History of Social Structure in the University of Cambridge.

1 See Peter Laslett, *The World We Have Lost* (London, 1971; 2nd ed.), 89, where I refer to sixteenth- and seventeenth-century England.

would push our knowledge of these particulars further back. But, for the moment, it looks as if the history of age at menarche—the age in time when a woman is first capable of conception—will have to stand for the whole phenomenon of sexual maturation in men and women.

We have to be satisfied, however, with the small things which we can do in historical sociology, and the little insight we have into the secular trend of age at menarche is certainly intriguing. Most of it seems to confirm the tendency toward a progressive decline in the age at which women became mature. Tanner, who is the established authority on this complex subject, and the only contemporary medical writer who appears to be collecting information on the long-term and short-term trends, estimates that "menarche in Europe has been getting earlier during the last hundred years by between three and four months per decade."[2] To its level in Great Britain in the 1960s of about 13.25 years, it has fallen from about 14.5 in the 1920s, 15.5 in the 1890s, 16.5 in the 1860s, and 17.5 in the 1830s. He prints a series of figures from observations going back over the past 125 years.[3] Though they come from a variety of northern and western European countries (Denmark, Finland, Sweden, Germany, and Great Britain), these observations plot a noticeably regular line.[4] This line slopes downward from an age of a little over 17 for Norway in the 1840s, through the range 15.5–16.2 in the 1880s for Norway, Finland, Sweden, and Germany, down to 14.5–15.0 in the 1920s, and so down to its present level. Starting at 1900, records for the United States show a consistently lower age at menarche, which fell to 12.5–13.0 in 1940–45 (white girls). But the curve is roughly parallel in America, and all series show the same downward tendency for the twentieth century.

The literature provides little critical examination of the sources of these figures, but Tanner has said that the data are sketchy and not entirely reliable for all of the earlier recordings. (It has not been possible to investigate the documentation which lies behind these conclusions.[5]) My object is to call attention to such possibilities as are open

2 J. M. Tanner, "The Secular Trend Towards Earlier Physical Maturation," *Tydshrift voor geneeskunde*, XLIV (1966), 531.

3 *Ibid.*, 532. Cf. J. M. Tanner, *Growth at Adolescence* (Oxford, 1962; 2nd ed.), 152.

4 *Ibid.*, 153.

5 Since this paper was written, some of Tanner's early nineteenth-century evidence has been reviewed. Its imperfections are evident but it appears that it can be used and extended in interesting ways. Results will be published in due course.

to the sociological historian, and, particularly, to the historical demographer, for the examination of this important problem. In particular, I use the very imprecise but nevertheless illuminating evidence of an individual document—that of a list of the Christian Orthodox inhabitants of Belgrade, the capital of what was once Serbia, now Yugoslavia, for the year 1733–34. We shall see that estimates of the maximal age at sexual maturity for women recoverable from that document point to a period at which menarche occurred earlier than it apparently did in Norway in the 1840s or in Finland in the 1850s.

Although the evidence of actual observations is difficult to obtain and tricky to use, literary evidence is obtainable and is beginning to be published. It also tends to confirm the probability that age at menarche may have been about fourteen in medieval and early modern times, so that it must have risen later on to reach the ages which have been recorded for the nineteenth century. Tanner himself quotes interestingly from Shakespeare and from an early seventeenth century writer named Quarinonius or Guarinonius. But literary evidence of this kind should be handled with great care, even with some suspicion.[6]

Nevertheless, it is useful to cite the materials from medieval literature collected and discussed in an interesting note by Post.[7] They bear more weight as empirical evidence, being the writings of medieval gynecologists. At their strongest, the statements quoted by Post imply that age at menarche was observed by these physicians to occur in the thirteenth or fourteenth year. Of course, the accuracy of these observations is somewhat impaired by the further claim, which Post quotes from Avicenna and such splendidly entitled works as *Trotula Major* and *Trotula Minor*, that menstruation lasts "until the fiftieth year if the woman is thin; until sixty or sixty-five or fifty-five if she is moist; until thirty-five if moderately fat." Though Post suggests that these absurdities about the cessation of menstruation, the menopause, may be due to the paucity of cases, as few women lived into the higher ages, they seem to me to be unfortunately typical of the literary sources, even when medical. They are

6 See Laslett, *The World We Have Lost*, 57, where I discuss the notorious case of Juliet's marriage age in *Romeo and Juliet* being used as an indication of mean age at marriage for women in Elizabethan England.

7 J. B. Post, "Ages at Menarche and Menopause: Some Medieval Authorities," *Population Studies*, XXV (1971), 83–87.

ordinarily incapable of yielding anything which is, properly speaking, numerical.[8]

The one way to obtain figures would appear to be by working backward from marriage recordings. Since a marriage within the universal Christian church could only be celebrated if both parties were sexually mature, figures for the age at first marriage for women can be taken as figures for *maximal* age at menarche. Care must be taken, however, to distinguish between a promise to marry (a *spousal*), and marriage itself. A person could become engaged at any age, before puberty or after, and the undertaking was regarded as binding by the church like any other promise. This engagement became a valid marriage when sexual intercourse took place, quite apart from a church ceremony. But spousal itself was not a marriage. Indeed, as is well known, inability to copulate in either partner was a proper ground for ending an engagement, or even of annulling a "marriage."[9]

A marriage could exist which had not been celebrated in church and so, presumably, had never been registered. Nevertheless, both partners to such a union were, by definition, sexually mature at the time it began. If, therefore, the date of a woman's marriage is known, then it can be assumed that she was sexually mature at the time. But it remains uncertain as to how long she had been mature. Mean age at first marriage as an indication of maximal age at menarche is of little use even if it falls below the age of 21 unless it tells us something over and above what is known on general grounds, for a mean age at menarche of much above twenty can be discounted. Unfortunately it turns out that women only rarely were married before twenty in Western Europe before the nineteenth century. No mean age at first marriage, as calculated from parish registers by the complex process of family reconstitution,[10] ever falls as low in England, France, or even eighteenth century Canada, where the age was lowest.[11] It seems,

8 *Ibid.* The evidence of family reconstitution may finally establish something like a mean age of cessation of fertility, which would, in its turn, presumably be a firm indicator of the age of menopause. If there is any necessary relationship between menopause and menarche, then it would follow that such a figure could be used to establish the earlier event, too.

9 On spousals, see Laslett, *The World We Have Lost,* 140–145.

10 See E. A. Wrigley, "Family Reconstitution," in E. A. Wrigley (ed.), *An Introduction to English Historical Demography from the Sixteenth to the Nineteenth Century* (London, 1966), 96–159; *idem.,* "Family Limitation in Pre-Industrial England," *The Economic History Review,* XIX (1966), 82–109; *idem.,* "Mortality in Pre-Industrial England," *Daedalus,* XLVII (1968), 546–577.

11 Jacques Henripin, *La population Canadienne au début du XVIIIe siècle* (Paris, 1954).

after all, that nothing useful can be learned about age at menarche from the study of ecclesiastical marriage registrations in Western Europe—certainly there is nothing to help us decide whether sexual maturity came earlier or later in the eighteenth century than in the nineteenth.

Some women married and had children before twenty, even in England and France. An intense study of the baptismal registers might add to the impression gained from the many miscellaneous sources which bear upon the problem that conception was certainly possible in the teens among the English or French peasantry and townsfolk of earlier times. Little more can be expected of the parochial registers in these countries.[12] Nevertheless, there is an independent documentary source of an "observational" kind in such census-type documents as have survived from before the nineteenth century. If such a list of inhabitants specifies ages and familial relationships, then it is possible to see how many women were married before twenty, and how many at the crucial ages were accompanied by children. This last observation enables us, by subtracting the ages of eldest resident children from those of their mothers, to obtain something like a mean age of first conception for all mothers in the community.[13]

Among the 780 inhabitants of the Warwickshire agricultural and mining village of Chilvers Coton in the year 1684, for example, there were three married women whose ages are given as below twenty. None of these had an accompanying child incontrovertibly her own, though one (aged eighteen) had two present with her who looked as if they belonged to her husband (aged fifty) and had been born to a previous wife. Nevertheless, subtraction shows that one wife living in the village had conceived at fourteen, two at fifteen, one at sixteen,

12 It might be thought that information about ages of mothers at the birth of bastards might provide some useful information, and a few such figures are beginning to be available to us from family reconstitution; indeed, one of these appears below. Nevertheless, the first indications are that the proportion of all illegitimate births which took place among women under twenty was low, less than 6 per cent of all those occurring in one English village between the sixteenth and nineteenth centuries, where the women's birth dates are known. This compares with over 35 per cent in the United States in 1959. See Peter Laslett and Karla Oosterveen, *Illegitimacy in England, Sixteenth to Nineteenth Centuries* (forthcoming), for details.
13 See Peter Laslett, "The Work of the Cambridge Group for the History of Population and Social Structure," in Mattei Dogan and Stein Rokkan, *Quantitative Ecological Analysis in the Social Sciences* (Cambridge, Mass., 1969) and "Mean Size of Household in England Since the 16th Century," *Population Studies*, XXIII (1969), 199–223, for sources of this kind and their exploitation.

two at eighteen, and four at nineteen.[14] Only 31 out of the 229 cases of women with children are described well enough to count, and although it may seem surprising that ten of these women apparently conceived before the age of twenty, it must be remembered that the recently married are the most likely to provide the precise information that makes subtraction possible.

These facts from Chilvers Coton illustrate sufficiently the difficulties of such data. Among the thirty-one whose particulars we can analyze in this way, the mean apparent age at first conception turns out to be well over twenty-two. No estimate for a maximum age of menarche for all women of the village at this time could be based on this handful of cases. If it had been possible to check the census-type document with the parish register, we would at least have had some independently sanctioned dates of first birth, and some reliable marriage ages. But the registers of Chilvers Coton are defective for this period, and, even if we had both good parochial registration and a listing giving ages, the small numbers marrying under twenty in any English village would ensure that no decent maximal figure for age at menarche could be obtained. This is why it is so fortunate that a listing of inhabitants has appeared which clearly belongs to an area and an epoch where mean age at marriage for women was below the age of twenty, and where the possibilities of working out a useful estimate of something like a maximal age at menarche are accordingly much better.

It is true that a much more accurate result would have been obtainable for maximal age at menarche in that region and at that time were there a full and well kept set of Serbian parish registers covering the years from 1650 to 1750 and preferably earlier and later years as well. Family reconstitution based on such a record can yield a mean

14 It is to be expected that the numbers of conceptions below twenty for the whole group of women should be much higher than those for women actually below that age at the time of the count, since the first figure represents those belonging to all the age cohorts present, and the second only to one of them. Nevertheless, in view of the probable loss from the sample of children already dead and those who had left home, which must have been considerable, the difference looks rather large, as it does in Belgrade and in all of the examples we have studied, including official nineteenth-century census documents. The explanation may lie partly in the fact that the very youngest are the least well recorded in all counts of this kind, and in the wish to conceal illegitimate births or births conceived before marriage, a motive which is less important when reporting children's ages later on. More important is the fact that no child born in the year of the count after the date of the count will appear, but all subsequent births which occurred in that year will be referred later on to the year in which the count was made.

age of first marriage for women, and so a maximal age at menarche, for any chosen sub-period of, say, twenty-five, thirty-five or fifty years, depending on the size of the community concerned. It can also yield a mean age of first conception, including pre-marital and extra-marital conceptions, which might suggest a significantly lower age at menarche than the maximum indicated by the mean age at first marriage.

The census-type document from Belgrade which the Cambridge Group for the History of Population and Social Structure has been given the opportunity to work upon is, however, of great interest for many purposes, in addition to the present one.[15] With the expected shortcomings and imperfections, it provides the names, most of the ages and sexes, and indications of relationships within the household, of 1,357 Serbian Orthodox Christians living in Belgrade at a date given by the scholar who had the document printed as being 1733-34. The naming system makes it possible to infer the sexes of nearly all persons and to check the relationship of children to their biological fathers, though not to their mothers.[16]

An examination of the distribution of this population by age, sex, and marital status shows that its marriage habits were very different from those we have found in England and France at the same period, and, in particular, in Chilvers Coton in 1684. Whereas in Belgrade nearly 70 per cent of all women in the age group 15-19 were married or widowed, the proportion at Chilvers Coton was under 10 per cent. Stated a little differently, 87 per cent of all women above the age of fifteen, 96 per cent above twenty, and 98 per cent above twenty-five, were married or widowed in Belgrade. In Chilvers Coton, however, these figures were 54 per cent, 65 per cent, and 77 per cent. In a group of six preindustrial English parishes, the proportion married above the age of fifteen was only 60 per cent, and only a mere six out of the 402 women in these villages aged between fifteen

15   See Peter Laslett and Marilyn Clarke, "Household and Familial Structure in Belgrade, 1733/4," paper presented at the International Conference on the Comparative History of the Family (Cambridge, September, 1969).

16   This rare manuscript appears to have been drawn up by the clergy and was published by D. J. Popović, "Gradja za istoriju Beograda, 1711–1739," *Proceedings of the Royal Serbian Academy*, LXXVIII, fascicule 61 (Belgrade, 1935) 59–65. The reference was supplied to the Cambridge Group by Joel Halpern of the University of Massachusetts, and the work of transliteration from the Cyrillic and of translation was done by Stojana Burton of Newnham College, Cambridge. Marilyn Clarke has done the intricate work of disentangling ages, etc., on this list, and Michael Prentice the statistical work.

and nineteen were married at all. Although in the absence of marriage recordings for the women at issue in Belgrade we cannot know their mean age at first marriage, it must have been well below twenty. This in itself is a hint that they reached maturity in the early rather than the late teens.

The high marriage rate among young women is brought out by the first of the three tables printed below, which together present the numerical evidence from the Belgrade list as it bears on the question of the age of sexual maturation. As might be expected in an unsettled population living in a region characterized by a state of military confusion and low material standards, with presumably a modest level of education throughout the community, the figures are approximate in detail and incomplete overall. Sex information is missing for 13.5 per cent of the people, and age information for 11.6 per cent. Some of these persons appear, from their position in their families and the ages of their close kin, to have been eligible for consideration if proper particulars had been present. The peculiarities of the data are plain enough from the figures below, at least in respect of the clustering at various ages.

In Table 1 the numbers and ages of all women up to the age of twenty-one are given with information as to their marital status and the presence of children. In Table 2 mothers only are listed by age from twenty-two upwards. In Table 3 the ages of mothers at the birth of their first child are given. These were obtained by subtracting the number of years given for the eldest resident son or daughter from that of his or her own mother.[17]

The rough and arbitrary character of this series of numbers will convince the reader that very little in the way of reliable detailed inference can be expected of them, though general inferences of a fair probability seem permissible. The figures of Table 3—the ages at the birth of the first child—naturally interest us the most, but some are impossible. Girls of six and eight cannot have had babies. But, before we tackle these and other oddities, let us make what we can of the figures in the first table concerning the number of women married at various ages. They demonstrate that, insofar as women knew their

17 It is not always clear whether a child mentioned after a woman's name is, in fact, her offspring, though in nearly all cases the relationship is made unambiguous by the presence of the words *his* or *her*, or by the naming system which, in Serbian usage, links all offspring to their fathers. The uncertainty is greatest in the case of widows, especially those of more advanced years.

Table 1 Women 10–21, by age, marital status, and presence of offspring

	AGE	NUMBER	MARRIED		WITH CHILDREN	
			NUMBER	%	NUMBER	%
	10	25	0	0	0	0
	11	9	0	0	0	0
	12	19	1	5.3	0	0
	13	16	0	0	0	0
	14	8	0	0	0	0
Totals	10–14	77	1	1.3	0	0
	15	9	3	33.3	0	0
	16	9	5	55.5	0	0
	17	10	8	80.0	1	10.0
	18	15	11	73.2	2	13.3
	19	10	10.	100.0	5	50.0
Totals	15–19	53	37	69.8	8	15.1
Totals	10–19	130	38	29.3	8	6.1
	20	31	30[a]	96.6	12	38.7
	21	10	9	90.0	6	60.0
Totals	10–21	171	77[a]	45.0	26	15.2
Totals	15–21	94	76[a]	80.9	26	27.6

a Including one widow.

ages, and had them accurately recorded by the Christian Orthodox priest who seems to have drawn up the census, marriage did in fact come very early. A third of all girls of the age of fifteen, and over half of those of sixteen, already had husbands. These young wives must have been sexually mature if the Christian rule on the point were being observed. Nothing can be said, of course, about the maturation of the six girls of age fifteen, the four aged sixteen, and the two aged seventeen who were not married, and it is possible that their late development was the reason why some of them were still celibate. Nevertheless it would seem out of the question to suppose that their backwardness was the sole reason, or even a major one, for their being spinsters.

For this would imply that sexual maturity was not simply an essential qualification for marriage, but was universally and immediately

Table 2 Mothers, 21 and over, by age

AGE	NUMBERS	AGE	NUMBERS
22	6	40	14
23	4	43	1
24	1	45	2
25	20	46	1
26	11	47	1
27	2	50	15
28	16	55	1
30	38	58	1
31	1	60	8
32	3	63	1
33	1	65	1
34	4	70	2
35	8	78	1
36	6	80	1
37	2	Totals:	22–80 = 177
38	3		0–80 = 203
39	1	Of whom widows =	31

followed by marriage. In the case of Belgrade, where husbands were, on average, nearly ten years older than their wives, such an unlikely rule would present a picture of the men waiting until their late twenties or early thirties to get themselves partners, and then seeking out the youngest nubile girls they could find to marry. Every woman would be offered on the marriage market as soon as she became physiologically capable of mating, and taken up with the shortest possible delay. No market can be as efficient, even with "buyers" and "sellers" as eager as those just described.

Eugene Hammel, of the University of California, Berkeley, a student of present and past Serbian familial life, tells me that nothing in the Serbian social structure or familial custom indicates any tendency toward such extraordinary precipitation. These considerations can be taken to justify the assumption that the non-marriers were not markedly later in maturing than those who did marry, although it is always possible that the really poorly fed and badly developed did follow the others partly because they were still unfit. In general, it would seem that wives in any age group can be taken as representative in these respects of all women in the age group, with some allowance made in the earliest years—say up to sixteen—but none later.

The considerable numbers of cases studied in our own time show

Table 3 Mothers by age at birth of eldest resident child (from subtraction)

	AGE	NUMBERS
	6	1
	8	3
	10	1
	11	1
	12	2
	13	5
	14	10
	15	13
	16	12
	17	16
	18	16
	19	13
	20	20
	21	3
Total	6–21	116
	22	17
	23	9
	24	9
	25	5
	26	5
	27	9
	28	7
	29	3
	30	5
	31	1
	32	3
	33	1
	35	1
	36	1
	37	1
	38	2
	40	4
	42	2
	44	1
	50	1
Total	6–50	203

that ages at menarche are normally distributed and that the range between the earliest and latest ages is relatively short. There does not seem to be much discussion of this range in the literature, nor more than a passing reference to the important possibility that it was greater in the case of the poor and undernourished than in that of the rich and well-fed, the humble not only maturing later, therefore, but over a wider spread of ages. Tanner simply says that a standard deviation of a value of "1.1 years is characteristic of most series studied."[18] If this value of 1.1, or even a somewhat higher one, is applied to the figures in our Table 1, and the assumption of normal distribution is retained for them, then a further and more specific, though still very inexact, numerical indication of the maximal menarcheal age can be obtained. Since over 95 per cent of all cases in a normal distribution will lie within four standard deviations of a value at the extreme, then it follows that practically all girls in Belgrade became fit to marry within four years after the first recorded age at marriage. Since twelve is the lowest age in Table 1, then 12–16 would be a first estimate of the range of ages at issue. This is to place a great deal of weight on a single value, especially as no bride of thirteen or fourteen is present, but the general shape of the distribution certainly implies that the ages between thirteen and fifteen were the years when girls reached marriageability and the years between seventeen and nineteen look very unlikely.[19] This statement is true, even allowing for the possibility of the unmarried being slower developers, and for the half-year which has to be added to the ages in Tables 1 and 2 because they are declared ages, not ages in years and months actually attained.

When we turn finally to the numbers in Table 3 we are at last in a position to work out single numerical estimates for our statistics, but it has to be said that the figures themselves look so haphazard that the ill-defined range just given might be thought of as preferable as a result. Beginning with the whole number of mothers—that is, all women of known age in the sample, accompanied by a child whose age has been subtracted from hers—gives a total of 203 (set out in Tables 2 and 3). The means and medians are as follows:

Mean age at birth of first resident child: 21.40, less 0.75.
Mean age at first conception: 20.65 years.
Median age at birth of first resident child: 20.40, less 0.75.
Estimated maximal median age at first conception: 19.65 years.

18 J. M. Tanner, *Growth at Adolescence*, 154.
19 Some support for the youngest ages being perfectly genuine can be gained even from English evidence, quite apart from Table 3 above. There is the Countess of Leicester who, in 1589, had a child at age thirteen (Laslett, *World We Have Lost*, 91); a girl at Colyton in Devonshire had a bastard in the eighteenth century when she was thirteen. Though ages at marriage from family reconstitution yield so little, the

The half year does not have to be added here, since the finding of the difference between the ages of the mothers and the eldest resident child has taken care of it, and the 0.75 represents the period of gestation. These ages are absolute maxima for the average number of years lived before first conception, and they accord well enough with the facts already reviewed. But, as must be expected, they add almost nothing in the way of positive information.

For more useful single statistics we must turn to ages below twenty-one years. This is on the assumption that all women must have reached menarche by the beginning of the twenty-second year, and, therefore, first conceptions—or apparent first conceptions—can be disregarded at higher ages.

> Mean age at birth of first resident child of all mothers of twenty-one or under at that birth: 16.69, less 0.75.
> Estimated maximum mean age at first conception: 15.91 ± 0.11 years
> Median age: 17.66, less 0.75
> Estimated maximum median age at first conception: 16.91 years
> Interquartile range 13.94–19.20
> Quartile deviation 2.63.
> 50 per cent of all cases within 2.63 of 16.91 years.

With figures such as those in Table 3, it is obvious that the median is likely to be a better indication of central tendency than the mean, especially with the impossible ages below ten. Our best estimate must therefore be the last set of results given above.

"Best" must here perhaps be read as "least misleading", but this outcome does not correspond to the statistics usually worked out from good data. This estimate is derived from the attributes of the normal distribution, and, for what it is worth, mean age at first conception thus arrived at comes to 16.3 ± 0.11 years, using the standard deviation of 1.1 already referred to. We could allow for the possibility that in the case of this population the spread of ages at menarche might be double what is now usual, and the result would then be 16.7 ± 0.22 years.[20]

---

much rougher ages given in marriage license records for much larger samples are more helpful. Vivien Elliott, working with the Cambridge Group, finds six brides of fifteen, six of sixteen, and nineteen of seventeen among 363 mariners in the London area between 1660 and 1694, and one of twelve, one of fifteen, and three of seventeen among sixty yeomen between 1679 and 1694.

20 Allowance for the proportion of women in the population not married and providing for random variation would raise the figure above seventeen years and perhaps as high as eighteen, but the quality of the data does not warrant such refinements.

In considering these and the other estimates, it must be remembered that they suppose that the interval between becoming mature and conceiving a child within marriage is roughly constant, although that interval is unknown to us. We can only suggest limits for the average time taken for the location of potential partners, courtship, and marriage in that society, but it seems unlikely that it could be less than a year, and was very probably two years and more. If the age data from the listing from Belgrade in 1733–34 are at all reliable, and if the women in that city were representative of a wider population in that area at that time, it would seem that age at menarche must have been below fifteen years in early eighteenth-century Serbia.

My own impression of the evidence, from Table 1 more particularly than from Table 3, is that it may have been even lower, but that the spread of ages at which maturity was attained was wider than that observed in contemporary women. But these suggested inferences would be falsified if it could be shown that the entire distribution of the population by age was seriously distorted by the vagaries in the figures of our tables. They would only be misleading if a downward bias were present, but it must be remembered that the margins are quite narrow. A general upward shift of two years would do much to eliminate the difference we have tried to establish between the eighteenth-century Balkans and nineteenth-century Scandinavia or England.

In lieu of unavailable space to discuss all of the possible sources of error, I include the full figures. This will permit readers to decide whether the pronounced heaping at ages ten and twenty in Table 1 or at twenty-five, thirty, and all higher decennial years in Table 2 results from a rounding downward rather than upward. Critical examination would appear to show that some upward effect must be contemplated, but it would affect the measures for the whole population rather than for those under twenty-one, where the revision would at most have to be a month or two.

Some confidence in the age figures for the Belgrade population as a whole can be gained from comparing them with similar distributions for other preindustrial European societies. Mean overall age at Belgrade was 24.5, whereas in the six English communities mentioned above it was 25.73; medians 20.83 and 21.70. For males, the mean at Belgrade was 26.05 (a median of 21.09) and, in the English sample, 25.26 and 20.23; females 23.47 and 20.42 against 26.17 and 22.59. The population was a little younger and the gap is greatest for women, but the discrepancy is no greater than is found between communities in England. The really disconcerting figures come in Table 3, with its impossible ages at birth of the first accompanying child. Though it can be shown that all of these cases were probably the results of a woman marrying a widower with children, and though the errors even in this table offset each other, at least to some extent, the statistics from this set of figures are of problematic value and have been treated as such here.[21]

This rough, preliminary exercise in the numerical study of age at maturity in earlier times may imply two principles. The first is that it cannot be assumed of the persons living in traditional societies, where they were immured for so long in their families of origin and kept under discipline for a good part of their lives, that they were necessarily more likely to be reconciled to their situation for physiological reasons. When we contemplate the patriarchal household in Stuart England, Colonial America, or in France under the *ancien régime*, where marriage was so much later than it was in Belgrade, and where —in England especially but in France, and perhaps the Colonies, as well—so many young people were in subjection as servants (compulsorily celibate like the children), we must think of the long years when young people were capable of fully adult roles, sexual fulfilment, and the direction of a family. If fathers were concerned about the chastity of their daughters, it was because they were probably often quite as capable of producing bastards in their middle teens as they are today. Fathers also faced their teenage sons as grown up persons, as strong as they were themselves in a society where personal, physical violence was more formidable than now.

The second principle is still scarcely established, and it may take many years to decide about it: age at menarche and maturation generally could vary, over time, as well as from social class and place to place. We cannot attempt to go into the reasons for this variation, even if it were within our competence. We may notice that the experts now no longer suppose that climate explains a great deal of the differences in menarcheal age in various parts of the world, so this factor would not account for the contrast between Belgrade and northern Europe.

21 No doubt a difference table of this kind might yield valuable data, given better recordings. No attempt was made to amend these figures because so little was known about the method of registration or the population itself. It may be worth pointing out that the very low and unacceptable values due to remarriage have to be offset in Table 3 against an unknown but assuredly very large proportion of high values which are missing because the child concerned had either died or left home.

Nothing can be said from this haphazard evidence about the extent to which it was due to genetical heritage, just as the body shape of Latin American peoples is different from that of Asian peoples, for reasons of what was once called race. But Frisch and Revelle[22] have recently published evidence that seems finally to bear out the view that "the attainment of a specific body weight at the peak of the adolescent spurt...may be critical for menarche."[23] And such attainment of critical weight is due, as they show, and as Tanner and others have supposed for many years, to nutrition in the early and especially the earliest years. As historical demographers, we know something already about variations in food supply and its effect on demographic rates, its extreme effects in the crisis of subsistence which the French have delineated, and its long term effects in the control of population size. It is interesting to have to recognize that differences in nutrition may have caused variations in the internal balance of the domestic group as well, as it definitely must have influenced the physiological relationships between classes. Finally, let the American readers of this article reflect on the consequences of the fact that from their very beginnings the American people, and especially American children, have been better fed than Europeans.

22 Rose Frisch and Roger Revelle, "Variation in Body Weights and the Age of the Adolescent Growth Spurt Among Latin American and Asian Populations in Relation to Calorie Supplies," *Human Biology*, XLI (1969), 185–212, *idem.*, "The Height and Weight of Adolescent Boys and Girls at the Time of Peak Velocity of Growth in Height and Weight: Longitudinal Data," *Ibid.*, 536–559.
23 *Ibid.*, 558.

Journal of Interdisciplinary History, VIII:2 (Autumn 1977), 183–220.

Susan Grigg

Toward a Theory of Remarriage: A Case Study of Newburyport at the Beginning of the Nineteenth Century

When a marriage ends in one spouse's death, the widow or widower is apt to survive for years and even decades. This was true in the eighteenth century as it is in the twentieth, and the age of the survivor has only secondary importance.[1] A knowledge of influences on the likelihood of remarriage is therefore essential to an appreciation of the personal and social consequences of widowhood. Yet historians of the family have seldom given the subject much attention, despite the implications of failure to remarry for the welfare of the widow or widower and the survival of the household. This essay will begin redressing that neglect through a case study of remarriage in Newburyport, Massachusetts, at the beginning of the nineteenth century.[2] It will examine the personal attributes of a cohort of newly widowed men and women and use that information to explain why some remarried and others failed to do so. The argument will follow a model developed from the findings of published case studies of the correlates of remarriage in a number of European and North American communities between the sixteenth and eighteenth centuries. There will be no systematic study of the communal characteristics that affected aggregate remarriage

Susan Grigg is an archivist at the Yale University Library.

The research for this article was supported by an Adelia A. Field Johnston Fellowship from Oberlin College and a Woodrow Wilson Fellowship in Women's Studies. The author is indebted to Allan G. Bogue, James Sweet, Constance H. Berman, and Margaret Thompson for their thoughtful criticisms. They bear no responsibility, however, for the methods used or the conclusions drawn.

1 "The Increasing Chances of Widowhood," Metropolitan Life Insurance Company *Statistical Bulletin*, XVII, 6 (June 1936), 6; Jessie Bernard, *Remarriage: A Study of Marriage* (New York, 1956), 11; John Knodel, "Two and a Half Centuries of Demographic History in a Bavarian Village," *Population Studies*, XXIV (1970), 363–364; Robert V. Wells, "Demographic Change and the Life Cycle of American Families," *Journal of Interdisciplinary History*, II (1971), 282; *idem*, "Quaker Marriage Patterns in a Colonial Perspective," *William and Mary Quarterly*, XXIX (1972), 425.

Twentieth-century studies differ from historical works in that they must consider divorce as well as widowhood as an important source of candidates for remarriage.

2 Newburyport in this period was a thriving center of trade, shipbuilding, and other manufacturing. For more economic background, see Samuel Eliot Morison, *The Maritime History of Massachusetts, 1783–1860* (Boston, 1921), 151–155.

*

rates; the goal, rather, is to develop a procedure for ranking individuals according to their relative likelihood of remarriage.

Historians of family life in colonial America have emphasized two ideas about remarriage: that it was forced by necessity and prevented by lack of opportunity. These assumptions can be combined with demographic information to yield predicted remarriage rates, but few scholars have gathered the data to test such predictions or asked appropriate questions about published remarriage statistics. The usual practice has been to emphasize the rapidity of remarriage and fail to determine its frequency, perhaps on the assumption that great rapidity implies high frequency.[3] Even the recent advances in historical demography have made little difference, possibly because the discovery of remarkably low mortality invites the assumption that widowhood and remarriage were mainly the experience of those who were no longer economically important or biologically productive.[4] The familiar impression that there were many poor widows in the colonies, especially during the eighteenth century and in the cities, is at last being supplemented with systematic investigation of the frequency of remarriage.[5] No one, however, has challenged the assumption that remarriage was determined primarily by the interplay of opportunity and necessity, nor fully appreciated the importance of asking who remarried as well as how many. This essay is intended both to pose a broader set of questions and to provide some tentative answers.

Notwithstanding its limited range of inquiry, scholarly literature on colonial families has much to contribute to a study of the correlates of remarriage. The early interpretations, based primarily on narratives of courtship, call attention to property's effect on

3 Alice Morse Earle, *Customs and Fashions in Old New England* (New York, 1893), 36; Arthur W. Calhoun, *A Social History of the American Family from Colonial Times to the Present* (Cleveland, 1917), I, 69–70; Curtis P. Nettels, *The Roots of American Civilization: A History of American Colonial Life* (New York, 1938), 445; John Demos, *A Little Commonwealth: Family Life in Plymouth Colony* (New York, 1970), 66–67.

4 Demos, *Little Commonwealth*, 65–66; Philip J. Greven, Jr., *Four Generations: Population, Land, and Family in Colonial Andover, Massachusetts* (Ithaca, 1970), 26–28, 109–110, 191–196.

5 Carl Bridenbaugh, *Cities in Revolt: Urban Life in America, 1743–1776* (New York, 1955), 87, 124; Rowland Berthoff, *An Unsettled People: Social Order and Disorder in American History* (New York, 1971), 85, 92; Robert V. Wells, *The Population of the British Colonies in America before 1776: A Survey of the Census Data* (Princeton, 1975), 76–77. The innovator is Alexander Keyssar, "Widowhood in Eighteenth Century Massachusetts: A Problem in the History of the Family," *Perspectives in American History*, VIII (1974), 88–94.

the marital prospects of widows. Recent research in the vital records of Massachusetts towns has produced evidence of variations in remarriage rates according to sex and age, and the importance of these demographic variables is confirmed by a number of case studies of Old and New World communities since the sixteenth century. Much of this material is exclusively empirical, but a consideration of the effect of remarriage on household economy can be made to furnish a theoretical framework. The resulting synthesis will provide a broad range of testable hypotheses about the correlates of remarriage.

Although rarely offered as such, historical evidence on the frequency of failure to remarry can be extracted from certain published statistics by comparing the actual number with the maximum possible number of second marriages in a particular population. If every surviving spouse were to remarry, the total number of persons marrying a second time would equal the number of first marriages. When this rule is applied to the marital experience of the Plymouth Colony in the seventeenth century, it appears that between 53 and 66 percent of all possible second marriages occurred. There were also six third marriages for every hundred men and one third marriage for every hundred women.[6] Thus, remarriage was the norm for survivors of first marriages in seventeenth-century Plymouth, but it was far from universal, and long successions of marriages were less common than may have been supposed.[7] One might expect to find an unusually high remarriage rate in a newly settled farming area with widespread ownership of land. The discovery that so many of Plymouth's widows and widowers failed to remarry therefore suggests that remarriage was at least as infrequent in many other populations.

Comparison between the Plymouth findings and other series

6 Demos, *Little Commonwealth*, 194. The upper limit of 66 percent is based on the numbers for ever-married persons aged fifty and over. The lower limit of 53 percent is derived by using the distribution of ages at death (193) to estimate the proportion of ever-married persons who died before the age of fifty. If none of them remarried, the new proportions married more than once are .35 for men (i.e., 40/[100(1 + 13/87)]) and .18 for women (i.e., 26/[100(1 + 30/70)]). Some probably did survive their first spouses and marry again, however; this is why the calculations merely produce lower limits. The contamination of the statistics on age at death by the inclusion of people who died unmarried can safely be ignored, in view of the low average age at first marriage for women, the small fraction of men who died before the age of thirty (193), and the likelihood of a very high marriage rate for single men and women.

7 *Ibid.*, 67; Earle, *Customs and Fashions*, 36; Alice Morse Earle, *Colonial Dames and Goodwives* (Boston, 1895), 32.

of remarriage statistics confirms this supposition. Table 1 shows the proportion of widows and widowers among all marriage partners in various North American and European communities between the sixteenth and eighteenth centuries. Two of the three highest values for men are for Plymouth and for the first generation in Andover, Massachusetts; the third (for Geneva between 1550 and 1599) should be set aside on the grounds that it reflects a pattern of early and almost universal marriage that apparently vanished from Western Europe before the end of the seventeenth century.[8] The values for women are in slightly different order, but once more the Plymouth figure is unquestionably high. The studies are too few in number and too irregular in their geographical distribution to guarantee their representativeness, but there are two plausible generalizations: an average remarriage rate of less than two-thirds was probably the maximum both in Europe and in North America in the seventeenth and eighteenth centuries, and that level may have been achieved only in the early years of colonial settlement. Here is justification for a broadly based study of the reasons for failure to remarry.

Age is the most obvious and familiar predictor of remarriage. In the Plymouth Colony, almost as many men and women had been married only once among persons aged seventy and over as among those aged fifty and over; the decrease with advancing age was from 60 to 55 percent for men and from 74 to 69 percent for women. Under any reasonable assumption about mortality, the proportion of persons married only once among men and women aged fifty to sixty-nine must have been only a few points higher than for everyone aged fifty and over. The implication is that most remarriage occurred long before the age of seventy, despite life expectancies that made early widowhood relatively rare.[9] Greven does not provide comparable information for Andover, but he seems to have found that age and remarriage were inversely related, and he endorses a similar association in the work of other

8 J. Hajnal, "European Marriage Patterns in Perspective," in D. V. Glass and D. E. C. Eversley (eds.), *Population in History: Essays in Historical Demography* (Chicago, 1965), 101–117.

9 Demos, *Little Commonwealth*, 192, 194. If there had been just as many people aged seventy and over as there were aged fifty to sixty-nine, the proportion married only once in the second group would have been 65 percent for the men and 79 percent for the women. The proportions would have been lower if there had been more people aged fifty to sixty-nine than there were aged seventy and over.

Table 1 Proportion of Remarriages among All Marriages in Certain Communities between the Sixteenth and the Eighteenth Centuries

PLACE	PERIOD	PROPORTION OF REMARRIAGES	
		MEN	WOMEN
Plymouth Colony	17th c.	max .32	.21
		min. 29	.16
Andover, Mass. (records begin 1651)	1st generation	.28	
	2nd generation	max .21	
		min .20	
	3rd generation	max .22	
		min .20	
middle colonies (Quaker)	18th c.	.11	.02
N. J. (Dutch Reformed)	18th c.	.10	.08
French Canada	18th c.	.19	.13
Bas–Quercy (France)	18th c.	.11	.05
Geneva	1550–1599	.26	max .23
			min .18
	1600–1649	.21	max .10
			min .09
	1650–1699	.13	max .05
			min .04
	1700–1749	.12	max .07
			min .03
	1750–1799	.10	max .04
			min .01
Tourouvre-au-Perche (France)	1665–1770	.21	.17
Remmesweiler (Saar)	18th c.	.15	.03

SOURCES: Demos, *Little Commonwealth,* 193-194 (see text, n. 6, for calculation of the minimum); Greven, *Four Generations,* 29, 111; Robert V. Wells, "Quaker Marriage Patterns in a Colonial Perspective," *William and Mary Quarterly,* XXIX (1972), 423-434; Jacques Henripin, *La Population canadienne au début du XVIIIe siècle: nuptialité, fecondité, mortalité infantile* (Paris, 1954), 98; Pierre Valmary, *Familles paysannes au XVIIIe siècle en Bas-Quercy: étude démographique* (Paris, 1965), 102; Louis Henry, *Anciennes Familles genevoises: étude démographique: XVIe-XXe siècle* (Paris, 1956), 57 (the maxima are for wives, the minima for daughters); Hubert Charbonneau, *Tourouvre-au-Perche aux XVIIe et XVIIIe siècles* (Paris, 1970), 78; Jacques Houdaille, "La Population de Remmesweiler en Sarre aux XVIIIe et XIXe siècles," *Population,* XXV (1970), 1186.

historians. Keyssar, discussing the widows of eighteenth-century Woburn, generalizes that the few who remarried were relatively young.[10] None of this evidence is perfectly suited to the purpose, but it suggests consistently that remarriage occurred early in colonial Massachusetts despite the infrequency of early widowhood.

The findings for Plymouth can also be construed to suggest that the likelihood of remarriage varied according to sex; but some preliminary definitions are in order. Let the remarriage ratio be the ratio of remarriages to first marriages for either sex. Let the remarriage rate be the likelihood that a widowed person will remarry. The latter is a more discriminating measure, but it can only be estimated from the published information. The argument has two parts. Consider, first, that the difference between the remarriage ratios for persons aged seventy and over and for those aged fifty and over was greater for men (55.5 versus less than 47 per hundred) than for women (32 versus 27 per hundred). Since older women were apt to outlive their husbands, the remarriage rate must have been higher for men than for women after the age of fifty. The comparison is less satisfactory for younger people. The substantial difference between the remarriage ratios for men and women aged fifty and over (46 or 47 versus 27 per hundred) may indeed reflect lower age-specific remarriage rates for younger as well as older widows, but it must also owe something to the high mortality of married women in their childbearing years.[11] If most married people who died young were women, few young women can have had the opportunity to marry a second time. It is almost certain, then, that the older widows in Plymouth were less apt to remarry than widowers of the same age, and this may have been true of younger people as well.

That remarriage should favor youth over age and men over women is a literary convention and a social commonplace, and several other studies confirm the implications of the Massachusetts data. Table 2 provides age-specific remarriage rates by sex for small populations in several European communities in the seventeenth and eighteenth centuries. Table 3 offers the same informa-

10 Greven, *Four Generations,* 29, 110–111; Keyssar, "Widowhood," 94.
11 Demos, *Little Commonwealth,* 193–194. Thirty percent of the women but only 13 percent of the men who lived to age twenty-two died before age fifty. Wives tended to be younger than their husbands, but the gap narrowed in the course of the seventeenth century.

Table 2 Remarriage Rates by Sex and Age in Certain European Communities in the Seventeeth and Eighteenth Centuries

PLACE	PERIOD	AGE	PROPORTION OF WIDOWED PERSONS WHO REMARRIED	
			MEN	WOMEN
Tourouvre	1665–1714	under 30	.83	.80
(France)	(n=96,84)	30 to 39	.80	.48
		40 to 49	.59	.25
		50 to 59	.29	.08
		60 to 69	.12	.03
	1715–1770	under 30	.82	.78
	(n = 75,38)	30 to 39	.67	.47
		40 to 49	.37	.18
		50 to 59	.30	.04
		60 to 69	.12	.00
Ile-de-	18th c.	under 30		max 1.00
France				min .86
		under 40	1.00	max .75
				min .62
		40 to 49		.11
		40 to 59	max .50	
			min .44	
Anhausen	1692–1799	under 40	1.00	.73
(Bavaria)	(n = 44,38)	40 to 49	.87	.40
		50 to 59	.42	
		50 and up	.26	.05
		60 and up	.00	

SOURCES: Charbonneau, *Tourouvre-au-Perche,* 81; Jean Ganiage, *Trois Villages d'Ile de France au XVIIIe siècle: étude démographique* (Paris, 1963), 62; Knodel, "Two and a Half Centuries," 364.

tion for France between 1943 and 1952 and for the United States in 1940. As one would expect with such a range of times and places, the five pairs of distributions differ substantially from one another, but nonetheless they have two essential features in common: a strong inverse relationship between age and the proportion who remarried and a much lower remarriage rate for women than for men except among the very young. No doubt the distinctive pattern of American population growth has produced many local exceptions to the second generalization, but the Plymouth finding puts these hypothetical cases in perspective by suggesting how

Table 3 Remarriage Rates by Sex and Age for France (1943-1952) and the United States (1940)

AGE	FRANCE		U.S.	
	WIDOWERS	WIDOWS	WIDOWERS	WIDOWS
20–24	.86	.87		
25			.97	.78
25–29	.78	.69		
30			.92	.60
30–34	.77	.48		
35			.79	.43
35–39	.66	.32		
40			.66	.29
40–44	.50	.20		
45			.50	.18
45–49	.42	.13		
50			.35	.11
50–54	.33	.07		
55			.23	.07
55–59	.25	.03		
60			.12	.04

SOURCES: Roland Pressat, "Le Remariage des veufs et des veuves," *Population,* XI (1956), 52; "The Chances of Remarriage for the Widowed and the Divorced," Metropolitan Life Insurance Company *Statistical Bulletin,* XXVI, 5 (May 1945), 2. The French rates are a composite of national vital statistics. The U.S. rates are based on the vital statistics of certain states.

readily biological processes could overcome an initial excess of men when heavy immigration was not sustained.[12]

12 Herbert Moller, "Sex Composition and Correlated Culture Patterns of Colonial America," *William and Mary Quarterly,* II (1945), 113–131. Widowers could compensate for a shortage of women their own age by competing with younger men for younger wives. Demos, *Little Commonwealth,* 151, 193, shows a convergence in average age at first marriage that may reflect a relaxation in such competition as women became less scarce. Of course, men may prefer younger women even when the sexes are roughly balanced. Insofar as they succeed in attracting younger wives, the opportunities of younger men and older women will be diminished (unless they marry one another). Whatever the sex ratio among older people, rapid natural population growth is apt to favor the remarriage of widowers over widows by creating a relatively large pool of young marriageable women.

Daniel Scott Smith, "Population, Family and Society in Hingham, Massachusetts, 1635–1800," unpub. Ph.D. diss. (University of California, Berkeley, 1973), 281–284; Linda Auwers Bissell, "Family, Friends, and Neighbors: Social Interaction in Seventeenth-Century Windsor, Connecticut," unpub. Ph.D. diss. (Brandeis University, 1973), 56, present corroborative evidence on age-specific and sex-specific remarriage rates in colonial New England that came to my attention after this essay was written. Smith thoughtfully offered me his findings.

Variations in remarriage rates according to sex and age acquire fresh significance in the context of the developmental cycle of the family. Berkner, drawing on a census of certain Austrian peasant villages made in 1763, observes that remarriage was very common for both sexes while all the children were young but that widows were much less apt to remarry once they were old enough to have grown children. He connects this pattern with a system of impartible inheritance of land, whereby the oldest son would probably marry and set up housekeeping only when his parents were willing to retire in his favor.[13] The argument is that both men and women remarried out of need when the son was too young to take his father's place but that women were more apt to choose retirement when that option became available. In this view, the sexes differed fundamentally in their attitude toward remarriage, but the apparent effect of age was at least partly a consequence of the necessity of having a married couple at the head of every household. Berkner offers no explanation for the difference between the sexes.

This argument rests on tendencies, not on perfect patterns of association. It would be remarkable if it were otherwise, and most of the irregularities are theoretically inconsequential. A possible exception is the presence of twenty-one retired widowers and twenty-six retired widows aged fifty-eight or more. The rough equality in numbers may mean that men of this age were no more apt to remarry than women of the same age. When one considers that two-fifths (38) of the ninety-eight married men in this category were also retired, it becomes obvious that many older men had decided in favor of retirement, whether the choice was freely made or dictated by disability. The widowers' failure to remarry may have resulted from such a decision, or been imposed by their inability to find a suitable woman willing to marry an old man with grown children. In either case, the result merely qualifies the original argument. The claim that the sexes differed in attitude toward retirement and remarriage remains tenable because of the

---

13 Lutz K. Berkner, "The Stem Family and the Developmental Cycle of the Peasant Household: An 18th-Century Austrian Example," *American Historical Review*, LXXVII (1972), 404. Michael Drake, *Population and Society in Norway, 1735–1865* (Cambridge, 1969), 116–117, reports a similar excess of women among retired persons in three Norwegian communities and cautiously suggests that sons were more successful in persuading mothers than fathers to retire.

virtual absence of retired widowers aged forty-eight to fifty-seven when there were twenty-five retired widows of the same age. The qualification is that sex may be of little value as a predictor of re-marriage among the oldest men and women.

Another important exception is the presence of thirteen widows among the several hundred heads of household aged twenty-eight to forty-seven.[14] Perhaps these women were resist-ing the economic pressure to remarry, an explanation that merely qualifies the assumption that married couples were necessary to the survival of these Austrian peasant households, and as such pos-sesses only local interest. But they may have failed for lack of opportunity—an explanation with important theoretical implica-tions. If younger widows found it difficult to remarry, older women may well have had the same experience, and the distinc-tion between widows with and without grown sons would be-come less crucial. The objection may be trivial because of the small number of women involved, but it deserves recognition because it demonstrates the potential importance of allowing for both oppor-tunity and desire in identifying and explaining patterns of remar-riage. Notwithstanding a strong desire to remarry among women under the age of fifty, for example, opportunity might in some in-stance be so constricted as to produce a relationship between age and remarriage much like those shown in Table 2, with remarriage rates under 50 percent for widows in their thirties and hardly any remarriage at all among older women. This was not necessarily happening in the Austrian villages, but merely suggests how easily one ideal pattern could slip into the other.

Berkner's reasoning is valid only for the particular economic and legal system that he studied. If, for example, his work is to point the way toward a model of remarriage for nonagricultural communities, at least one further modification is required. Histo-

14 Berkner graciously provided the hitherto unpublished information in this paragraph and the one preceding in a letter to the author, April 1975. Here is the distribution of widowed persons by sex, age, and position in household:

AGE	WIDOWERS		WIDOWS	
	ACTIVE	RETIRED	ACTIVE	RETIRED
28–47	1	0	13	3
48–57	3	2	5	25
58 and up	1	21	1	26

rians who discover an important incentive to remarry in the necessity of having a couple at the head of every household do not limit
the generalization to farmers, but that may be their intention; in
any case, it is doubtful whether many urban residents felt the same
pressure. First, there is the character of most urban property. It
was more common and more convenient to separate home from
workplace and ownership from use of property in cities than in
rural places. A widower could easily live as a boarder unless he
wanted to provide a home for young children, and a widow would
be less apt to require a husband to assist her in exploiting her
dower right.[15] Second, many urban dwellers depended mainly on
their own labor for their support.[16] For them, even more than for
the well-to-do, marriage would probably increase prosperity only
by providing new sources of income, not by facilitating the improvement of present property. Nor was the widowed parent's
remarriage so crucial to the prospects of the oldest son; urban
households could be multiplied indefinitely, property could
readily be divided, shared, or transported, and economic opportunity was more likely to expand with the population.

Ganiage's study of three eighteenth-century villages in the
Ile-de-France suggests a more flexible approach to the effect of
children on remarriage. He finds that widows who remarried had
an average of 1.5 unmarried children under the age of twenty,
while those who remained widowed (and belonged to age
categories some of whose members did remarry) had more than
twice as many children. Widowers' children, by contrast, had no
such effect on their fathers' likelihood of remarrying.[17] Since the
number of minor children probably increased with the mother's
age for women young enough to have any likelihood of remarrying, it is arguable that the negative effect of age on the remarriage
rate for widows (which is shown in Table 2) was the underlying
cause of the negative effect of the presence of children, but this

15 Keyssar, "Widowhood," 114-115, argues that rural widows sometimes had difficulty
producing income from farm property but suggests that in the eighteenth century it was
becoming easier to find more satisfactory forms of investment when the probate court
would authorize the sale of unprofitable dower rights.
16 Berkner, "Stem Family," 400, limits the sample to peasants. Drake, *Population and
Society,* 96-132, distinguishes between farmers and crofters (whose widows could be
evicted) in many contexts, including the discussion of remarriage.
17 Jean Ganiage, *Trois Villages d'Ile de France au XVIII*ᵉ *siècle: étude démographique* (Paris,
1963), 62.

would require that the children of widowers showed the same pattern. A more serious weakness of the argument is the failure to consider whether women with children were less apt to remarry than those with none because their children's current or prospective earnings protected them from the necessity. The argument assumes either that all minor children made remarriage less feasible or else that all widows wanted to remarry. Whatever the shortcomings of the interpretation, the evidence is sufficient to demonstrate that minor children affected the likelihood of remarriage and to warrant further study of such relationships.

An economic approach to the influence of children raises the possibility that wealth itself is a correlate of remarriage. This hypothesis has received little attention since it first appeared more than half a century ago. Calhoun, still the most ambitious interpreter of the history of the American family, had little sense of the demographic context of colonial remarriage but laid great stress on its economic aspects. Drawing on Earle's concept of the "belleship" of widows, he generalized that widows in the colonies were in extraordinary demand as wives. The historian's only problem was to explain why men preferred them to younger single women. Applying his theory of the preeminence of property considerations in arranging marriages before the Revolution, he concluded that widows occupied a strong position in the marriage market because they tended to have more wealth.[18] Nevertheless, a recent student of colonial Massachusetts found only weak evidence that wealthy widows were more apt to remarry than poor ones.[19]

18 Calhoun, Social History, I, 41, 57–58, 247–248; II, 13–14; Earle, Colonial Dames, 29–30; in median age at death between husbands and wives was roughly the same for the two Century New England (New York, 1966), 56–58.
19 Keyssar, "Widowhood," 109. He rejects the argument that widows were matrimonial prizes on two grounds: the husband could not very well work his new wife's estate if he already had one of his own, and many bequests were limited to the term of widowhood. On the other hand, Bernard Farber, Guardians of Virtue: Salem Families in 1800 (New York, 1972), 138, reports that while sea captains and wives of sea captains were almost equally likely to marry more than once (16 versus 12 percent), laborers, mariners, and fishermen were less than a third as apt to do so as their wives (9 versus 31 percent). Because the difference in median age at death between husbands and wives was roughly the same for the two occupational categories (19 versus 16 years), 45, these findings suggest an inverse relation between wealth and remarriage for the women. Salem had an economy similar to that of Newburyport.

An adequate test of Calhoun's thesis would have at least three elements: a search for evidence that wealth made remarriage of widows more likely, a consideration of whether most widows needed to remarry, and a parallel study of remarriage among men. Necessity is especially important because it challenges the most vulnerable point in his reasoning. If it was practical for women to choose to remain widowed, it is no longer obvious that remarriage rates were higher for rich women than for poor ones. That expectation rests on the idea that the relation between wealth and remarriage resulted exclusively from men's efforts to marry the wealthiest women who would have them. All widows (as well as all single women) were potential mates, and rich women were more apt to remarry because they were more apt to be chosen. But if widows did not need remarriage to secure their economic well-being, they could play a more active part in the bargaining. They could make their decisions exclusively on noneconomic grounds or they could strike a balance between the advantages or disadvantages of matrimony and the advantages or disadvantages of marrying the wealthiest men who were willing to marry them. In some times and places, virtually all widows may have concluded that even the least attractive offer of marriage was better than none, in which case competition should have produced a higher remarriage rate for the wealthy; but the interpreter of actual remarriage patterns should begin by supposing that significant numbers of women (and men as well) preferred continued widowhood to their own prospects for remarriage or even to any remarriage whatsoever.

All these arguments can be combined in a reformulation of Berkner's model of remarriage to suit the Newburyport economy. The relation between the widowed parent's age and the likelihood of remarriage will no longer echo the coming of age of the oldest son. But insofar as age is an index of desire or opportunity to remarry, the association will persist. Nor will the oldest son's age be independently important; instead, the children's net contribution, if any, will make remarriage more or less likely depending on whether or not the widowed parent wants to remarry. The same reasoning will accommodate the idea that wealthier widows are in greater demand as wives, with one qualification: if remarriage is not necessary in order to maintain the household, the surviving spouse may use wealth to avoid remarriage rather than to achieve it. The resulting model predicts the likelihood of remarriage for both sexes using three independent variables—age, wealth, and the presence of children—to represent collectively the interplay of necessity, opportunity, and desire.

A different approach to the study of remarriage would stress the sex ratio, which measures the relative number of males and females in a particular population at a particular time. The application of this concept to the study of remarriage is at root an exercise in arithmetic. The number of men marrying must equal the number of women marrying. The likelihood of remarriage for either sex is apt to vary inversely with its numbers relative to the other sex, although the number of marriages between single men and widowed women may be different from the number between single women and widowed men. The relation has special significance in United States history because of the importance of migration in American population growth. More men than women were in each wave of settlement, but in each newly settled region the balance shifted first toward rough equality in numbers and then toward an excess of women as natural increase overwhelmed the early imbalance and was then undermined by emigration.[20] Doubtless there have been many similar developments in modern European and American history, and the identification of such patterns will play a major part in any comprehensive study of widowhood and remarriage. There is, however, a limit to the value of the sex ratio as a predictor of remarriage rates: it controls the difference between the rates for the two sexes, but it does not determine whether both were relatively high or relatively low. Attempts to infer remarriage rates from the sex ratio, or vice versa, must begin with the premise that opportunity is a necessary but not sufficient condition for remarriage. To complete the analysis, one must discover the extent to which need and desire for remarriage encouraged widows and widowers to take advantage of such opportunities as they encountered.

The sex ratio has been omitted from the model just developed, not because it is unimportant but because it has no bearing on the relative likelihood of remarriage of individuals living in

---

20 Moller, "Sex Composition," 113–131; Wells, "Quaker Marriage Patterns," 434–436; Keyssar, "Widowhood," 95–99.

the same community at the same time. Those specifications imply an identical sex ratio for every candidate for remarriage, in which case the variable must have the same value for every observation. The sex ratio would be valuable only in a model designed to explain differences in remarriage rates among different communities or among different cohorts of widows and widowers in the same community. Such a model would also feature such variables as the economic organization, the legal system, and the conventions of male and female behavior. These possibilities are beyond the scope of this essay, which is why the emphasis has been on the common elements in published remarriage statistics. When the model for determining the relative likelihood of remarriage is applied to the Newburyport data, the influence of the sex ratio will be measured indirectly as an adjunct to the main part of the analysis, but that is possible only because the period of the study is long enough to permit distinctions among persons widowed at different times.

The hypothetical population for this case study is all white marriages existing in Newburyport on May 1, 1800 that ended in one spouse's death there before May 1, 1810.[21] These couples were identified by screening the resident male taxpayers in the 1800 valuation list and the white male-headed households in the 1800 United States census. Vital records and advertisements by administrators of estates provided a few additional names. The result is a list of 276 marriages (omitting doubtful cases) in a white population of 5876 persons comprising 1041 households.[22] Circumscribed research in the sources just named, the Essex County probate records, and published genealogical material produced information about these couples that reduces to four variables: sex

21 Blacks—1.2 percent of the population in 1800—were excluded because the records cover them so poorly.
   Beginning the year on May 1 conforms to the assessors' practice.
   The two-stage screening process favors geographically stable marriages of long duration; but working with a cohort of married couples reduces the risk of wrongful omissions. For a scheme of analysis that begins at the moment of marriage, see Louis Henry, *Démographie: analyse et modèles* (Paris, 1972), 91–92.
22 *Town Records and Tax Records of Newburyport, Massachusetts* ([Salt Lake City, 1972]); *Population Schedules of the Second Census of the United States, 1800*, National Archives Microcopy, 32, roll 14, Massachusetts (Washington, 1959); *Vital Records of Newburyport, Massachusetts, to the End of the Year 1849* (Salem, Mass., 1911); *Newburyport Herald* (May 1800–June 1810).

and age of the surviving spouse, number of minor children by age, and husband's valuation in the year of his or his wife's death.[23] The object is to discover how these attributes affected the likelihood of remarriage of the survivor.

Table 4 shows the distribution of the 276 widows and widowers by sex and age.[24] There are two outstanding features: a substantial excess of women over men (163 to 113) and a concentration of women under the age of fifty. Although there were roughly equal numbers of widows and widowers aged fifty and over, there were almost twice as many women as men under fifty. The preponderance of women overall is not surprising, but the surplus of younger widows is remarkable. One might have expected to find women underrepresented in the childbearing years.[25] Ordinarily, furthermore, one would not predict a dearth of young men due to natural causes alone.

The large number of young widows can be traced to the frequent exposure of mariners to premature death by drowning or disease.[26] Of 124 late husbands for whom any information could

23 Among the genealogies for old Newbury families are James Edward Greenleaf (comp.), *Genealogy of the Greenleaf Family* (Boston, 1896); Thomas S. Lunt (comp.), *Lunt: A History of the Lunt Family in America* (Salem, Mass., [1914]); Gilbert Merrill Titcomb, *Descendants of William Titcomb of Newbury, Massachusetts, 1635* ([Ann Arbor, 1969]).

The Essex Institute and the Topsfield Historical Society have published vital records for all towns in Essex County. Research farther afield is more difficult. For Boston, see Registry Department, *Records Relating to the Early History of Boston* (Boston, 1876–1909), XXIV, XXVIII, XXX. The marriage records are helpful for the entire eighteenth century, but the birth records have little value after 1750. The best source for Portsmouth has a geographical and cultural bias: Albert Gooding (comp.), "Records of the South Church of Portsmouth, N.H.," *New England Historical and Genealogical Register*, LXXXI (1927), 419–453; *ibid.*, LXXXII (1928), 25–33, 138–146, 281–302.

24 In two hundred five cases, both years of birth were known ("age" being the difference between the fiscal year of widowhood and the fiscal year of birth). In sixty-five cases (involving nineteen widows and six widowers), one year had to be derived from the other by computing the regression of the last two digits of the wife's fiscal year of birth on the last two digits of the husband's fiscal year of birth for the marriages for which both were known. The result was this equation, for which $r = .94$:

wife's year $= 7.78 + .915$ (husband's year)

In six cases (five widows, one widower) both years were missing, and the information was supplied by subtracting the average age at most recent marriage for the other observations (thirty for men, twenty-six for women) from the year of widowhood.

25 For conflicting evidence for rural Massachusetts in the colonial period, see Demos, *Little Commonwealth*, 193; Greven, *Four Generations*, 192, 195.

26 Bridenbaugh, *Cities in Revolt*, 124; (more tentatively) Keyssar, "Widowhood," 98–99, connect the large number of widows in mid-eighteenth-century Boston with the hazards of seafaring. On the general subject of maritime mortality, see Morison, *Maritime History*, 111–112.

Table 4 Disposition of Widows and Widowers by Age (the proportion of the column is given in parentheses.)

SEX	DISPOSITION	AGE						
		24–29	30–39	40–49	50–59	60–65	66–84	Total
Male	Remarried	5(.83)	16(.67)	17(.59)	13(.62)	6(.60)	0	57(.50)
	Died late[1]	1(.17)	4(.17)	12(.41)	7(.33)	4(.40)	18(.78)	46(.41)
	Died early[1]	0	0	0	1(.05)	0	5(.22)	6(.05)
	Disappeared late	0	3(.12)	0	0	0	0	3(.03)
	Disappeared early	0	1(.04)	0	0	0	0	1(.01)

When the second through fifth rows are combined, chi square = 26.06 (significant at .0001) and gamma = .55.

SEX	DISPOSITION	21–29	30–39	40–49	50–59	60–83	Total
Female	Remarried	8(.57)	15(.30)	10(.21)	2(.09)	0	35(.22)
	Died late	3(.21)	23(.46)	26(.54)	17(.77)	18(.62)	87(.53)
	Died early	0	4(.08)	1(.02)	0	9(.31)	14(.12)
	Disappeared late	3(.21)	7(.14)	7(.15)	0	0	17(.10)
	Disappeared early	0	1(.02)	4(.08)	3(.14)	2(.07)	10(.06)

When the second through fifth rows are combined, chi square = 18.28 (significant at .001) and gamma = .62.

1 See text, n. 7, for a definition of early and late death and disappearance.
SOURCES: See text, n. 22 and n. 23.

be discovered, the deaths of at least twenty-nine were related to seafaring: these men were younger than the average. More than 70 percent of all of the men of known occupation died after the age of forty, but 59 percent of those who died at sea or in another port were between twenty-four and thirty-nine.[27] Part of the association between seafaring and early death is explained by a pattern of retirement to less dangerous work in middle age.[28] But the fact that the victims of maritime hazards died younger than the marin-

27 Farber, *Guardians*, 45, shows a difference of eighteen years in median age at death between two classes of occupations—merchants, professionals, and artisans (63.6 to 66.3) versus sea captains, laborers, mariners, and fishermen (45.2 to 49.5). He stresses wealth rather than occupation as the point of contrast.
28 Kenneth Wiggins Porter, *The Jacksons and the Lees: Two Generations of Massachusetts Merchants, 1765–1844* (Cambridge, Mass., 1937), 7–9, describes career patterns by which a young man began as a mariner or a supercargo and then became a merchant ashore. Wesley Brooke [George Lunt], *Eastford; or, Household Sketches* (Boston, 1855), 255, portrays a seaman who became an occasional fisherman and then a doer of odd jobs and recipient of charity ashore as his physical capacity declined. Lunt was born in Newburyport in 1803, lived there much of his life, and made the town the setting for his book.

Table 5 Index of Occupation by Age at Death for Late Husbands of Widows (the proportion of the row is in parentheses.)

INDEX OF OCCUPATION	AGE				Total
	24–39	40–49	50–59	60–84	
Died at sea or in another port	17(.59)	10(.34)	2(.07)	0	29
"Mariner"; manner of death unknown	5(.26)	8(.42)	4(.21)	2(.10)	19
Employed on land	11(.16)	17(.25)	15(.22)	25(.37)	68
"Captain"; last occupation unknown	1(.12)	0	3(.38)	4(.50)	8
Total	34(.27)	35(.28)	24(.19)	31(.25)	124

Chi-square = 28.96 (significant at .0007). Gamma = .65. If the third and fourth rows are reversed, gamma = .57.
Note: Thirty-nine men were omitted for want of information.
SOURCES: Essex County Probate Records; *Vital Records of Newburyport,* II.

ers whose cause of death is unknown should answer this objection. More detailed findings appear in Table 5.

The surplus of widows promises a higher remarriage rate for the men, but the actual difference exceeds expectations. Half the widowers eventually remarried, while only a fifth of the widows did, so that remarried men outnumbered remarried women by 63 percent.[29] The discrepancy may reflect discrimination against widows (or their dependent children) by single and widowed men alike, but there are also two arithmetical explanations. Even in sea-

29 Computation of remarriage rates is complicated by the fact that some widows and widowers died or disappeared (from the town or from the records) before they had enjoyed much opportunity to remarry. Table 4 allows for this by distinguishing between those who died or disappeared rather rapidly and those who certainly remained eligible to remarry for a longer period of time. Everyone whose death or remarriage could not be established is recorded as "disappeared." Those recorded as having died or disappeared early are those who did so within the time in which half the persons of that sex who ever remarried actually did so. Thus, each man who died or disappeared early did so less than two fiscal years after his wife's death, and each woman in the same category left the population less than six years after her husband's death. (Using the mean rather than the median produces the same divisions.) Table 4 shows that early death and disappearance had little effect on age-specific remarriage rates. Early death was rare except in the age category in which no remarriage occurred. Early disappearance was negligible except among women aged forty and over, and the relatively large number of cases for that group probably has more to do with the problem of establishing the continued presence of widows than with departure or unrecorded death.

faring places, the ratio of single women to widows probably decreased with age, and an effective preference for young wives on the part of men would have put the widows at a disadvantage. It is also conceivable that the ratio of men to women was even lower for single persons than for widowed ones, in which case marriage could have occurred indiscriminately between the two categories and yet resulted in fewer remarriages for widows than for widowers.

The first section of the essay cites the abundant historical evidence that remarriage declined with age, and Table 4 reveals the same phenomenon among the widows and widowers of Newburyport. Remarriage was most likely for people under the age of thirty and did not occur at all among the oldest 18 percent of either sex. Beyond these broad similarities the findings for men and women differ. The small number of observations makes the boundaries somewhat arbitrary, but the difference in pattern is unmistakable. Remarriage became progressively less likely for women as the age at widowhood increased, but among widowers the remarriage rate did not vary with age except at the extremes (about 60 percent for that vast majority of men who lost their wives between the ages of thirty and sixty-five).

The pattern of age-specific remarriage rates is theoretically important because it may help to determine whether the widowed parent's likelihood of remarriage was substantially lower with a grown son in the family. The goal is to test the prediction that urban places like Newburyport did not experience the generational cycle in remarriage that Berkner discovered among Austrian peasant widows. Two proofs would be required to verify a generational cycle: an abrupt decline out of trend in age-specific remarriage rates and an increase in the average number of grown children at roughly the same threshold age. The evidence is ambiguous for the widows. We have seen that there was no threshold age in remarriage for women except in the narrow sense that none of the oldest widows remarried, but this evidence is satisfactory only from an empirical point of view. The problem is that the remarriage rates for middle-aged widows are too low to provide an adequate theoretical test. Table 6 shows that the average number of grown children per widow probably became greater for widows over the age of fifty, but there is no room left for a corre-

Table 6 Upper Limits for the Mean Number of Children Aged 21
and Over by the Age of the Widowed Parent

PARENT	AGE					
	40–44	45–49	50–54	55–59	60–64	65–69
Widower	0	.57	1.77	3.15	4.15	4.81
Widow	.35	1.28	2.70	3.30	3.63	3.93

SOURCES: See text, n. 22 and n. 23.

sponding collapse in the remarriage rate.[30] The 9 percent rate (2
out of 22) for widows aged fifty to fifty-nine happens to extend
the linear relation between age and remarriage for women aged
thirty to forty-nine; but if none of the women aged fifty and older
had remarried, the difference between two and zero would have to
be considered too small to carry any weight. Thus, from these
data, there is no means of determining whether the theoretical argument for a generational cycle in remarriage draws support from
the findings for the Newburyport widows.

Evidence for the widowers is more conclusive. Remarriage
fell off abruptly around the age of sixty-five, but Table 6 demonstrates that this threshold has no equivalent in the distribution of
grown children by the age of the widowed father. If the eldest
son's coming of age had discouraged remarriage among men, the
remarriage rate would decline sharply around the age of fifty-
five—a decade earlier than it actually does. Some allowance must
be made for the small population in making this distinction; but
since nothing in the literature suggests a generational cycle for
widowers, the obvious conclusion is that its effect on remarriage
in Newburyport was confined to widows if it existed at all. There,
as in the Austrian villages, widowers were apt to forego remarriage only rather late in life.

Interpreting the influence of minor children requires a similar
line of reasoning. On the premise that they must have made a
great difference in the well-being of many households, they probably had a corresponding impact on their parents' likelihood of

30 Projections are based on the average maximum number of children aged sixteen to
twenty belonging to widows who were multiples of five years younger than those in the
appropriate category.

remarriage. Once it is accepted that children's economic significance is being measured, the rest of the argument falls into place. According to this assumption, a child's influence on remarriage is compounded of costs and benefits to its widowed parent (and its prospective stepparent). When current income is the major consideration, there must be a more or less gradual shift in favor of remarriage as the child grows older and contributes some income to the parent.

The original ordering of the data provides for testing this hypothesis by having the minor children divided into four categories by age—under five, between five and nine, between ten and fifteen, and between sixteen and twenty.[31] When these four variables are used simultaneously in a linear regression analysis of remarriage, their partial correlation coefficients ought to reflect the evolution of the children's earning capacities. The coefficients should increase with the central ages for the respective categories of children, and there may be a change of sign from negative to positive in the middle of the range.[32] Alternatively, one can partition the population by age and then calculate the average number of children per widow or widower. The difference between the number of children belonging to persons who remarried and the number belonging to those who did not should vary with the age of the children in the same way as the partial correlation coefficients.

The reasons for performing the regression analysis and the cross-tabulation are to demonstrate that the results of the two methods confirm one another and to show the pattern in a tabular form that is immediately accessible to readers who are not familiar with regression.

31 The term "minor" is used throughout as a synonym for "under 21," which was the criterion used in gathering the data. Massachusetts, *Revised Statutes* (1836), 494, shows that male apprentices were free at this age but females were free at eighteen.
32 See Robert W. Fogel and Stanley L. Engerman, *Time on the Cross: The Economies of American Negro Slavery* (Boston, 1974), 74, 76, for evidence that the net earnings of slaves in the Old South around 1850 began increasing from their minimum value after the age of two or three and passed into the positive range after the age of eight. Presumably the parents of Federalist Newburyport had neither will nor opportunity to work their children this effectively.

The first section of Table 7 shows the results for widowers of the regression of remarriage on five independent variables—parent's age and the four age categories of children.[33] The correlations are moderately negative for the second and third categories and weakly positive for the first and last. Children aged five to fifteen reduced the likelihood of remarriage; older and younger offspring increased it. The last three categories may show the expected progression toward a positive influence of children on remarriage, but there is a clear discrepancy in the positive correlation for the youngest children. The first section of Table 8 makes the same point by means of cross-tabulation. A comparison of age-specific remarriage rates shows consistently that widowers who remarried had fewer children aged five to fifteen and roughly the same number in the other two categories. Once again, the evident discrepancy is in the absence of a negative effect on remarriage of children under five.

Perhaps the number of observations is too small to support such a fine reading of the results, and one should instead emphasize that all the relationships involving children are weak, only one being significant at the .10 level. An alternative explanation of the irregular coefficient for the youngest children is that fathers of infants and toddlers were more apt to remarry because they were more eager to do so. Otherwise they would have had to pay heavily for child care.[34] But with some risk of additional expense, they could combine the personal advantages of married life with an assurance of good care for their children. The argument is especially apt in a town where large numbers of men were away at sea for many months out of every year. Here is a plausible exception to the hypothesis that town-dwellers felt less pressure for remarriage than farmers.

33 One naturally questions the propriety of performing regression analysis with independent variables so obviously correlated with one another. The largest correlation coefficient (r) for a pair of independent variables is .45 for the men (between children aged ten to fifteen and children aged sixteen to twenty), .54 for the women (in absolute value, between age and children under five), which is not large enough to discredit the procedure.

34 Minute Book of the Newburyport Overseers of the Poor, Newburyport Public Library, shows that the Female Charitable Society charged the overseers 75 cents per week board for a six-year-old girl in 1805. Morison, *Maritime History*, 110–111, reports monthly wages for able seamen ranging from 17 to 21 dollars between 1799 and 1811, while common laborers received from 80 cents to a dollar per day. Neither could expect year-round full employment.

Table 7 Regression of Remarriage on Age and the Maximum Number of Minor Children by Age

WIDOWERS

Number of Observations	113			
Standard Error of Estimate	.43			
Multiple Correlation Coefficient	.55			
Coefficient of Determination	.30			
Corrected Coefficient of Determination	.27			

VARIABLE	REGRESSION COEFFICIENT	STD. ERROR OF REGRESSION COEFFICIENT	STANDARDIZED REGRESSION COEFFICIENT	PARTIAL CORRELATION COEFFICIENT	SIGNIFICANCE LEVEL
Constant	.72	.08		.66	.00
Age[1]	-.71	.12	-.57	-.50	.00
Child 0–4	.03	.05	.06	.06	.51
Child 5–9	-.06	.05	-.11	-.12	.23
Child 10–15	-.07	.04	-.16	-.16	.10
Child 16–20	.03	.06	.04	.04	.65

WIDOWS

Number of Observations	163			
Standard Error of Estimate	.37			
Multiple Correlation Coefficient	.49			
Coefficient of Determination	.24			
Corrected Coefficient of Determination	.21			

VARIABLE	REGRESSION COEFFICIENT	STD. ERROR OF REGRESSION COEFFICIENT	STANDARDIZED REGRESSION COEFFICIENT	PARTIAL CORRELATION COEFFICIENT	SIGNIFICANCE LEVEL
Constant	1.03	.14		.51	.00
Age	-.01	.00	-.50	-.42	.00
Child 0–4	-.07	.04	-.14	-.13	.10
Child 5–9	-.07	.04	-.15	-.14	.07
Child 10–15	-.06	.04	-.11	-.10	.19
Child 16–20	-.09	.04	-.17	-.18	.03

1 For widowers, this variable is dichotomous (up to age 65 versus age 66 and over).
SOURCES: See text, n. 22 and n. 23.

Table 8 Remarriage by Average Maximum Number of Children by Age

		WIDOWERS (113 observations)				
REMARRIAGE	AGE OF CHILDREN	AGE OF WIDOWER				
		24–29	30–39	40–49	50–65	66–84
Yes	0–4	1.20	1.25	1.00	0	
	5–9	0	1.25	.94	.21	
	10–15	0	.44	1.47	.68	
	16–20	0	0	1.00	1.00	
No	0–4	1.00	.88	1.08	.17	0
	5–9	0	1.12	1.75	.33	0
	10–15	0	.88	1.75	1.17	.13
	16–20	0	0	.75	1.17	.09

		WIDOWS (163 observations)				
		21–29	30–39	40–49	50–59	60–83
Yes	0–4	1.62	.73	.20	0	
	5–9	.38	.60	.70	0	
	10–15	0	.20	.40	0	
	16–20	0	0	.30	0	
No	0–4	1.67	1.23	.63	0	0
	5–9	.67	1.37	1.05	.05	0
	10–15	0	.60	1.10	.40	.07
	16–20	0	.23	1.34	.50	.17

SOURCES: See text, n. 22 and n. 23.

The results of regression analysis for widows, appearing in the second section of Table 7, do not conform to the prediction. The partial correlation coefficients for the four categories of children are strongly negative and roughly equal, and such irregularities as do appear do not suggest that widows were more apt to remarry when they had children old enough to provide for themselves. Cross-tabulation in the second section of Table 8 shows the same consistency in the difference between the average numbers of children belonging to widows who did and did not remarry. One can account for these findings by supposing that many widows would have preferred not to marry again. Under this assumption, the economic incentive to remarry would be strongest when the children were most dependent on their mother and weakest when they were contributing most toward their own support. Their appeal to prospective stepfathers would follow the opposite course. In such circumstances, mothers of older children would be inclined to apply their increasing earnings to sustaining themselves in widowhood rather than to advancing their chances of remarrying, and there might result the actual pattern of a negative correlation between remarriage and the presence of children that is roughly invariant with respect to the children's ages.

Published remarriage statistics provide no foundation for investigating the influence of relatives other than children on remarriage, but it is reasonable to speculate that a widow whose children were too young to provide for her or even for themselves might turn instead to her own family. A systematic test of this hypothesis is out of reach, but there is an extraordinary demonstration of what parents and siblings might contribute to a widow's well-being in the experience of Lois Foss, nee Tenney of Rowley (the second town south on the road to Boston), whose husband Captain John died in Cuba in the summer or fall of 1800. There is no proof of her residence between 1801, when she finished her work as administratrix of her husband's estate, and 1814, when she remarried as a resident of Rowley, but close relations probably played an important part in her life in the intervening years. The first clue is the listing for her sister's husband Joseph Young in the Newburyport census for 1810. He headed a household whose ten members correspond by sex and age category with himself and his wife, their five surviving children, and Lois Foss and her two sons. Her older boy John named his second son after this same uncle. The migration to Rowley probably occurred in 1812, shortly after the probate of her father's will, in which he bequeathed her part of his house for as long as she should remain unmarried. A final sign of her close ties with the Young household is her having died in Newburyport in 1836, eleven years after her second husband's death in Rowley. The Tenney family genealogist claims that she died in her sister's house, but the 1830 census has no room for her there.[35]

35 *Vital Records*, I, 426–447; II, 170, 632, 665, 841–842; *Vital Records of Rowley* (Salem, 1928), 77, 295, 473; *Herald*, 24 October 1800; M. J. Tenney, *The Tenney Family* (Concord, N.H., 1904), 96; Essex County Probate Reocrds (hereafter PR), Probate Record Office, Salem, Mass., 27365; *Population Schedules of the Third Census of the United States*, National Archives Microcopy, 252, roll 18, Massachusetts (Washington, 1960); *Fifth Census of the United States: 1830: Population Schedules: Massachusetts*: III, File Microcopies of Records in the National Archives, 19, roll 61 (Washington, 1947). Neither son's birth is recorded. The

Lois Foss's experience is clearly unrepresentative in certain respects. She remarried despite the support of her relatives, but only
after fourteen years' widowhood.[36] The more important question
is whether she was also atypical in receiving so much assistance
from her family. Many shared households may be hidden in the
census returns, and other widows doubtless received cash contributions from kin; but extensive research in contemporary probate records suggests that such assistance was not very important.
A widow whose father had outlived her husband could anticipate
receiving her proportional share of the father's estate at the time of
his death if he had not given all he thought proper at the time of
her marriage, but Oliver Tenney's acknowledgment of a special
obligation toward a widowed daughter seems to have been exceptional. Nor did a widow have much prospect of receiving a bequest from any other relative. The prevalence of intestacy shows
that many men were inclined to let the laws of inheritance take
their course; when a husband did make special provision by will,
his usual purpose was to add to his widow's share, to deal with the
complexities introduced by multiple marriages, or to distinguish
among his children. Probate records for men whose widows were
living in Newburyport between 1808 and 1812 reveal only a
sprinkling of provisions for more distant kin, and some of these
bequests were left to the discretion of the widow or made contin-
gent on the death without descendants of one of the natural
heirs.[37] These provisions may imply similar contributions during
the lifetime of the benefactor, but their small number suggests that

---

identification with the extra members of the Young household in 1810 assumes that the first
boy, John (who married in 1814), was born at least nine months after his parents' marriage
in November 1793, so that he was under sixteen in August 1810. The second child could
have been born after August 1800 (making him under ten at the time of the census). The
gap in the birth record probably occurs because their father was a captive of the "Algerines"
(John Foss, *A Journal of the Captivity and Sufferings of John Foss* [Newburyport, (1798)]); he
was first assessed in May 1799.

36   Thirty-two of the thirty-five widows who ever remarried did so in the first nine years
of widowhood. Only one was widowed longer than Lois Foss.

37   Only forty-four wills, most disposing of large estates, were proved for almost 400
men. Sixteen mention someone other than wife and children. Thomas Brown bequeathed
his grandson $100 from a $20,000 estate (PR 3851). Bishop Norton, worth more than
$15,000, provided that his sister and his brother (who had not been taxed for 16 years)
might continue living in the house they then occupied, a third of which was his (PR 19611).
Nicholas Tracy provided that if his younger son should die a minor, his share should go to
his father's brothers and sisters in Ireland (PR 27970).

such arrangements were infrequent or unimportant in the lives of the beneficiaries.[38]

Testamentary evidence cannot prove what relatives did for one another during their lifetimes, and the arguments just offered do not guarantee that widows derived comparatively little support from their parents, brothers, and sisters. But they do forbid the assumption that Lois Foss was typical in the amount of aid she received. Comprehensive knowledge of the availability of relatives would doubtless help explain the occurrence of remarriage; but in the absence of evidence to the contrary, it is questionable whether widows derived as much support from their families of origin as from their own children. Presumably more distant relatives made less difference in the likelihood of remarriage. Evidence to test this hypothesis might come from patterns of co-residence.[39] Or it might come from a strong association between lack of kindred and either likelihood of remarriage or dependence on charity for support. Until such research is accomplished, the question must remain unresolved.

The entire discussion of the influence of relatives on remarriage involves an analogy between wealth and children's income. The sign of the correlation between wealth and remarriage must, it seems, vary with the widowed person's attitude toward remarrying, wealth being an advantage in either case. Desire for remarriage should produce a positive correlation; preference for widowhood, a negative correlation. The effect on remarriage of children aged sixteen to twenty suggests that men tended to choose remarriage and women to prefer continued widowhood. The result should be a correlation between wealth and remarriage that is positive for widowers and negative for widows.

The first section of Table 9 shows the relation between a widower's likelihood of remarriage and his valuation for purposes of taxation in the year of his wife's death.[40] Contrary to the prediction, the two variables are unrelated. The one exception, in the zero valuations, is easily accounted for: thirteen of the sixteen

38 See, however, Farber, *Guardians,* 138–140, which connects a Salem resident's decline with the death of his brother-in-law, who may have been providing him with skilled employment.

39 Michael Anderson, *Family Structure in Nineteenth Century Lancashire* (Cambridge, 1971), argues that sharing households tended to be on a basis of mutual benefit, with a preference for immediate gain for both parties.

40 Valuation is different from wealth primarily because real estate was assessed against the occupier rather than the owner. At least, that is the only reasonable interpretation of the dis-

328 | SUSAN GRIGG

Table 9 Remarriage by Husband's Last Valuation (the proportion of the column is given in parentheses.)

SEX	REMARRIAGE	VALUATION (DOLLARS)						
		NO TAX	100–499	500–999	1000–1999	2000–4999	5000–200,000	TOTAL
Male	Yes	2(.12)	11(.73)	5(.50)	9(.47)	15(.56)	15(.58)	57(.50)
	No	14	4	5	10	12	11	56
Female	Yes	5(.17)	14(.52)	1(.04)	8(.33)	5(.15)	2(.10)	35(.22)
	No	25	13	24	16	28	19	125

Note: Three widows of ministers are omitted because their husbands were exempt from taxation by reason of occupation.
SOURCE: *Town Records.*

Table 10 Age of Widows by Husband's Last Valuation (The proportion of the column is given in parentheses.)

AGE	VALUATION (DOLLARS)						
	NO TAX	100–499	500–999	1000–1999	2000–4999	5000–200,000	TOTAL
21–39	7(.23)	16(.59)	12(.48)	9(.38)	16(.48)	3(.14)	63(.39)
40–49	8(.27)	10(.37)	7(.28)	7(.29)	7(.21)	7(.33)	46(.29)
50–83	15(.50)	1(.04)	6(.24)	8(.33)	10(.30)	11(.52)	51(.32)
Total	30	27	25	24	33	21	160

Note: Three widows of ministers are omitted because their husbands were exempt from taxation by reason of occupation.
SOURCE: *Town Records.*

widowers in this category were at least sixty years old. These men were excused from paying taxes, not because they occupied less property than poor young men but because the assessors were more disposed to grant exemptions to those they perceived as chronically poor and even beyond labor.[41] Since the effect of age on remarriage has been solidly demonstrated, it is permissible to set aside this category and thus remove all evidence of a correlation between remarriage and wealth.

The second section of Table 9 shows the relation between a widow's likelihood of remarriage and her husband's valuation in the year of his death. Some trace of the predicted inverse correlation occurs but it is necessary to allow for the effect of age before describing the actual pattern of association. The relation between age and valuation for these women is shown in Table 10. When the two distributions are compared, several correspondences stand out. Widows with the highest and lowest valuations were relatively old, and their remarriage rates are correspondingly low. At the other extreme, the high remarriage rate for women with valuations between $100 and $499 can be attributed to their relative youth. These associations suggest that for widows, as for widowers, the apparent relation between wealth and remarriage is a mere by-product of the relation between remarriage and age.

There is one irregularity, however, that cannot be accommodated from either point of view: the virtual absence of remarriage among the comparatively young women whose husbands' last valuations fell between $500 and $999. The discrepancy is too large to be ignored, and there is no economic reason why this

---

tribution of residential real estate in the valuation lists, and comparison of valuations with inventories in the probate records confirms the point. But the legal warrant for the practice is not explicit. Massachusetts, *General Laws,* I (1823), 222, passed in 1785, merely requires the inhabitants to submit lists of the estates "which they were possessed of." Massachusetts, *Revised Statutes* (1836), 75, enacted in 1830, provides that taxes on real estate "shall be assessed . . . to the person, who shall be either the owner or in possession thereof. . . ." The assessors of Newburyport exercised this discretion in the 1820s when they sometimes assessed a poor man for his poll and noted that his house was to be assessed to another person named. Assessing real estate to the occupier produces an appearance of a more equal distribution of wealth than actually existed, but it does not fundamentally affect the measured relationship between wealth and remarriage. The correlation between valuation and inventory of estate for the ninety-eight late husbands of widows for whom both figures are available is .94.

41 Massachusetts, *Revised Statutes* (1836), 76.

group, which may have achieved a modest level of comfort for the married couple and a limited margin of security for the widow, should have behaved differently from women slightly richer or poorer. Clearly, there is no simple inverse relationship between remarriage and wealth, but it is not evident that the two variables are as completely unrelated for widows as they appear to be for widowers.

One can account for a lack of association between wealth and remarriage by supposing that widows and widowers were reluctant to marry anyone poorer than themselves. This is to argue that remarriage opportunities were stratified with respect to wealth, with a rough pairing between acceptable candidates for remarriage. Under this constraint, remarriage rates would vary with wealth in much the same way for both sexes, even if their preferences worked in opposite directions. Some wealthy men would have difficulty finding acceptable wives, and some poor widows would be unable to attract husbands who offered any promise of improving their economic condition. The result would be little or no correlation between wealth and remarriage for either sex. This is roughly the pattern of Table 9 when allowance is made for the effect of age, and regression analysis confirms this reading by producing correlations that have the predicted signs but are so weak as to be inconsequential.[42] It is impossible to test this network of inferences without determining the wealth of persons who married widows and widowers.[43] But the argument has the merit of accounting for the empirical findings on valuation and remarriage without undermining the theoretical foundations laid for the other variables.

Evidence favoring this interpretation comes from a related study of dependent poverty among widows who lived in New-

42 Neither correlation between wealth and remarriage is significant at the .25 level.
43 In the case of the widows, the technique would be to consider the men who married them and try to relate their attributes to those of their new wives. One would look for a negative correlation between the number of children belonging to a widow and the difference in wealth between her two husbands. An affirmative result would suggest that there was a relation between wealth and remarriage, however difficult to measure. The failure to find such a correlation would suggest that wealth and remarriage were fundamentally unrelated and support the proposition that children had their influence within the constraint of a rough match by wealth between parent and stepparent. It would not be necessary that the new husband be as wealthy as his predecessor, but merely that the difference be insensitive to the presence of children.

buryport between 1808 and 1812. This population includes many of the women belonging to the study of remarriage, and regression analysis along the lines presented in Table 7 produces similar results. The new population has the advantage of offering data that include the additional variable "dependency," which tells whether the widow received aid from the overseers of the poor. Adding this variable, and the husband's last valuation, to the five independent variables listed in Table 7 reveals an important difference between wealth and dependency as predictors of remarriage. Valuation and remarriage are once more unrelated, but there is a negative correlation between dependency and remarriage that is significant at the .001 level.[44] In other words, widows who received public aid were less apt to remarry than those who did not, despite the lack of association between valuation and remarriage.

This relationship can be explained in two ways. It has already been suggested that poor widows were unable to find husbands who offered much prospect of improving their condition, and paupers would have carried a special onus in that regard. If dependency is taken to be a better measure of wealth than the late husband's last valuation, its negative correlation with remarriage may mean that poverty prevented the poorest widows from satisfying their economic need to remarry. Another possibility is that the public provision made it unprofitable to marry men who were poor providers, which suggests that dependent women actually had less need to remarry than those who barely supported themselves. Both arguments lead to the same conclusion: that poor widows remarried no more often than wealthy ones because they were prevented or discouraged from doing so by lack of good opportunity.

The same study of dependent poverty provides a partial explanation of the low remarriage rate for women with valuations between $500 and $999. As Table 11 demonstrates, wealth and dependency have the expectable inverse relation, but the proportion of dependents is actually higher for this category than for women with lower valuations. If the discrepancy is large enough to require explanation, it must be cultural rather than economic.

44 The women in the population subjected to this analysis meet three criteria: they were living in Newburyport as widows at least part of one winter (December through February) between the spring of 1808 and the spring of 1812; their husbands died in Newburyport between May 1780 and April 1812 and were assessed for estate in the year of death.

Table 11 Receipt of Poor Relief by Husband's Last Valuation for Certain Widows Living in Newburyport between 1808 and 1812

RELIEF	VALUATION (DOLLARS)				
	100–499	500–999	1000–1999	2000 AND UP	TOTAL
No	13(.46)	14(.42)	21(.88)	59(.98)	107(.74)
Yes	15(.54)	19(.58)	3(.12)	1(.02)	38(.26)
Total	28	33	24	60	145

Note: The population is the one described in text, n. 44, except that women whose husbands died before May 1800 were excluded.
SOURCES: *Town Records*; Minute Book of the Overseers of the Poor.

Perhaps the overseers of the poor thought that these widows, who may have enjoyed a measure of respectability as married women that their widows' thirds of their husbands' estates could not sustain, deserved aid more than women who had been extremely poor even when their husbands were alive. The decayed gentlewoman is a classic figure in the history of social welfare, and this may be one of her manifestations.[45] There is no other evidence that the Newburyport overseers used a cultural criterion in their almsgiving; but whether this explanation is correct or valuation is simply a poor indicator of wealth, these findings strengthen the hypothesis that any tendency toward an inverse relation between remarriage and valuation for widows was dampened by an association between dependency and failure to remarry.

With all the evidence in view on the effect of children and wealth, it is possible to examine more critically the relation between these two economic variables. The problem lies in the assumption that children had the same effect on remarriage at every level of wealth. Surely a better starting point would be to suppose that poor parents were more vulnerable to this influence than rich ones—that there was, in other words, an interaction between the two variables. Efforts to test this hypothesis failed. The finding that wealth is not useful as an interaction term in regression

45 John Prince, *Charity Recommended from the Social State of Man* (Salem, Mass., 1806), 30; Alden Bradford, *An Address Delivered before the Wiscasset Female Asylum* (Hallowell, Me., 1811), 6–7; *Address of the Hartford Female Beneficent Society* (Hartford, Conn., 1813), 10; *The Constitution of the Association for the Relief of Respectable, Aged, Indigent Females* (New York, 1815), [15].

analysis is inconclusive because the relation may be too weak to be detected this way. Nor does it help to divide the widows by wealth and perform separate analyses for the two fractions of the population. A lower limit on valuation as modest as $3000 distinguishes only thirty-six women as wealthy. As a result, findings for the poorer widows are inevitably similar to those for the entire population, and those for the wealthier ones are inconclusive. The computations for the widowers are still less useful because for them the effect of children on remarriage was very slight even for the population as a whole. Proof or disproof of the hypothesis of interaction must therefore await a study of remarriage based on samples several times as large as the ones used here.

Another assumption to query is that every person widowed between 1800 and 1810 faced exactly the same remarriage market. Did every individual's opportunity to remarry depend exclusively on personal characteristics and not at all on the time of the spouse's death? The ten-year span is long enough to raise some doubts and many remarriages did not occur until the following decade or even later. A comprehensive test of the stability of the remarriage market is out of reach; it is not even certain what characteristics of the town would have to be taken into account. The practical alternative is to test the narrower hypothesis that the relative likelihood of remarriage of individual widows and widowers was affected by change in the sex composition of the marriageable population and consequently by change in remarriage opportunity.

The special demographic history of Newburyport suggests that such a development did occur. The ratio between men and women aged twenty-six to forty-four was roughly the same in 1800 and in 1810, merely increasing from .87 to .91. In the next decade, however, economic decline and selective emigration reduced the figure to .70.[46] The result must have been to increase remarriage opportunity for men and decrease the chances for women. Since the shift in the ratio between the sexes in the prime years for remarriage did not begin until shortly after the last of these men and women was widowed, the plausibility of the hypothesis rests solely on the fact that several years often separated widowhood and remarriage. Because of this problem of timing,

46 *Return of the Whole Number of Persons within the Several Districts of the United States* ([Washington, 1801]), 8; *Aggregate Amount of Each Description of Persons within the United States* (Washington, 1811), 10a; *Census for 1820* (Washington, 1821), 6.

Table 12 Regression of Remarriage for Widows on Age, the Number of Children by Age, and the Year of Widowhood

Number of Observations 163
Standard Error of Estimate .36
Multiple Correlation Coefficient .51
Coefficient of Determination .26
Corrected Coefficient of Determination .23

VARIABLE	REGRESSION COEFFICIENT	STD. ERROR OF REGRESSION COEFFICIENT	STANDARDIZED REGRESSION COEFFICIENT	PARTIAL CORRELATION COEFFICIENT	SIGNIFICANCE LEVEL
Constant	1.06	.14		.53	.00
Age	−.01	.00	−.46	−.39	.00
Child 0–4	−.07	.04	−.16	−.15	.06
Child 5–9	−.07	.04	−.15	−.14	.08
Child 10–15	−.04	.04	−.08	−.08	.33
Child 16–20	−.09	.04	−.18	−.18	.02
Year of Widowhood	−.02	.01	−.14	−.16	.05

SOURCES: See text, n. 22 and n. 23.

there is no ideal measure of the effective sex ratio at the time of prime eligibility to remarry, but the year of the spouse's death should serve as a rough index of opportunity if the original generalization about the demographic history of Newburyport is correct.

As Table 12 demonstrates, the year of the husband's death is a moderately useful predictor of remarriage among women; it has a negative correlation with the likelihood of remarriage that is significant at the .05 level. The corresponding relation for men has the predicted positive sign, but it is not statistically significant and so does not appear to support the hypothesis. The difference between the sexes in the average duration of widowhood prior to remarriage is the likely explanation for these mixed results. In this case, as in all others in the literature, widowers remarried much more rapidly than widows.[47]

In the ninety-two instances of remarriage, the average duration of widowhood was 5.6 years for women but only 1.9 years for men, with a corresponding difference in the median values. This means that a larger proportion of women than men widowed late in the ten-year period of the study enjoyed most of their opportunity to remarry after the sex ratio had begun to decline. It follows that the year of the spouse's death should show a stronger association with the likelihood of remarriage for them than for the widowers.

The findings for Newburyport are generally compatible with those of previous case studies, but the agreement is clearest with regard to the influence on remarriage of the variables sex and age. A comparison between the remarriage rates for Newburyport in Table 4 and the corresponding figures for European villages in Table 2 reveals a common pattern with remarriage inversely re-

---

47 Etienne Gautier and Louis Henry, *La Population de Crulai, paroisse normande: étude historique* (Paris, 1958), 89; Knodel, "Two and a Half Centuries," 364; Valmary, *Familles paysannes,* 103; Hubert Charbonneau, *Tourouvre-au-Perche aux XVIIe et XVIIIe siècles* (Paris, 1970) 82; Pierre Girard, "Aperçus de la démographie de Sotteville-les-Rouen vers la fin du XVIIIe siècle," *Population,* XIV (1959), 490; Jacques Henripin, *La population canadienne au début du XVIIIe siècle: nuptialité, fecondité, mortalité infantile* (Paris, 1954), 99–100; Jacques Houdaille, "La Population de Boulay (Moselle) avant 1850," *Population,* XXII (1967), 1064; *idem,* "La Population de Remmesweiler en Sarre au XVIIIe et XIXe siècles," *Population,* XXV (1970), 1186; Bernard, *Remarriage,* 213; Smith, "Population, Family and Society," 281; Wells, "Quaker Marriage Patterns," 425.

lated to age and less likely for women than for men of the same age. It would have been surprising to find anything else. The larger purposes of this essay required emphasizing such common ground, but further study of these relationships might better stress the circumstances—economic, demographic, legal, and cultural—that produced different patterns in age-specific and sex-specific remarriage rates in different communities and at different times.

Direct comparison of numerical results is less effective in confirming the conclusions about the effect of wealth and children on the likelihood of remarriage. The superficial obstacle is the lack of similar findings in other case studies. There is nothing comparably detailed on the effect of wealth, and the only examination of the effect of minor children has limited value in this context because it does not distinguish between children of different ages. But a modest increase in the available data would not necessarily make a great difference. The more fundamental difficulty is that direct comparison would be appropriate only in special cases. The goal, after all, is to show how the effect of wealth and children on remarriage depends on local conditions, especially on the practical and legal constraints on the improvement and transmission of property. This means that comparison would have to begin with communities, or with cohorts drawn from the same community, that were closely matched in such respects, and a comprehensive view would require several such comparisons representing a variety of economic types. The more times it proves possible to argue persuasively for a relation between the likelihood of remarriage and the presence of children or the possession of wealth, the more confidence one will have in each separate piece of reasoning toward that end, but there is no easier way of confirming the Newburyport findings.

The greater significance of this case study is that it demonstrates a certain method for the study of remarriage. This approach has two essential ideas: there are variations in desire as well as in need and opportunity to remarry, and those variations have an effect on the likelihood of remarriage that can be interpreted and measured in economic terms. The first proposition is a teaching of social experience, and if historians have failed to give it much attention, it may be because they have not recognized its susceptibility to analysis. That potential lies in the dual nature of wealth and the presence of children as determinants of the likelihood of re-marriage. Not only do those characteristics affect opportunity to remarry, as do age and the sex ratio, but they can also make it practical not to remarry. The way in which the possession of wealth and the presence of children of different ages affect the de-cision about remarriage can be expected to vary with time and place, but such differences are less important, in the present state of our knowledge, than the generalization that patterns in remar-riage can be identified and accounted for in such terms.

This essay has emphasized personal attitudes toward remar-riage because that subject has been neglected by historians of colo-nial America. Students of traditional European societies may find this preoccupation naive and misplaced: to them, it may seem more urgent to inquire in what circumstances widows and widow-ers felt constrained not to act on their desire to remarry. There is some justification for such an inquiry in our knowledge of the charivari, a noisy gathering of youth in protest against (among other things) the marriage of a widow or widower.[48] Such dem-onstrations, familiar in most parts of Europe for many hundred years, may well have been common in the very French villages whose remarriage patterns have been examined here, and the at-titudes toward remarriage that they embodied were probably far more pervasive than the disturbances themselves. The community

---

48 These are among the principal surveys and interpretations of the charivari against re-marriage: Arnold Van Gennep, *Manuel de folklore français contemporain* (Paris, 1946), I, 202, 614–628; Violet Alford, "Rough Music or Charivari," *Folklore*, LXX (1959), 506–507, 512–513, 518; Claude Lévi-Strauss, (trans. John and Doreen Weightman), *The Raw and the Cooked: Introduction to a Science of Mythology* (New York, 1969), I, 286–289; E. P. Thompson, " 'Rough Music': Le Charivari anglais," *Annales: Économies, Sociétés, Civilisa-tions*, XXVII (1972), 294–301, 310–312; Natalie Z. Davis, *Society and Culture in Early Modern France: Eight Essays* (Stanford, Calif., 1975), 105–107; Edward Shorter, *The Making of the Modern Family* (New York, 1975), 220–227. The writers agree, although with varying emphasis, that a charivari was especially likely if the widow or widower was marrying a younger single person. Insofar as this was so (and the choice of victims could have varied with time and place, as Thompson demonstrates in another context), it would reduce the importance of the charivari as an obstacle to remarriage.

Davis provides further reason for questioning its demographic significance when she implies that the object was less to make remarriage impossible than to express concern about the difficulties such unions might cause for the widow's or widower's children and for the young people in the neighborhood who were about to marry for the first time. There is some evidence, but relatively little, that old widows and widowers as such were a special object of attention, and it is not clear whether one sex faced more opposition than the other.

at large could have expressed hostility in more discreet but equally compelling ways, and widows and widowers themselves could have accepted such criticism as a legitimate assertion of a standard of decorum or an obligation to succeeding generations. But studying remarriage with these possibilities in mind would not require discarding the model offered here. The difference would come in interpreting the numerical results, at which time the historian, drawing on literary as well as demographic evidence, would want to determine whether "desire" to remain widowed resulted from a widespread opinion that remarriage should be foregone when it was not economically necessary. It might even prove worthwhile to explore this possibility for colonial America.[49]

49 J. William Frost, *The Quaker Family in Colonial America: A Portrait of the Society of Friends* (New York, 1973), 161–162, points out that American Quakers, interpreting the teachings of George Fox, required widows and widowers to wait a year before remarrying. This regulation, so much at odds with the practice in contemporary Europe and in Puritan New England, raises the question of whether the underlying attitudes discouraged remarriage in general.

Journal of Interdisciplinary History, v : 4 (Spring 1975), 537–570.

Daniel Scott Smith and Michael S. Hindus

Premarital Pregnancy in America 1640-1971: An Overview and Interpretation

Sexual expression is a basic human drive and its control, a ubiquitous feature of all societies. Although all cultures prescribe sexual intercourse within marriage, in Western and especially American society sex has been proscribed without. Since behavior obviously does not always conform to norms, essential to uncovering the history of sex is some objective measure of the extent of non-marital intercourse. As Schumpeter once put it, "we need statistics not only for explaining things but also in order to know precisely what there is to explain." [1] Since children are a measurable, if not inevitable, result of intercourse, premarital pregnancy—operationally defined as the conception, before marriage, of the first post-maritally born child—provides an index of change in sexual behavior. This measure has the advantages of coverage (since nearly all adults marry), reliability (since the births are legitimate and more likely to be recorded than illegitimate births), objectivity (since its measurement depends on the matching of records collected for other purposes), and sensitivity to change in the underlying phenomenon (since premarital pregnancy is a relatively minor violation of the prevailing ban on non-marital intercourse).

What has to be explained in the white American premarital pregnancy record is the cyclical pattern of troughs in the seventeenth century (under 10 percent of first births) and mid-nineteenth century (about 10 percent) and peaks in the second half of the eighteenth century (about 30 percent) and in contemporary America (between 20 and 25 percent) (Fig. 1). This cycle cannot be explained away by changes in the variables intermediate between premarital coitus and

Daniel Scott Smith is Assistant Professor of History at the University of Illinois, Chicago Circle, and Associate Director of the Family History Program at the Newberry Library.
Michael S. Hindus is a Fellow at the Center for the Study of Law and Society, University of California, Berkeley.

An earlier version of this analysis was presented to the annual meeting of the American Historical Association in 1971. We are indebted to John Demos, Michael Gordon, Kenneth Lockridge, Susan Norton, Edward Shorter, and Etienne van de Walle for criticism of the original paper.

1 Joseph A. Schumpeter, *History of Economic Analysis* (New York, 1954), 14. For a general introduction to the sociology of sex, see Kingsley Davis, "Sexual Behavior," in Robert K. Merton and Robert A. Nisbet (eds.), *Contemporary Social Problems* (New York, 1966; 2nd ed.), 322–372.

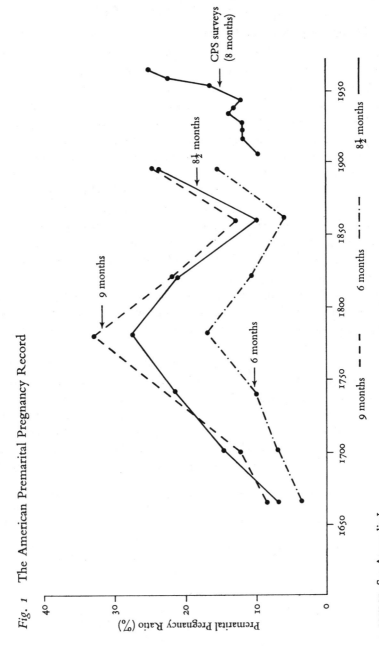

Fig. 1   The American Premarital Pregnancy Record

SOURCE: See Appendix I.

post-marital birth—fecundability and pregnancy wastage, contraceptive usage, induced abortion, and illegitimacy. Although these variables influence the level, we are concerned with the direction of the trend. It is unlikely that the underlying biological bases of American reproduction have varied enough to account for the magnitude and timing of the fluctuations in the premarital pregnancy ratio. Although contraceptive use obviously lowers fertility, since World War II both illegitimacy and premarital pregnancy have increased. Historically the trend in premarital pregnancy has paralleled that in illegitimacy.[2] Although the proportion of bridal pregnancies in all non-maritally conceived births is not constant over time and space, it appears to be a rule that when the overall level of non-marital conception increases, the proportion of non-marital pregnancies born outside of wedlock also rises.[3] To explain the major swings in premarital pregnancy, primary emphasis must rest on an analysis of the variation in the proportion of women who have engaged in premarital coitus. A similar long cycle also exists in West European illegitimacy and premarital pregnancy data (Fig. 2). Superficially at least the cyclical variation in premarital pregnancy is a striking regularity of early modern and modern social history.[4]

The basic strategy of this analysis is to distinguish between the periods with high ratios by comparing differentials in premarital

2   These are international phenomena; see Sidney Goldstein, "Premarital Pregnancies and Out-of-Wedlock Births in Denmark, 1950–1965," *Demography*, IV (1967), 925–936; K. G. Basavarajappa, "Pre-marital Pregnancies and Ex-Nuptial Births in Australia, 1911–66," *Australian and New Zealand Journal of Sociology*, IV (1968), 126–145; Shirley M. Hartley, "The Amazing Rise of Illegitimacy in Great Britain," *Social Forces*, XLIV (1966), 533–545; Daniel Scott Smith, "The Dating of the American Sexual Revolution: Evidence and Interpretation," in Michael Gordon (ed.), *The American Family in Social-Historical Perspective* (New York, 1973), 321–335. For the long-run European pattern see Edward Shorter, "Illegitimacy, Sexual Revolution, and Social Change in Modern Europe," *Journal of Interdisciplinary History*, II (1971), 237–272; Shorter, John Knodel, and Etienne van de Walle, "The Decline of Non-Marital Fertility in Europe, 1880–1940," *Population Studies*, XXV (1971), 375–393.
3   This rule is derived from the postwar experience of Great Britain (Hartley, "Amazing Rise," 540, Table 3), Denmark (Goldstein, "Premarital Pregnancies," 930), Australia (Basavarajappa, "Pre-marital Pregnancies," 141), and the cross-national relationship in Phillips Cutright, "Illegitimacy in the United States, 1920–1968," in Charles F. Westoff and Robert Parke, Jr. (eds.), *Demographic and Social Aspects of Population Growth* (Washington, D.C., 1972), 405.
4   The American and West European cycles are not identical. The early nineteenth-century American decline occurred a half-century or more before the corresponding downturn in Western Europe. Although a reduced incidence of premarital coitus seems central to the American decline, the use of contraception is the principal variable in the European decrease.

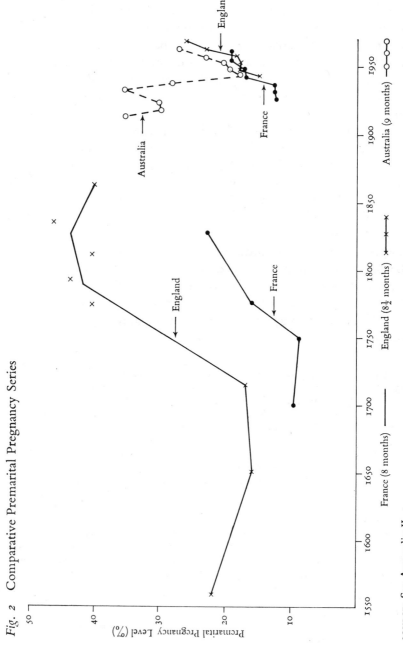

Fig. 2   Comparative Premarital Pregnancy Series

SOURCE: See Appendix II.

pregnancy between groups, and then to assess eras with lower ratios by focusing on differences in the social control of sexuality. The social relationships underlying similar premarital pregnancy levels are strikingly dissimilar. The analysis of the transitions thus concentrates on the changing relationships between sexual behavior and the social mechanisms controlling it. Throughout we will be concerned with individual behavior, the role of the family as the principal regulator of sexual expression, and the larger societal context.

PERIODS WITH HIGH RATIOS   The family of orientation (family of birth) played a much more direct role in the high premarital pregnancy level of the late eighteenth century than it does in the modern peak. This contrast is apparent in the incidence of premarital pregnancy by age; the incidence by class; the relative incidence among interclass unions; and the transmission and support of the tendency toward premarital pregnancy.

Age   In contrast to the relatively constant age-specific pattern among pre-industrial women, modern premarital pregnancy is increasingly concentrated among teen-agers (Table 1). Although the low teen-age rates for seventeenth-century Hingham, Massachusetts and pre-industrial West European samples may be attributed to adolescent subfecundity, the relative stability after age 20 can best be explained by the absence of a clear demarcation between youth and maturity in pre-industrial society.[5] Couples in their late 20s entered into marriage in the same social context as those marrying at an earlier age. In contemporary populations, by contrast, teen-agers do not employ contraceptives as often and as effectively as women in their 20s. Aging in modern society from 15 to 25 involves qualitative changes in the context of behavior which did not occur two centuries earlier.

Economic strata   Although family income had little impact on the incidence of premarital coitus of white 15–19 year-old unmarried females surveyed in 1971, parental economic status was inversely related to the frequency of premarital pregnancy in the eighteenth-century case (Table 2). Based on a Detroit sample of 1960, parental

5   Since a low age at menarche is related to diet, particularly protein consumption, the American age historically may have been below that in Europe. For this suggestion see Peter Laslett, "Age at Menarche in Europe since the Eighteenth Century," *Journal of Interdisciplinary History*, II (1971), 236.

Table 1   Relationship of Female Age at First Marriage to Premarital Pregnancy

DESCRIPTION OF SAMPLE PLACE AND PERIOD OF MARRIAGE	AGE AT MARRIAGE OF WOMAN				
	15–19	20–24	25–29	30–34	35 AND OVER
Hingham, Mass. (rate)					
–1720	2.4 (100)	11.4 (475)	3.9 (162)[a]		
1721–1800	40.9 (100)	23.8 (58)	21.6 (53)		
1801–1840	23.9 (100)	15.5 (65)	13.5 (56)		
1841–1880	15.4 (100)	11.0 (71)	2.7 (17)		
Andover, Mass. (ratio)[1]					
1685–1744	19.0 (100)	15.8 (83)	6.7 (35)[a]		
United States (ratio)[2]					
1964–1966	29.8 (100)	14.7 (49)	5.9 (20)[a]		
Northwest France (ratio)[3]					
1670–1769	3.7 (100)	6.4 (175)	6.8 (184)	6.3 (171)	6.5 (177)
France (rate)[4]					
1925–1929	18.4 (100)	11.9 (65)	8.6 (47)	7.1 (39)	6.0 (33)
1955–1959	33.0 (100)	18.2 (55)	14.4 (44)	11.3 (34)	3.7 (11)
Australia (rate)[5]					
1911	58.8 (100)	34.5 (59)	20.3 (34)	15.2 (26)	6.8 (12)
1965	44.6 (100)	16.2 (36)	13.5 (30)	10.8 (24)	3.9 (9)

a 25 or more.

SOURCES:

1 We are indebted to Philip J. Greven, Jr. for these unpublished data.

2 Mary Grace Kovar, "Interval from First Marriage to First Birth: United States, 1964–66 Births," unpub. paper, (1970), Table A.

3 Louis Henry, "Intervalle entre le mariage," 277, Table 9.

4 Jean-Claude DeVille, Structure, 91, Table 35.

5 K. G. Basavarajappa, "Pre-marital Pregnancies," 143, Table A.

Table 2 Economic Status, Premarital Pregnancy in Eighteenth-Century Hingham, Mass., The United States, 1964–66, and Premarital Coital Incidence for White American 15–19 Year-Olds, 1971

DESCRIPTION OF SAMPLE	WEALTH CRITERION AND INCIDENCE OF PREMARITAL PREGNANCY					
	IN QUINTILES					
	TOP 20%	U-M 20%	M 20%	L-M 20%	POOR 20%	TOTAL
WEALTH OF HUSBAND, HINGHAM RECONSTITUTED FAMILIES OF 1721–1800	19.8% (91)	22.5% (89)	29.1% (103)	43.8% (105)	29.2% (130)	29.3% (518)
Children of taxpayers on 1767 first parish list						
Sons	24.7% (81)	35.2% (54)	34.6% (26)	47.9% (48)	50.0% (34)	36.2% (243)
Daughters	16.4% (67)	37.3% (67)	44.2% (43)	37.8% (45)	22.2% (27)	31.3% (249)
United States, 1964–66[1]	FAMILY INCOME (IN THOUSANDS OF DOLLARS)					
	$10+ 8.2%	7–9.9 11.5%	5–6.9 17.6%	3–4.9 23.3%	<3 37.5%	21.6%
Premarital coital experience of unmarried white	FAMILY INCOME (IN THOUSANDS OF DOLLARS)					
15–19 year old females, 1971[2]	$15+ 25.6%	10–14.9 23.6%	6–9.9 22.1%	3–5.9 23.4%	<3 28.5%	23.4%

SOURCES:
1 Kovar, "Interval from first Marriage," Table F.
2 John F. Kantner and Melvin Zelnik, "Sexual Experience of Young Unmarried Women in the United States," *Family Planning Perspectives*, IV (1972), 10–11, Tables 1, 2.

status also has relatively little effect on the frequency of premarital pregnancy.[6] Higher economic status no longer provides parents with leverage over the sexual behavior of their children.

Heterogamy In the Detroit sample, premarital pregnancy ratios were markedly higher when the wife's father was of higher status than the husband's father; pregnancies in which the male's family had higher status presumably ended in illegitimate births. Interclass marriages in Hingham show the same lower pattern of premarital pregnancy exhibited by marriages within the wealthier 40 percent of the population (Table 3). Since behavior followed the pattern of the higher status partner, parental control is more evident. The absence of a differential in interclass marriages suggests that community coercion overcame the more serious consequences of pregnancy for women. Further suggestive detail on the roles of parental and community authority is available for the reconstituted Hingham families established between 1761 and 1780. Men who married daughters of wealthier parents were penalized most by premarital pregnancy, implying that there was no necessity for the girl's father to contribute economically to a marriage that had been made inevitable by pregnancy.[7] For the children of poorer parents, premarital pregnancy seemed to have involved no economic setback. Lacking economic resources, less wealthy fathers could not restrain the sexual activity of their unmarried children.[8]

Sexually Restrictive and Permissive Groups Continuity is apparent in the institutional basis of the sexually more restrictive subculture. In both eras, religious involvement is associated with lower levels of pre-

6 Lolagene C. Coombs, Ronald Freedman, Judith Friedman, and William F. Pratt, "Premarital Pregnancy and Status before and after Marriage," *American Journal of Sociology*, LXXV (1970), 810, Table 3.
7 Premaritally pregnant couples, whose fathers both ranked in the upper 40 percent by wealth, were 1.9 quintiles lower in wealth with respect to the husband's father than couples of similar status who were not pregnant at marriage. When the husband's father was wealthy and the wife's father less so, the difference was 0.6 quintiles; in the reverse case, the premaritally pregnant were 1.5 quintiles poorer on the average. Finally, if both fathers ranked in the poorer 60 percent of the population, the premaritally pregnant were 0.4 quintiles higher in comparison with the husbands' fathers than the non-premaritally pregnant.
8 In both the eighteenth century and today, couples who had a child on the way at the wedding have lower subsequent economic status than those not pregnant at marriage (see the first and fourth row of Table 2). Curtailment of education is the major reason for the modern differential.

Table 3 Proportions Pregnant at Marriage by Status of Parents

DESCRIPTION OF SAMPLE	STATUS OF WIFE'S FATHER	STATUS OF HUSBAND'S FATHER %			
		GRADE SCHOOL	HIGH SCHOOL	COLLEGE	TOTAL
Detroit marriages of 1960 (father's education)[1]	Grade school	16.0	16.7	16.1	
	High school	17.5	20.7	16.9	
	College	31.3	24.5	15.9	

		WEALTHIER 40%	POORER 60%	TOTAL
Hingham reconstituted families of 1761–1780 (father's wealth)	Wealthier 40%	31.0 (29)	35.7 (14)	32.6 (43)
	Poorer 60%	33.3 (18)	50.0 (38)	44.6 (56)
	Total	31.9% (47)	44.6% (52)	39.4% (99)

1 Coombs et al., "Premarital Pregnancy and Status," 810.

Table 4 Church Membership (1717–1786), Wealth,[1] Premarital Pregnancy Status of Parents, and Premarital Pregnancy Status of Children

CATEGORY	WEALTH STATUS		
	WEALTHIER 40%	POORER 60%	TOTAL
Persons taxed in 1767			
One or both spouses members	9.4% (53)	32.3% (34)	18.4% (87)
Neither spouse member	27.3 (33)	35.3 (68)	32.7 (101)
Parents pregnant at marriage			
Sons			
Both or spouse member	36.4% (11)	0.0% (2)	30.8% (13)
Neither church member	25.0 (12)	46.9 (32)	40.9 (44)
Daughters			
Both or spouse member	50.0% (4)	50.0% (12)	50.0% (16)
Neither church member	40.0 (20)	69.2 (13)	51.5 (33)
Parents not pregnant at marriage			
Sons			
Both or spouse member	25.4% (63)	50.0% (20)	31.3% (83)
Neither church member	23.1 (39)	44.7 (38)	33.8 (77)
Daughters			
Both or spouse member	23.8% (63)	36.0% (25)	27.3% (88)
Neither church member	28.6 (28)	33.3 (48)	31.6 (76)

1 Hingham first parish list of 1767.

marital sexual activity, On the Hingham first parish tax list of 1767, only 18.4 percent of the cases where the property holder or his spouse were church members involved premarital conceptions; in 30.3 percent of the cases where neither spouse was identified as a church member, there was a premarital pregnancy (Table 4, top two rows). This relationship holds, however, only for the wealthier stratum.[9] In the 1971 survey of teen-age sexual experience, females who attended church on less than three occasions in the previous month were, depending on denomination, two to three times more likely to be non-virgins than those who attended four or more times. Active religious participation is also closely related to restrictive sexual attitudes.[10]

The association of religiosity and premarital sexual restrictiveness does not automatically imply a causal relationship. In more than 80 percent of the Hingham cases from the 1767 list, church membership followed marriage, often by five or more years. Arguing from chronology, premarital pregnancy deterred religious affiliation among the wealthier rather than vice versa. Although the children of Hingham church members were less likely to be pregnant at marriage, this minor effect disappears when one controls for wealth (Table 4). Since beginning sexual intercourse and abandoning church attendance are part of a general change in life style of maturing teen-agers, the association of religiosity and premarital sexual restrictiveness in cross-sectional surveys may be largely spurious. Religion can be said to have an impact on the overall incidence of premarital sex only when it is an encompassing and controlling force in the lives of the young and not merely an option.

The more impressive relationship in Table 4 is the consistent difference between the daughters whose mothers were pregnant at marriage and those whose mothers were not. Inasmuch as there existed a sexually permissive subculture in eighteenth-century Hingham, its continuity depended on the female line and on the less wealthy section of the population. The former relationship did not pass unnoticed by

9 In the town of Groton only 11.3 percent of persons admitted to full communion between 1761 and 1775 confessed to premarital fornication while 33 percent of those owning the baptismal covenant did so. Since formal church membership is probably related to wealth, the causation here is uncertain. For the Groton figures see Henry Reed Stiles, *Bundling: Its Origins, Progress and Decline in America* (Albany, 1871), 78.
10 Kantner and Zelnik, "Sexual Experience," 16, Table 11; Ira L. Reiss, *The Social Context of Premarital Sexual Permissiveness* (New York, 1967), 42–44, 99–100.

contemporaries, as is evidenced by the subtitle and following lines of an anonymous poem published around 1785:

> Some maidens say, if through the nation,
> Bundling should quite go out of fashion,
> Courtship would lose its sweets; and they
> Could have no fun till wedding day.
> It shant be so, they rage and storm,
> And country girls in clusters swarm,
> And fly and buz like angry bees,
> And vow they'll bundle when they please.
> Some mothers too, will plead their cause,
> And give their daughters great applause,
> And tell them 'tis no sin nor shame,
> For we, your mothers did the same.[11]

In summary, intergenerational family relationships are deeply involved in the great boom of premarital pregnancy in the eighteenth century.

Premarital sexual activity in modern society is structured through the peer group and more broadly through a youth subculture, which is reinforced by age-stratified institutions such as schools and promoted by other forces such as marketing and the mass media. Although objective family background characteristics such as income, education, or religious preference have little impact on the incidence of teen-age intercourse, higher familiar status, especially parental education, is associated with the more frequent use of contraception by sexually active teen-agers.[12] Modern parents generally lack the power to be oppressive in an effective way. This absence of parental control and influence is strikingly demonstrated by the low correspondence between the political opinions of parents and children.[13] If teen-agers are not controlled by their parents, neither are they autonomous. The adolescent way station between dependent childhood and independent adulthood is characterized by an alienation but not a separation from

11   Anon., "A New Bundling Song; Or a reproof to those Young Country Women, who follow that reproachful Practice, and to their Mothers for upholding them therein," in Stiles, *Bundling*, 81–82.

12   Reiss, *Social Context*, 171–180; James J. Teevan, Jr., "Reference Groups and Premarital Sexual Behavior," *Journal of Marriage and the Family*, XXXIV (1972), 283–291; Kantner and Zelnik, "Sexual Experience," Tables 2, 3, 4, 10; "Contraception and Pregnancy: Experience of Young Unmarried Women in the United States," *Family Planning Perspectives*, V (1973), 21–35, esp. Tables 2, 3, 9.

13   See the summary article by R. W. Connell, "Political Socialization in the American Family: The Evidence Re-Examined," *Public Opinion Quarterly*, XXXVI (1972), 322–333. The median correlation in a range of studies was only 0.2.

parental values and culture. Survey research suggests that premarital coitus is directly related to the extent of this estrangement.[14] Although the modern family fails to restrict successfully the sexual activity of children, it and the other institutions involving youth limit the possibilities of a rational separation of sex and procreation.

PERIODS WITH LOW RATIOS   Just as the peaks in premarital pregnancy when examined in detail reflect quite different underlying patterns, so the troughs of the seventeenth and nineteenth centuries result from different systems of control. Although a sexually repressive ideology characterized both centuries, the emphasis in the Puritan seventeenth century was on external controls, while internal control or self-repression was the central feature of Victorian morality. Premarital sexual restraint was possible both in the seventeenth-century community and in nineteenth-century society, but not during the transition. Maintenance of morality, however, shifted from direct to indirect, from being based primarily on social control to resting principally on socialization.

The importance of external controls in the seventeenth century may be readily demonstrated. Premarital pregnancy ratios were low not just in North America but in England and France as well. English premarital pregnancy, for example, was 26 percent below the sixteenth-century figure, and illegitimacy ratios between 1651 and 1720 were less than half of those prevailing between 1581 and 1630 and from 1741 to 1820. English North America shared the organized religious intensity that pervaded Western Europe during the seventeenth century.[15] With a premarital pregnancy level less than half that of England, mid-seventeenth-century New England, as Governor Bradford of Plymouth was "verily persuaded," was a society "with not more evils in this kind [sexual deviation], nor nothing near so many by proportion as in other places; but they are here more discovered and seen and made public by due search, inquisition and due punishment; for the churches look narrowly to their members, and the magistrates over all, more

14 For example, 43.4 percent of white 15–19 year-old females who "strongly agreed" with the statement, "I don't confide very much in my parents," had had intercourse, while only 13.5 percent of those who strongly disagreed were not virgins (Kantner and Zelnik, "Sexual Experience," 15, Table 9).
15 For English bridal pregnancy data, see Appendix II. For illegitimacy trends see Peter Laslett, *The World We Have Lost* (London, 1971; 2nd ed.), 142. John Bossy, "The Counter-Reformation and the People of Catholic Europe," *Past & Present*, XLVII (1970), 51–70.

strictly than in other places."[16] Instead of the Puritans becoming "inured to sexual offenses, because there were so many," as Morgan puts it, they prosecuted their comparatively few sexual offenders vigorously. Morgan was right in his now classic reading of the court records, however, when he emphasized the calm, matter-of-fact approach of the Puritans toward even the most extreme manifestations of sexual deviance. Although this composure had its roots in the theological belief in original sin, the elaborate structure of social repression maintained by the Puritans suggests that they did not expect the population at large to have internalized sexual control. Broadly speaking, Puritanism may be characterized as a communal response to the strains accompanying the disintegration of the bases of medieval society.[17]

Nineteenth-century morality was forged in a new social matrix and constructed with different materials. The reappearance of premarital sexual restraint in the nineteenth century was based on the autonomy of the young adult and the incorporation of the groups tending toward premarital pregnancy into a new social order. By the early nineteenth century, people were generally independent in life at a younger age than ever before.[18] Although there were objective changes, such as the economic shift from the apprentice to the wage system and the substitution of boarding for service as the transitional living arrangement for young people, most significant was the social acceptance of youthful autonomy.

The new independence of nineteenth-century youth was recognized in various ways. The practical impact of the introduction of universal male suffrage was not so much the enfranchisement of a permanent proletariat as the granting of political rights to young adults. Proponents of manhood suffrage presented their arguments in terms of the reality of allowing young men the political autonomy commensurate with their social and economic status.[19] During and after the

16 William Bradford (ed. Samuel Eliot Morison), *Of Plymouth Plantation, 1620–1647* (New York, 1959), 317.

17 Edmund S. Morgan, "The Puritans and Sex," *New England Quarterly*, XV (1942), 595; Michael Walzer, "Puritanism as a Revolutionary Ideology," *History and Theory*, III (1961), 59–90.

18 Joseph F. Kett, "Growing Up in Rural New England, 1800–1840," in Tamara K. Hareven (ed.), *Anonymous Americans* (Englewood Cliffs, N.J., 1971), 9–10. For the comments of European travelers on the freedom of antebellum youth, see Frank F. Furstenberg, Jr., "Industrialization and the American Family: A Look Backward," *American Sociological Review*, XXXI (1966), 329–330, 335.

19 For examples of this argument, see Chilton Williamson, *American Suffrage from Property to Democracy* (Princeton, 1960), 139, 147, 171, 177, 187–188, 195.

Second Great Awakening, religious conversion became a common experience for teen-agers. Not unrelated to early religious involvement
is the fact that youths began to play important roles in reform
movements.[20]

The early nineteenth century also witnessed the social incorporation of the groups previously prone to premarital pregnancy. The
erosion of the social base of the sexually permissive segment of the
population was partly the result of a dramatic expansion of religious
participation. Estimated formal church membership in America
tripled from 7 to 23 percent between 1800 and 1860.[21] With younger
conversion, religion could have a more effective impact on premarital
sexual choices. The concomitant splintering of American Protestantism
meant that each stratum had one or more denominations tailored to its
particular condition and needs. Although denominations differed in
social base and religious style, the regulation of individual morality
was a central concern of nineteenth-century Protestantism.[22] Although
seventeenth-century Puritanism stressed external controls, antebellum
religious enthusiasm rejected Calvinist determinism in favor of free
will doctrines. The basic social support of nineteenth-century sexual
restraint—religion—rested on the centrality of autonomy and individual
choice. Finally, nineteenth-century Protestantism incorporated women,
the apparent source of the intergenerational transmission of premarital
pregnancy in the eighteenth century, into the social order. If women
did not entirely dominate religion symbolically and organizationally in
the nineteenth century, the churches did provide an important outlet
for a wide range of female needs.[23] A more active part of the churches,
nineteenth-century women absorbed the message of sexual restraint
more completely.

Since the supporting social restraints involved voluntary action,
the new anti-sexual ideology of the nineteenth century was necessarily
more total than the Puritan hostility to non-marital sexual expression.

20   Joseph F. Kett, "Adolescence and Youth in Nineteenth-Century America, "*Journal
of Interdisciplinary History*, II (1971), 289–291; Lois W. Banner, "Religion and Reform
in the Early Republic: The Role of Youth," *American Quarterly*, XXIII (1971), 677–695.
21   N. J. Demerath III, "Trends and Anti-Trends in Religious Change," in Eleanor B.
Sheldon and Wilbert E. Moore (eds.), *Indicators of Social Change: Concepts and Measure-
ments* (New York, 1968), 353.
22   Timothy L. Smith, *Revivalism and Social Reform* (New York, 1965), esp. 33–44,
148–162. See also Alexis de Tocqueville (ed. Phillips Bradley), *Democracy in America*
(New York, 1945), I, 313–318.
23   Barbara Welter, "The Feminization of American Religion: 1800–1860," in
William L. O'Neill (ed.), *Insights and Parallels: Problems and Issues of American Social
History* (Minneapolis, 1973), 305–332.

Intellectually intertwined with the entire system of liberal bourgeois ideology, Victorian morality was more than a functional system for the control of premarital sexual behavior. The exaggerated aversion to masturbation, for example, is inexplicable if the system were merely designed to prevent premarital pregnancy.[24] Victorian morality was relevant to the immediate needs and social position of both young men and women. Tocqueville emphasized the free marriage market as the structural determinant of the high degree of sexual restraint among young American women. "No girl," observed the aristocratic visitor, "then believes that she cannot become the wife of the man who loves her, and this renders all breaches of morality before marriage very uncommon."[25] Since women were on their own in the marriage market but lacked economic resources thereafter, Victorian morality raised the price of sex and thus substantially increased the bargaining power of both single and married women.[26]

Because sexual restraint was compatible with the norms of thrift and abstinence required of the upwardly striving young capitalist, the morality advantageous to women also appealed to the rationality, if not the passion, of males. The early age of independence from the family of orientation prepared young middle-class men not for early marriage but for a period of capital accumulation and entry into a career, the two prerequisites to marriage. Having internalized the mechanism of deferred gratification in terms of his economic life, the nineteenth-century American male would not risk the consequences of a marriage precipitated by a premarital pregnancy. Although not every man was making it in nineteenth-century America, more and more were caught up in the competition. Most importantly, the obstacles to advancement in society were seen as within the capacity of the individual to overcome.

THE TRANSITIONS AND THEIR IMPLICATIONS   Have basic American institutions changed gradually and easily? Have the external forms

24   Peter Cominos, "Late Victorian Sexual Respectability and the Social System," *International Review of Social History*, VIII (1963), 18–48, 216–250; Steven Willner Nissenbaum, "Careful Love: Sylvester Graham and the Emergence of Victorian Sexual Theory in America, 1830–1840," unpub. Ph.D. diss. (University of Wisconsin, 1968), 3–32.
25   Tocqueville, *Democracy*, II, 216; generally, 215–221.
26   For a more extended discussion of the role of nineteenth-century women in promoting Victorian morality, see Daniel Scott Smith, "Family Limitation, Sexual Control and Domestic Feminism in Victorian America," *Feminist Studies*, I (1973), 40–57.

of control been painlessly modified to conform to new or more freely expressed desires of individuals? Or did "crises" arise in the older social arrangements before new patterns of behavior appeared? With more than three centuries of data on the key aspect of human behavior which is under examination here, some insights are possible concerning this fundamental problem in American history. Since two thirds of white women were not pregnant at marriage throughout the course of American history, continuity in the efficacy of control is obviously apparent. Yet, since premarital pregnancy is at least a mild form of deviancy, the magnitude of the cyclical fluctuation is impressive. Our contention is that rising premarital pregnancy is a manifestation of a collision between an unchanging and increasingly antiquated family structure and a pattern of individual behavior which is more a part of the past than a harbinger of the future. The downturn in premarital pregnancy follows as a necessary but not sufficient consequence of a transformation in the family's role as a regulator of the sexual behavior of the young. Neither the old institutional pattern of control nor the rebellion against it can predict the subsequent sexual behavior of the young. The sexual revolutionaries of the eighteenth century, if the premarital procreators may be so labeled, were obviously not the vanguard of a sexually liberated nineteenth century.

The increase in premarital pregnancy in late seventeenth-century New England provides empirical evidence for the notion of the declension of Puritanism from a "golden age." At first the authorities attempted to maintain their vigilance in the face of increased sexual deviance (Table 5). As late as the 1670s, at least by a rough estimate of the number of premarital pregnancies in Essex County, well over half of the guilty couples were being convicted.[27] Before any marked socio-economic change occurred in New England, cracks surfaced in the sexually repressive order. During the last third of the century punishment declined from corporal to monetary, and individuals were given the choice between fines or whippings.[28] Although illegitimacy

27 Direct matching of premarital pregnancy cases from the vital records to prosecutions in court records yields a similar estimate. Three of five couples in Ipswich (1657–1682), and three of five in Hingham (1670–1682) with a birth within six complete months of marriage were found in the published court records.

28 See Table 5. Even with this amelioration in penalties, punishment and prosecution were more severe in New England than in English church courts. See Ronald A. Marchant, *The Church under the Law: Justice, Administration and Discipline in the Diocese of York, 1560–1640* (Cambridge, 1969), 27, 215–219, 240–243; George Elliott Howard, *A History of Matrimonial Institutions* (Chicago, 1904), II, 180–200.

Table 5. Crime and Punishment for Fornication in Essex County, Massachusetts, 1643–1682

CONVICTIONS	1643–1652	1653–1667	1668–1682	TOTAL
Married couples	4	19	85	108
(known early birth)	3	3	13	19
Women only	6	30	69	105
(known pregnancy)	2	18	38	58
Men only	4	22	46	72
(bastardy cases)	2	7	26	35
Total incidences[a]	11	54	161	226
Mean population[b]	4,100	6,000	11,000	
Incidence rate (per 1000 per decade)	2.7	6.0	9.8	
KNOWN PUNISHMENTS				
fine	5	22	66	93
whipping	4	27	17	48
whipping or fine	2	8	95	105
child support only	1	22	17	40
other	2	2	1	5
Total known	14	81	196	291

ESTIMATE OF PERCENTAGE OF PREMARITAL PREGNANCIES CONVICTED:

MARRIED COUPLES CONVICTED, 1671–80	POPULATION ESTIMATE	MARRIAGE RATE[c]	PREGNANCIES EXPECTED[d]	PERCENT CONVICTED
65	11,000	12/1000	106	61%

a   The total of incidences is obtained by adding the number of married couples convicted, the number of single women convicted, and the small number of single men (thirteen for the forty year period) who were prosecuted without a partner being arraigned.

b   From William I. Davisson, "Essex County Wealth Trends," *Essex Institute Historical Collections*, CIII (1967), 292.

c   From Susan Norton, "Population Growth in Colonial America: A Study of Ipswich, Massachusetts," *Population Studies*, XXV (1971), 451.

d   Premarital pregnancy ratio of 8% based on three Essex County towns— Ipswich (7.3% before 1700), Salem (8.2%, 1671–1700), and Topsfield (7.7%, 1660–1679). To be conservative, a nine-month standard was used.

prosecutions continued after 1700, civil punishment for premarital pregnancy gradually disappeared. Although the churches then picked up the burden of repression by requiring confessions for baptism and admission, individuals, typically, were ready to join only after their premarital experience had passed. As premarital pregnancy continued to increase during the eighteenth century, the churches dropped or diluted the confession requirement.[29] In short, the severity of active social repression is inversely related over time to the level of premarital pregnancy.

The removal of the communal controls of Puritanism left exposed a set of traditional relationships. Although pressures in the direction of the substantive autonomy of youth may have been inherent in the American wilderness from the beginning, environmental forces were more than blunted by traditional familial, social, and ideological arrangements. Nearly a century passed before the customary high male age at marriage was lowered. Other indices of traditionalism in family patterns persisted well past the middle of the eighteenth century.[30] Even the modernity of the influential *Some Thoughts Concerning Education* may be questioned.[31] Although Locke stressed affection between mature sons and their fathers (who handily reserved the right to disinherit), the psychological basis for this rational relationship developed in the context of a severe, but not total, crushing of the son's will as an infant. "Fear and awe," proclaimed Locke to fathers, "ought to give you the first power over their minds," and thus compliance "will seem natural to them."[32]

Alternative explanations do not account adequately for the transition to higher premarital pregnancy levels in the eighteenth century. Premarital sex was never normatively approved, even during engagement. Most premaritally pregnant couples (from two thirds to three fourths of those marrying in Hingham between 1741 and 1780) were also pregnant at the time of legal engagement—the filing of the intention to marry.[33] On the other hand, over 40 percent of women not

29 Emil Oberholzer, Jr., *Delinquent Saints: Disciplinary Action in the Early Congregational Churches of Massachusetts* (New York, 1956), 136.

30 Philip J. Greven, Jr., *Four Generations: Population, Land, and Family in Colonial Andover, Massachusetts* (Ithaca, 1970); Daniel Scott Smith, "The Demographic History of Colonial New England," *Journal of Economic History*, XXXII (1972), 176–180; *idem*, "Parental Power and Marriage Patterns: An Analysis of Historical Trends in Hingham, Massachusetts," *Journal of Marriage and the Family*, XXXV (1973), 419–428.

31 For the mixture of patriarchalism and consent in Locke, see Gordon J. Schochet, "The Family and the Origins of the State," in John W. Yolton (ed.), *John Locke: Problems and Perspectives* (Cambridge, 1969), 81–98; M. Seliger, *The Liberal Politics of John Locke* (New York, 1968), 209–226.

32 John Locke, *Some Thoughts Concerning Education* in James E. Axtell (ed.), *The Educational Writings of John Locke* (Cambridge, 1968), 146–147. In the introduction to his recent documentary collection (*Childrearing Concepts, 1620–1860* [Itasca, Ill., 1973], 1–6), Greven stresses the continuity of repressive ideas until the 1820s and 1830s.

33 Of the thirty-six children born within 4 complete months of marriage, thirty-three (91.7%) were born within 8½ months of the intention to marry; of the thirty-seven born in the fifth and sixth month after marriage, twenty-nine (78.4%) were born within

pregnant at marriage had been legally engaged for three months or longer. If betrothal licence is an unsatisfactory explanation, the custom of bundling is even less adequate. Although an environmental explanation (cold weather and poorly heated houses) has been seriously advanced, the low seventeenth-century incidence of premarital pregnancy and its seasonal pattern contradict this argument. Premarital conceptions occurred year-round with a slight bulge during the warmer months.[34] Bundling was an eighteenth-century compromise between persistent parental control and the pressures of the young to subvert traditional familial authority.

As a system with contradictory elements, eighteenth-century courtship was not dominated by the newer theme of romantic love. If interpersonal affection and attraction—resulting in premarital pregnancy—had been replacing the old criteria of property and status in mate selection, then one would expect that "love matches" would be more heterogamous than "property matches." To the contrary, however, premaritally pregnant couples were as similar in wealth origins as non-pregnant couples.[35] The eighteenth-century surge in premarital pregnancy did involve a revolt of the young, but it was constrained within the framework of traditional motivation. The generational interpretation is not, of course, new. Eilert Sundt, the most astute observer of courtship practices in nineteenth-century rural Europe, saw the phenomenon as "a form of protest against inordinate parental authority; its decline was in part explained by the moderating of familial controls which young people sought to subvert."[36] And an

---

8¼ months of the intention; of the thirty-eight born between the beginning of the seventh and 8¼ months of marriage, only thirteen (34.2%) were born within 8¼ months of the intention. Overall, 67.6% of the births within 8¼ months of marriage came within 8¼ months of the intention, and 73.9% were born within 9 months of the intention.

34 Stiles, *Bundling*, 53. Of premarital conceptions in Hingham between 1721 and 1800, 27.2%, 26.5%, 23.1%, and 23.1% (N = 147) occurred respectively in the quarters April–June, July–Sept., Oct.–Dec., and Jan.–March. Post-marital first conceptions (N = 363) were distributed in the same quarters as follows—19.0%, 21.5%, 26.7%, and 32.8%.

35 Comparing the wealth of the wife's father and the husband's father in Hingham reconstituted marriages between 1761 and 1780, we find no difference between the relative origins of the pregnant and nonpregnant couples. (Gamma for the pregnant couples was 0.70 (N = 39) and 0.69 (N = 60) for the nonpregnant).

36 Arthur Hillman, "Eilert Sundt: Pioneer Student of Family and Culture," in Thomas D. Eliot et al. (eds.), *Norway's Families* (Philadelphia, 1960), 40. On the work of Sundt, see Michael Drake, *Population and Society in Norway, 1735–1865* (Cambridge, 1969), 19–29.

Anglican polemicist in 1763 anticipated Sundt's conclusion. "Among dissenters, when a married pair happen to have a child born too soon after marriage," he noted, "they do not repent but if they were again in the same circumstances, they would do the same again, because otherwise they could not obtain their parent's consent to marry."[37]

The transference of this generational conflict to the political domain during the pre-Revolutionary crisis with Great Britain was not, as two scholars have recently maintained, because the contractual, Lockean, and republican nature of the family was a settled issue in everyday experience. Rather, power relationships within the family were being challenged, and the very ambiguity of the relationship between parents and children heightened the salience of the familial analogy for the parallel struggle that was developing between the colonies and the mother country.[38] Nor did the leaders of the resistance to England wish to incite a revolution in the family. For example, among the other evils which Jefferson cited in the preamble to the Virginia bill to abolish entail was that this custom "sometimes does injury to the morals of youth, by rendering them independent of, and disobedient to their parents."[39] The Revolution did signal, however, a general shift from passive to active consent on the part of the people; although an analogy is necessarily vague, it is not unreasonable to assume that a similar shift occurred in intergenerational relations. By the 1830s this new republican consensus on the family was firmly established. The father, according to Tocqueville, "exercised no other power than that which is granted to the affection and experience of age. . . . . The master and the constituted ruler have vanished, the father remains."[40] The sexual expression underlying the eighteenth-century peak in premarital pregnancy was a product of a situation of profound social disequilibrium, not an end in itself. Once the familial and social context had altered, sexual restrictiveness reappeared.

37 John Beach, *A Friendly Expostulation with all persons concern'd in publishing a late Pamphlet, Entitled, The real Advantages which Ministers and People may enjoy, especially in the Colonies, by conforming to the Church of England* (New York, 1763), 38. (We are indebted to Samuel Haber for this reference.)

38 Edwin G. Burrows and Michael Wallace, "The American Revolution: The Ideology and Psychology of National Liberation," *Perspectives in American History*, VI (1972), 167–306, esp. 255–267.

39 Paul Leicester Ford (ed.), *The Works of Thomas Jefferson* (New York, 1904), II, 269.

40 Tocqueville, *Democracy*, II, 205–206, and generally Ch. 8 "Influence of Democracy on the Family," 202–208

The crisis in traditional family structure was resolved by a republican solution—the acceptance of the maturity of young adults. Men and women in the nineteenth century responded to the risks of premarital freedom by constraining their sexual drives. Yet, the ideology of the participant-run courtship system emphasized romantic affection and love. Although elaborate dichotomies between pure love and evil sex were developed, the potential for premarital sexual intimacy was built into the Victorian system of courtship. As the Victorian cultural synthesis collapsed in the late nineteenth and twentieth centuries, the dominant themes in premarital sexuality continued to be commitment, love, and marriage. For the young adults who had become autonomous as a result of the transformation in age roles in the family a century earlier, higher rates of sexual intercourse did not produce proportional increases in premarital pregnancy. Contraception made possible the temporary separation of sex and procreation. Teen-agers, on the other hand, remained psychologically enmeshed in but not controlled by their families of orientation. With the extension of schooling in the twentieth century, the trend toward youthful autonomy perhaps has been reversed.

The dependence-independence ambivalence is crucial in the explanation of the high premarital pregnancy ratios of contemporary teen-agers. With an estimated decline in the age of menarche of 2.5 to 3.3 years during the twentieth century, American females are biologically mature earlier but socially immature as long or longer than in the nineteenth century.[41] Not independent in society (and therefore not responsible for the consequences of their actions), teen-aged girls accept the risk of pregnancy rather than consciously separate sexual intercourse from procreation. The rational use of contraception requires a teen-aged girl to adopt a self-definition inconsistent with her own assumptions.[42] The "problem," then, is not an absence of "morality" among teen-agers, but rather the persistence of a morality based on the sexual restraint of women presumed to be independent and responsible. In modern America, teen-age sexual behavior is

41 J. M. Tanner, "Earlier Maturation in Man," *Scientific American*, CCXVIII (Jan. 1968), 24–27.
42 For example, roughly two thirds of 13–19 year olds agreed with statement, "If a girl uses birth control pills or other methods of contraception, it makes it seem as if she were *planning* to have sex" (Robert C. Sorenson, *Adolescent Sexuality in Contemporary America* [New York, 1973], 408, Table 185). Both the responses and the use of italics in the question convey the implicit values.

guided neither by the old standard of prohibition nor by a new one of rational expressiveness.[43]

SUMMARY   The historical variation in premarital pregnancy in America suggests a notable absence of a Malthusian constancy of passion. Sexual restraint before marriage typified eras in which inter-generational relationships were well defined, in which extrafamilial institutions reinforced familial controls, and in which the population was relatively well integrated into the central structure of values. Conversely, premarital sexual activity has been more prevalent when there was more ambiguity and uncertainty in the parent-child relation-ship, when the social supports of morality were weakened or not appropriate to the current realities of coming of age, and when there emerged a segment of the population outside the mainstream of the culture. Discontinuity is the central fact of the premarital pregnancy record. In this important area of behavior, American history has not been a "seamless web." The transitions, furthermore, have not in-volved the simple triumph of new behavioral patterns over outmoded institutions of control. During the crisis periods the actions of the "rebels" appear, ironically, to be well integrated into the old regime of sexuality and its control.

Perhaps the cycle in premarital pregnancy should not surprise social historians. It fits two well-known models of the discontinuities of modern history—the cultural and the structural stages. The first perspective is the familiar Puritan-Enlightenment-Victorian-Post-modern organization of the four centuries of American cultural history. The latter and more interesting model involves a sequence of equilibrium-shock-adjustment-new equilibrium. In this perspective, the eighteenth-century surge in premarital pregnancy is related to the disintegration of the traditional, well-integrated rural community and to the beginnings of economic and social modernization. Once the crisis of transition to modern society had passed, premarital pregnancy began to decrease. Expectations among individuals and groups were once again predictable, and the various parts of the social system

---

43 The sex education debate is revealing in this context. Both sides in the con-troversy oppose sexual autonomy for teen-agers. Although the opponents see it as a threat to parental authority, the supporters perceive it as a supplement to parental authority by presenting sex in a wider matrix of adult values. For an amusing and perceptive account of the struggle, see Mary Breasted, *Oh! Sex Education* (New York, 1970).

meshed together.[44] Contemporary Western societies also appear to be in a similar transitional phase. The proliferation of transitional terms, e.g., post-industrial, post-modern, post-Protestant, suggests an awareness that a social order is dead but a new one is not yet definable.

What, then, of the future of premarital pregnancy and sexuality? If sexuality and procreation do become separated in the future through the universal acceptance and use of contraception and abortion in premarital relations, and if teen-agers emerge as an autonomous age group in society, then premarital pregnancy will obviously decline. Whether sexuality will continue within the romantic boundaries of love and relatively permanent commitment between individuals or jump to the utopian sexuality envisioned by Herbert Marcuse and Wilhelm Reich is more problematic. Alterations in the social control of sexuality historically have had unanticipated consequences for sexual behavior. Thus the future qualitative meaning of sexuality cannot be categorized as either romantic or utopian. Evidence exists that the structural basis for such an option is being constructed at present. The eighteen-year-olds' vote, for example, is a symbolic recognition of a younger age at maturity. Less symbolic but more to the point at issue here is the sharp drop from 68 percent of Americans in 1969 to only 48 percent in 1973 who think that "it is wrong for people to have sex relations before marriage."[45] If the analysis in this essay has validity, such a redefinition of the family and age groups in society has a clear historical precedent.

44 Examples of the use of this model are numerous. See Charles Tilly, "Collective Violence in European Perspective," in Hugh Davis Graham and Ted Robert Gurr (eds.), *The History of Violence in America* (New York, 1969), 4–44, esp. 21–33; E. J. Hobsbawm, "Economic Fluctuations and Some Social Movements since 1800," in his *Laboring Men* (New York, 1967), 148–184, esp. 153–157. For the framework applied to the family, see Shorter, "Illegitimacy, Sexual Revolution, and Social Change"; Neil Smelser, *Social Change in the Industrial Revolution* (Chicago, 1959); Smith, "Parental Power and Marriage Patterns."

45 Gallup poll for national sample reported in the *Hartford Courant*, 12 Aug. 1973, 24. The trend toward a complete separation of premarital sex and conception is apparent in Western Europe. Between the mid-1960s and c. 1970 the premarital pregnancy rate increased in only one of nine countries examined in a recent study; during the first half of the 1960s, however, the rate increased in seven of the nine countries. See France Prioux-Marchal, "Les Conceptions Prénuptiales en Europe Occidentale Depuis 1955," *Population*, XXIX (1974), 63, Table 1.

APPENDIX I

Summary

PERIOD	UNDER 6 MONTHS		UNDER 8½ MONTHS		UNDER 9 MONTHS	
	%	N	%	N	%	N
–1680	3.3	511	6.8	511	8.1	663
1681–1720	6.7	445	14.1	518	12.1	1156
1721–1760	9.9	881	21.2	1146	22.5	1442
1761–1800	16.7	970	27.2	1266	33.0	1097
1801–1840	10.3	573	17.7	815	23.7	616
1841–1880	5.8	572	9.6	467	12.6	572
1881–1910	15.1	119	23.3	232	24.4	119

Individual Studies: For the efficient display of the maximum detail, the data are reported in the following order: sample description, marriage period, percent of marriages linked to first births, number matched, percentage born under 6, 8½, and 9 months.

Hingham, Massachusetts: reconstitution study (non-native-born excluded in the nineteenth century).

	%		%	%	%
1641–1660	n.a.	33	0.0	0.0	0.0
1661–1680	n.a.	80	5.0	11.2	11.2
1681–1700	n.a.	86	3.5	12.8	18.6
1701–1720	69	109	7.3	13.8	17.4
1721–1740	67	172	11.6	22.7	27.3
1741–1760	65	212	13.2	31.2	38.2
1761–1780	64	200	19.0	33.5	36.5
1781–1800	55	204	21.0	32.8	39.1
1801–1820	58	215	14.9	24.6	28.4
1821–1840	61	276	7.3	16.0	20.3
1841–1860	n.a.	235	4.7	8.5	10.2
1861–1880	n.a.	145	9.0	16.0	16.5

Watertown, Massachusetts: genealogy.

	%		%	%	%
–1660	n.a.	9	0.0	11.1	11.1
1661–1680	n.a.	35	0.0	8.6	8.6
1681–1700	n.a.	44	6.8	9.1	13.6
1701–1720	n.a.	76	7.9	19.8	25.1
1721–1740	n.a.	96	4.2	18.7	25.8
1741–1760	n.a.	110	10.9	21.8	23.6
1761–1780	n.a.	112	15.2	24.1	29.4
1781–1800	n.a.	111	15.3	26.1	32.5

Dedham, Massachusetts: vital record study.

	%		%	%	%
1662–1669	84	21	4.8	4.8	4.8
1671–1680	67	36	2.8	8.5	11.1
1760–1770	43	73	19.2	30.1	32.9

Topsfield, Massachusetts: vital record study.

	%		%	%	%
1660–1679	n.a.	13	7.7	7.7	7.7
1680–1699	n.a.	44	2.3	4.5	6.8
1738–1740	n.a.	25	12.0	24.0	24.0

Andover, Massachusetts: Greven, *Four Generations,* 113. (The figure for 1731–1749 comes from unpublished data kindly furnished by Greven.)

	%				%
1655–1674	41	21	—	—	0.0
1675–1699	55	64	—	—	12.5
1700–1730	41	115	—	—	11.5
1731–1749	8	29	—	—	17.3

Hollis, New Hampshire: vital record study.

	%		%	%	%
1741–1760	n.a.	39	2.6	12.8	17.9
1761–1780	n.a.	84	13.1	26.2	29.8
1781–1800	n.a.	57	10.5	31.6	35.1

Coventry, Connecticut: vital record study; Cheryl Krajcik, "The Trend in Premarital Pregnancy Ratios in Mansfield 1700–1849 and Coventry, 1711–1840," unpub. undergraduate sociology paper (University of Connecticut, 1972). We are indebted to the author and to Michael Gordon for this reference.

	%				%
1711–1740	n.a.	84	—	—	20.2
1741–1770	n.a.	179	—	—	23.5
1771–1800	n.a.	104	—	—	25.0
1801–1840	n.a.	43	—	—	4.6

Mansfield, Connecticut: vital record study; Phyllis Schneider, "Premarital Pregnancy in Mansfield, Connecticut, 1700–1849," unpub. undergraduate sociology paper (University of Connecticut, 1972.) We are indebted to the author and to Michael Gordon for this reference.

	%				%
1700–1739	n.a.	73	—	—	12.3
1740–1769	n.a.	265	—	—	19.2

	%				%
1770–1799	n.a.	296	—	—	20.6
1800–1819	n.a.	154	—	—	12.3
1820–1849	n.a.	88	—	—	5.7

Christ Church Parish, Middlesex County, Virginia: vital record study of marriages and baptisms.

	%		%	%	%
1720–1736	64	191	9.4	15.2	16.8

Kingston Parish, Gloucester County, Virginia: vital record study of marriages and baptisms, letters A–I.

	%		%	%	%
1749–1760	n.a.	36	2.8	13.9	13.9
1761–1770	n.a.	66	12.1	22.7	24.2
1771–1780	n.a.	63	12.7	25.4	30.1
1749–1780	64	165	10.3	21.8	24.2

Bergen, New Jersey: Reformed Dutch Church, vital record study of marriages and baptisms.

	%		%	%	%
1665–1680	64	18	0.0	5.6	5.6
1681–1700	55	31	19.4	19.4	19.4
1701–1720	47	16	18.7	25.0	25.0

New Paltz, New York: Reformed Dutch Church, vital record study of marriages and baptisms.

	%		%	%	%
1801–1803 } 1808–1812 }	37	82	8.5	28.0	33.0

Boston, Massachusetts: vital record study.

	%		%	%	%
1651–1655	62	84	3.6	6.0	14.3
1690, 1692	52	39	0.0	17.9	23.1

Ipswich, Massachusetts: reconstitution; Susan Norton, "Population Growth in Colonial America: A Study of Ipswich, Massachusetts," *Population Studies,* XXV (1971), 636; (1650–1687 from our own study).

	%		%	%	%
–1700	n.a.	68	—	—	7.3
1701–1725	n.a.	143	—	—	5.6
1726–1750	n.a.	100	—	—	6.3
1650–1687	76	182	3.8	6.0	8.2

Bristol, Rhode Island: vital record study; John Demos, "Families in Colonial Bristol, Rhode Island: An Exercise in Historical Demography," *William and Mary Quarterly,* XXV (1968), 56.

	%				%
1680–1700	c.33	19	—	—	0.0
1700–1720	c.14	8	—	—	0.0
1720–1740	c.40	42	—	—	10.0
1740–1760	c.23	35	—	—	49.0
1760–1780	c.14	23	—	—	44.0

Salem, Massachusetts: reconstitution (based on unpublished data kindly supplied by James Somerville).

	%				%
1651–1670	n.a.	131	—	—	5.3
1671–1700	n.a.	123	—	—	8.2
1701–1730	n.a.	239	—	—	5.8
1731–1770	n.a.	176	—	—	12.5

Lexington, Massachusetts: vital record study.

	%		%	%	%
1854–1866	n.a.	56	3.6	3.6	12.5
1885–1895	n.a.	119	15.1	19.3	24.4

Willimantic, Connecticut: vital record study; John P. Sade, "Premarital Conception and Social Change in Willimantic, Connecticut, 1850–1910," unpub. undergraduate history paper (University of Connecticut, 1973). We are indebted to Sade for these data.

	%				%
1850, 1870	26	31	—	—	19.3
1890	48	41	—	—	31.7
1910	46	72	—	—	25.0

Washentaw County, Michigan: vital record study. Data for 1867–1870 and 1886–1890 include Ann Arbor and Ypsilanti only. Overall, 34.2% of marriages were linked to births (Samuel Gorsline and Harold Smith, "A Study of Premarital Pregnancy in Washentaw County, 1867–1900," unpub. undergraduate history paper [University of Michigan, 1972]). We are indebted to the authors and to Kenneth Lockridge for these data.)

			%		%
1867–1870 } 1876–1880 }	—	136	5.1	—	11.8
1886–1890 } 1896–1900 }	—	162	8.0	—	16.0

Utah County, Utah, vital record study. Percent born within 196 and 251 days of all first births coming in first 48 months of marriage; 1670 cases. Harold T. Christensen, "The Time between Marriage of Parents and the Birth of Their First Children: Utah County, Utah," *American Journal of Sociology,* XLIV (1939), 521.

	196 days (%)	251 days (%)
1905–1907	11.9	20.1
1913–1915	14.8	29.1
1921–1923	9.6	20.4
1929–1931	8.0	19.3

Tippecanoe County, Indiana: vital record study. Percent born within 196 and 251 days of all first births coming within the first 48 months of marriage. Harold T. Christensen and Olive P. Bowden, "Studies in Child-Spacing, II: The Time-Interval between Marriage of Parents and Birth of Their First Child, Tippecanoe County, Indiana," *Social Forces,* XXXI (1953), 348.

	%		196 days (%)	251 days (%)
1919–1921	39	487	11.9	19.6
1929–1931	28	352	14.8	28.2
1939–1941	37	692	9.8	20.0

Defiance County, Ohio: vital record study. Percent born within 196 days of marriage of those births coming within first 48 months of marriage. Harold T. Christensen, "Child-Spacing Analysis via Record Linkage: New Data plus a Summing Up from Earlier Reports," *Marriage and Family Living,* XXXV (1963), 275.

	%
1918–1922	10.9
1929–1931	14.1
1939–1942	6.9

Wood County, Ohio: vital record study; Samuel H. Lowrie, "Early Marriage, Premarital Pregnancy and Associated Factors," *Journal of Marriage and the Family,* XXVII (1965), 50.

		195 days (%)	265 days (%)
1957–1962	1,850	9.3	18.8

Massachusetts: vital record study. Elizabeth Murphy Whelan, "The Temporal Relationship of Marriage, Conception, and Birth in Massachusetts," *Demography,* IX (1972), 404.

	196 days (%)	265 days (%)
1966–1968	17.8	29.0

National surveys: See the discussion and data in Smith, "Dating of the American Sexual Revolution," 323–327.

APPENDIX II

I. *France* (within 7 complete months of marriage):

PLACE	SOURCE	PERIOD	RATIO (%)
A. Before the second half of the eighteenth century:			
Sainghin-en-Mélantois	5	1690–1769	15.2
Boulay	15	before 1749	9.1
Boulay (7 surrounding villages)	16	before 1760	8.6
Crulai	11	1674–1742	2.8
Meulan	19	1660–1739	7.7
Troarn	2	1661–1740	12.0
Tamerville	28	1624–1740	10.1
Tourouvre	4	before 1750	3.0
Bayeux	8	1600–1699	8.3
Lourmarin	24	1681–1750	15.1
Sérignan	22	1716–1750	20.0
Northwest France	13	1670–1769	5.8
Southwest France	14	1720–1769	6.4
Total of 13 samples			9.5
B. Encompassing the mid-eighteenth century:			
Saint-Méen	1	1720–1792	8.9
Bayeux	8	1700–1780	11.3
Blere	20	1677–1788	4.0
Bessin, three villages	8	1686–1792	17.1
Bas-Quercy	27	1700–1792	4.8
Saint-Agnan	17	1730–1792	9.1
Ingouville	26	1730–1770	14.7
Rumont	23	1720–1790	9.0
Tonnerrois	7	1720–1800	7.8
Villedieu-les Poëles	18	1711–1790	2.6
Saint-Pierre-Eglise	21	1657–1790	9.0
Total of 11 samples			8.9
C. Second half of the eighteenth century:			
Tamerville	28	1741–1790	20.0
Tourouvre	4	after 1750	10.0
Meulan	19	1740–1789	11.8
Lourmarin	24	1751–1800	18.1
Boulay	15	1750–1809	12.3
Boulay (7 surrounding villages)	16	1760–1799	7.4

PLACE	SOURCE	PERIOD	RATIO (%)
C. *Second half of the eighteenth century* (continued):			
Sainghin-en-Mélantois	5	1770–1799	15.8
Troarn	2	1741–1780	13.7
Saint-Auban	1	1749–1789	4.3
Bilhères	9	1740–1819	10.3
Ile-de-France	10	1740–1799	14.0
Sotteville-les-Rouen	12	1760–1790	30.2
Châtillon-sur-Seine	3	1772–1805	15.8
Southwest France	14	1770–1789	12.1
Serignan	22	1751–1792	40.9
Total of 15 samples			17.4
D. *First half of the nineteenth century:*			
Sainghin-en-Mélantois	5	1800–1849	50.5
Boulay	15	1810–	28.5
Boulay (7 surrounding villages)	16	1800–1862	18.3
Meulan	19	1790–1839	23.6
Bilhères	9	1820–1859	2.8
Lourmarin	24	1801–1830	23.9
Southwest France	14	1790–1819	11.2
Total of 7 samples			22.7

E. *Twentieth Century* (within 7 complete months per 100 marriages; sample of 240,000 families in the 1962 census):

France	6	1925–1929	12.3
		1930–1934	12.6
		1935–1939	12.6
		1940–1944	17.0
		1945–1949	17.2
		1950–1954	19.4
		1955–1959	19.5
		1960–1961	19.3

SOURCES

(1)   Yves Blayo, "Trois paroisses d'Ille-et-Villaine," *Annales de démographic historique*, VI (1969), 206.

(2)   Michel Bouvet and Pierre-Marie Bourdin, "A travers la Normandie des XVIIᵉ et XVIIIᵉ siècles," *Cahier des Annales de Normandie*, VI (1968), 191–202.

(3)   Antoinette Chamoux and Cécile Dauphin, "La Contraception avant la Révolution francaise: L'exemple de Châtillon-sur-Seine," *Annales: E.S.C.*, XXIV (1969), 680.

(4) Hubert Charbonneau, *Tourouvre-au-Perche aux XVIIe et XVIIIe siècles: Etude de démographie historique* (Paris, 1969), 142.

(5) Raymond Deniel and Louis Henry, "La population d'un village du Nord de la France, Sainghin-en-Mélantois, de 1665 a 1851," *Population*, XX (1965), 581.

(6) Jean-Claude Deville, *Structure des Familles* (Paris, 1972), 91.

(7) D. Dinet, "Quatre paroisses du Tonnerrois," *Annales de démographie historique*, VI (1969), 80.

(8) Mohamed El Kordi, *Bayeux aux XVIIe et XVIIIe siècles: Contribution à l'histoire urbaine de la France* (Paris, 1970), 91.

(9) Michel Fresel-Lozey, *Histoire démographique d'un village en Béarn: Bilheres-d'Ossau* (Bordeaux, 1969), 142.

(10) Jean Ganiage, *Trois villages d'Ile-de-France au XVIIIe siècle* (Paris, 1963), 92.

(11) Etienne Gautier and Louis Henry, *La population de Crulai, paroisse normande* (Paris, 1958), 257–264.

(12) Pierre Girard, "Aperçus de la démographie de Sotteville-les-Rouen vers la fin du XVIIIe siècle," *Population*, XIV (1959), 494.

(13) Louis Henry, "Intervalle entre le mariage et la première naissance. Erreurs et corrections," *ibid.*, XXVIII (1973), 263.

(14) Louis Henry, "La fécondité des mariages dans le quart sud-ouest de la France de 1720 a 1829," *Annales: E.S.C.*, XXVII (1972), 998.

(15) J. Houdaille, "La population de Boulay (Moselle) avant 1850," *Population*, XXII (1967), 1075.

(16) Jacques Houdaille, "La population de sept villages des environs de Boulay (Moselle) aux XVIIIe et XIXe siècles," *ibid.*, XXVI (1971), 1063.

(17) Jacques Houdaille, "Un village du Morvan: Saint-Agnan," *ibid.*, XVI (1961), 304.

(18) Marie-Hélène Jouan, "Les originalités démographiques d'un bourg artisan normand au XVIIIe siècle: Villedieu-les-Poeles (1711–1790)," *Annales de démographie historique*, VI (1969), 107.

(19) Marcel Lachiver, *La population de Meulan du XVIIe au XIXe siècle (vers 1600–1850)* (Paris, 1969), 175.

(20) Marcel Lachiver, "Une étude et quelques equisses," *Annales de démographie historique*, VI (1969), 220.

(21) Jacques Lelong, "Saint-Pierre-Eglise, 1657–1790," *ibid.*, 131.

(22) Alain Molinier, "Une paroisse du Bas-Languedoc, Sérignan, 1650–1792," *Mémoires de la société archéologique de Montpellier*, XII (1968), 164.

(23) Patrice Robert, "Rumont (1720–1790)," *Annales de démographie historique*, VI (1969), 36.

(24) Thomas F. Sheppard, *Lourmarin in the Eighteenth Century: A Study of a French Village* (Baltimore, 1971), 41.

(25) Edward Shorter, "Female Emancipation, Birth Control, and Fertility

in European History," *American Historical Review*, LXXVIII (1973), 638–639.
(26) Michel Terrisse, "Un faubourg du Havre: Ingouville," *Population*, XVI (1961), 286.
(27) Pierre Valmary, *Familles paysannes au XVIIIe siècle en Bas-Quercy* (Paris, 1965), 93.
(28) Phillipe Wiel, "Une grosse paroisse du Cotentin aux XVIIe et XVIIIe siècles," *Annales de démographie historique*, VI (1969), 161.

II. *Australia* (nine-month standard):

MARRIAGE PERIOD	PREMARITAL PREGNANCY INDEX	
	% OF MARRIAGES	% OF FIRST BIRTHS
1911–1915	29.1	35.0
1916–1920	25.2	29.9
1921–1925	25.0	29.8
1926–1930	26.7	32.5
1931–1935	26.4	35.1
1936–1940	19.3	27.7
1941–1945	13.8	17.9
1946–1950	16.7	19.2
1951–1955	18.1	20.2
1956–1960	21.9	23.2
1961–1965	23.6	28.3

SOURCE: Basavarajappa, "Pre-marital Pregnancies," 143, Table A; 145, Table C.

III. *Great Britain*

A. *England:* non-random sample of printed parish records; marriages traced to birth or baptism within 8½ months.

PERIOD	% MATCHED	NO. MATCHED	% PREGNANT
1500s	46	164	22.6
1600s	44	275	15.6
Late 1600s to 1749	50	199	17.6
1750 to c. 1800	50	713	40.2
1800 to 1819	43	388	40.2
1820 to 1843	45	95	46.3

SOURCE: P. E. H. Hair, "Bridal Pregnancy in Rural England in Earlier Centuries," *Population Studies*, XX (1966), 241–242.

III. (continued):

B. *England:* same description as above.

PERIOD	% MATCHED	NO. MATCHED	% PREGNANT
1500s	52	301	21.3
1600s	41	328	16.5
Late 1600s to 1749	42	79	16.5
1750 to 1836	48	288	43.4
1837 to 1887	52	50	40.0

SOURCE: P. E. H. Hair, "Bridal Pregnancy in Earlier Rural England Further Examined," *Population Studies,* XXIV (1970), 60.

C. *England and Wales:* To 1951, an interval of 8½ months was used; after 1951, 8 months.

MARRIAGE PERIOD	PREMARITAL PREGNANCY INDEX	
	% OF MARRIAGES	% OF LEGITIMATE FIRST BIRTHS
1941–1945	11.7	14.5
1946–1950	14.5	18.0
1951–1955	12.9	18.0
1956–1960	14.6	18.8
1961–1965	18.3	23.0
1966–1968	18.6	26.0

SOURCE: Great Britain, General Register Office, *The Registrar General's Statistical Review of England and Wales for the year 1968, Part II* (London, 1969), 192, Table UU; 12, Table Cl.

The Contributors

Reader on Marriage and Fertility

EMILY R. COLEMAN is Assistant Professor of History at the University of Pittsburgh.

BARBARA A. HANAWALT is Associate Professor of History at Indiana University and the author of *Crime and Conflict in English Communities, 1300-1348* (Cambridge, Mass., 1979).

STANLEY CHOJNACKI is Associate Professor of History at Michigan State University.

ROBERT V. SCHNUCKER is Chairman of the Department of Philosophy and Religion at Northeast Missouri State University. He is the author of *Modular Learning Program for World Civilization* (St. Charles, Mo., 1973).

WILLIAM ROBERT LEE is Senior Lecturer in the Department of Economic History, University of Liverpool, and the author of *Population Growth, Economic Development and Social Change in Bavaria, 1750-1850* (New York, 1977).

CISSIE FAIRCHILDS is Associate Professor of History at Syracuse University and the author of *Poverty and Charity in Aix-en-Provence, 1640-1789* (Baltimore, 1976).

GEORGE D. SUSSMAN is Assistant to the Deputy Commissioner for Higher and Professional Education, New York State Education Department, and is currently preparing a book on wet-nursing in France from the ancien régime to the twentieth century.

SUSAN GRIGG is an archivist at the Yale University Library.

WILLIAM L. LANGER was Archibald Cary Coolidge Professor of History at Harvard University. Among his last books was *Political and Social Upheaval, 1832-1852* (New York, 1969).

PETER LASLETT is Director of the Cambridge Group for the History of Population and Social Structure and the author, most recently, of *Family Life and Illicit Love in Earlier Generations* (New York, 1977).

EDWARD SHORTER is Professor of History at the University of Toronto and the author of *The Making of the Modern Family* (New York, 1975).

LOUISE A. TILLY is Associate Professor of History at the University of Michigan and the co-author with Joan W. Scott of *Women, Work and Family* (New York, 1978).

JOAN WALLACH SCOTT is Nancy Duke Lewis Professor and Professor of History at Brown University. She is the author of *Glassworkers of Carmaux: French Craftsmen and Political Action in a Nineteenth-Century City* (Cambridge, Mass., 1980) and the co-author of *Women, Work and Family* (New York, 1978) with Louise A. Tilly.

MIRIAM COHEN is Assistant Professor of History at Vassar College and the author of "Italian-American Women in New York City, 1900–1950: Work and School," in Milton Cantor and Bruce Laurie (eds.), *Class, Sex and the Woman Worker* (Westport, Conn., 1978).

DANIEL SCOTT SMITH is Associate Professor of History at the University of Illinois at Chicago Circle and Associate Director of the Family and Community History Center, The Newberry Library.

MICHAEL S. HINDUS is an associate attorney with McCutchen, Doyle, Brown, and Enersen in San Francisco and the author of *Prison and Plantation: Crime, Justice, and Authority in Massachusetts and South Carolina, 1767-1878* (Chapel Hill, 1980).